Hemocoagulative Problems in the Critically Ill Patient

Giorgio Berlot
Editor

Hemocoagulative Problems in the Critically Ill Patient

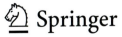
Springer

Giorgio Berlot
Cattinara Hospital
Anesthesia and Intensive Care
University of Trieste
Trieste
Italy

ISBN 978-88-470-2447-2   e-ISBN 978-88-470-2448-9
DOI 10.1007/978-88-470-2448-9
Springer Milan Heidelberg New York Dordrecht London

Library of Congress Control Number: 2012934249

© Springer-Verlag Italia 2012
This work is subject to copyright. All rights are reserved by the Publisher, whether the whole or part of the material is concerned, specifically the rights of translation, reprinting, reuse of illustrations, recitation, broadcasting, reproduction on microfilms or in any other physical way, and transmission or information storage and retrieval, electronic adaptation, computer software, or by similar or dissimilar methodology now known or hereafter developed. Exempted from this legal reservation are brief excerpts in connection with reviews or scholarly analysis or material supplied specifically for the purpose of being entered and executed on a computer system, for exclusive use by the purchaser of the work. Duplication of this publication or parts thereof is permitted only under the provisions of the Copyright Law of the Publisher's location, in its current version, and permission for use must always be obtained from Springer. Permissions for use may be obtained through RightsLink at the Copyright Clearance Center. Violations are liable to prosecution under the respective Copyright Law.
The use of general descriptive names, registered names, trademarks, service marks, etc. in this publication does not imply, even in the absence of a specific statement, that such names are exempt from the relevant protective laws and regulations and therefore free for general use.
Product liability: While the advice and information in this book are believed to be true and accurate at the date of publication, neither the authors nor the editors nor the publisher can accept any legal responsibility for any errors or omissions that may be made. The publisher makes no warranty, express or implied, with respect to the material contained herein.

Printed on acid-free paper

Springer is part of Springer Science+Business Media (www.springer.com)

This book is dedicated to all those patients who I treated during my first 30 years in Intensive Care Medicine and to those I shall treat in the coming years. Each of them taught or will teach me something

Preface

Libraries contain plenty of textbooks and manuals that are dedicated to the care of the critically ill and cover all aspects of treatment, with a particular focus on mechanical ventilation, cardiovascular and renal support, nutrition, and infection control. However, location of a text devoted to blood coagulation is more difficult, which seems surprising when one considers the growing interest in the multiple interactions linking the blood coagulation system to the inflammatory response and the difficulties in identifying and treating blood coagulation disturbances in patients with multiple organ dysfunctions. While large books on critical care and anesthesia typically include a chapter on this issue, it will inevitably be embedded among dozens of other chapters or sections and is likely to be difficult to look up at the bedside. We therefore wanted to fill this gap by providing the reader with a handbook which is both up-to-date and easy to consult. Its preparation passed through a variety of phases. Initially, we considered which are the most frequent issues to arise regarding blood coagulation during daily clinical rounds in the intensive care unit. Subsequently, we asked colleagues interested in the field to prepare one or more chapters relating to these issues. The choice of authors was based on their clinical experience, as we are convinced that only physicians with a hands-on attitude are able to recognize the needs of readers involved daily in the care of critically ill patients and to select those aspects essential to clinical practice. Individual sections are dedicated to the physiology of blood coagulation, laboratory evaluation, inborn defects, and alterations acquired under different conditions specific to critical diseases and the perioperative period. In addition, however, we wished to include chapters addressing (relatively) rare diseases such as the vasculitides, either because of the life-threatening multiple organ dysfunction that they cause or because of the difficulties encountered in their recognition.

Like everything in this era of rapidly growing knowledge, this book is destined to undergo rapid aging: as an example, the sad end of the saga of recombinant human-activated protein C prompted us to rewrite the section dedicated to this substance. Against this background, it will be up to readers to decide whether an updated edition of this text is needed in the next few years; should this be the case, we shall do our best to revise the text suitably and with the same enthusiasm and commitment that we have devoted to this book.

Trieste, March 2012

Giorgio Berlot

Contents

1 Physiology of Hemostasis 1
Paola Pradella, Federica Tomasella and Luca Mascaretti

2 Monitoring of Hemostasis 21
Carlo Giansante and Nicola Fiotti

3 Anticoagulation Therapy in ICU Patients 37
Emanuele Marras, Luigi Lo Nigro and Giorgio Berlot

4 Inborn Prothrombotic States 61
Nicola Fiotti and Carlo Giansante

5 Inborn Defects of the Coagulative System 73
Marinella Astuto, Nadia Grasso and Alessandro Trainito

6 Inflammation and Coagulation 85
Walter Vessella, Lara Prisco and Giorgio Berlot

7 Disseminated Intravascular Coagulation 93
Antonino Gullo, Chiara Maria Celestre and Annalaura Paratore

8 Coagulative Disturbances in Trauma 111
Giuliana Garufi, Maria Cristina Fiorenza and Giorgio Berlot

9 Hypothermia and Coagulation Disorders 125
Lara Prisco, Vincenzo Campanile and Giorgio Berlot

10 Hemostasis in Pregnancy and Obstetric Surgery 133
Marinella Astuto, Valentina Taranto and Simona Grasso

11 Hemostasis During Heart Surgery 163
Luigi Tritapepe, Sara Iannandrea, Michela Generali
and Maria Paola Lauretta

12 Hemocoagulative Aspects of Solid Organ Transplantation 181
Andrea De Gasperi

13 Antiphospholipid Antibody Syndrome 209
Marco Zambon, Davide Cappelli and Giorgio Berlot

14 Pulmonary-Renal Syndrome 217
Marco Zambon, Davide Cappelli and Giorgio Berlot

15 Coagulation Disorders After Central Nervous System Injury 227
Lara Prisco, Mario Ganau and Giorgio Berlot

Index 237

Contributors

Marinella Astuto Department of Anesthesia and Intensive Care, Pediatric Anesthesia and Intensive Care Section, "Policlinico" University Hospital, Catania, Italy

Giorgio Berlot Anesthesia and Intensive Care Unit, Cattinara Hospital, University of Trieste, Trieste, Friuli Venezia Giulia, Italy; Department of Neurosurgery, University of Trieste, Cattinara Hospital, Trieste, Italy; Department of Anaesthesiology, Intensive Care and Emergency Medicine, Cattinara Hospital, University of Trieste, Trieste, Italy

Vincenzo Campanile Department of Anaesthesiology, Intensive Care and Emergency Medicine, Cattinara Hospital, University of Trieste, Trieste, Italy

Davide Cappelli Anesthesia and Intensive Care, Cattinara Hospital, University of Trieste, Trieste, Italy

Chiara Maria Celestre Department of Anesthesia and Intensive Care, Medical School, "Policlinico" University Hospital, Catania, Italy

Andrea De Gasperi 2 Servizio Anestesia e Rianimazione Ospedale Niguarda Ca' Granda, Milan, Italy

Maria Cristina Fiorenza Anaesthesia and Intensive Care, Cattinara Hospital, University of Trieste, Trieste, Italy

Nicola Fiotti Unit of Clinica Medica, Department of DMS, University of Trieste, Trieste, Italy

Mario Ganau Department of Neurosurgery, University of Trieste, Cattinara Hospital, Trieste, Italy

Giuliana Garufi Anaesthesia and Intensive Care, Cattinara Hospital, University of Trieste, Trieste, Italy

Michela Generali Department of Anesthesia and Intensive Care, UOD Anesthesia and Intensive Care in Cardiac Surgery, University of Rome "La Sapienza", Rome, Italy

Carlo Giansante Unità Clinica Operativa di Clinica Medica Generale e Terapia Medica, University of Trieste, Trieste, Italy

Nadia Grasso Department of Anesthesia and Intensive Care, Pediatric Anesthesia and Intensive Care Section, "Policlinico" University Hospital, Catania, Italy

Simona Grasso Department of Anesthesia and Intensive Care, Pediatric Anesthesia and Intensive Care Section, "Policlinico" University Hospital, Catania, Italy

Antonino Gullo Department of Anesthesia and Intensive Care, Medical School, "Policlinico" University Hospital, Catania, Italy

Sara Iannandrea Department of Anesthesia and Intensive Care, UOD Anesthesia and Intensive Care in Cardiac Surgery, University of Rome "La Sapienza", Rome, Italy

Maria Paola Lauretta Department of Anesthesia and Intensive Care, UOD Anesthesia and Intensive Care in Cardiac Surgery, University of Rome "La Sapienza", Rome, Italy

Emanuele Marras Anesthesia and Intensive Care, Cattinara Hospital, University of Trieste, Trieste, Italy

Luca Mascaretti Hemostasis Laboratory, Transfusion Medicine Department, Cattinara Hospital, University of Trieste, Trieste, Italy

Luigi Lo Nigro Anesthesia and Intensive Care, Cattinara Hospital, University of Trieste, Trieste, Italy

Annalaura Paratore Department of Anesthesia and Intensive Care, Medical School, "Policlinico" University Hospital, Catania, Italy

Paola Pradella Hemostasis Laboratory, Transfusion Medicine Department, Cattinara Hospital, University of Trieste, Trieste, Italy

Lara Prisco Anesthesia and Intensive Care Unit, Cattinara Hospital, University of Trieste, Trieste, Friuli Venezia Giulia, Italy; Department of Anaesthesiology, Intensive Care and Emergency Medicine, Cattinara Hospital, University of Trieste, Trieste, Italy

Valentina Taranto Department of Anesthesia and Intensive Care, Pediatric Anesthesia and Intensive Care Section, "Policlinico" University Hospital, Catania, Italy

Federica Tomasella Hemostasis Laboratory, Transfusion Medicine Department, Cattinara Hospital, University of Trieste, Trieste, Italy

Alessandro Trainito Department of Anesthesia and Intensive Care, Pediatric Anesthesia and Intensive Care Section, "Policlinico" University Hospital, Catania, Italy

Luigi Tritapepe Department of Anesthesia and Intensive Care, UOD Anesthesia and Intensive Care in Cardiac Surgery, University of Rome "La Sapienza", Rome, Italy

Walter Vessella Anesthesia and Intensive Care Unit, Cattinara Hospital, University of Trieste, Trieste, Italy

Marco Zambon Anesthesia and Intensive Care, Cattinara Hospital, University of Trieste, Trieste, Italy

Physiology of Hemostasis

1

Paola Pradella, Federica Tomasella and Luca Mascaretti

1.1 A Brief History of Blood Coagulation

The unraveling of the mechanisms of one of the most remarkable characteristics of blood, its ability to clot, has taken almost one century.

The understanding of how coagulation works proceeded in a stepwise fashion as illustrated in Fig. 1.1, which shows some of the milestones in blood coagulation research. A considerable amount of basic work on protein chemistry and enzymology was conducted at the beginning of the last century in Europe and the USA. At that time, Morawitz described the conversion of prothrombin to thrombin by thrombokinase and the conversion of fibrinogen to fibrin by thrombin. In Morawitz's view, thrombokinase was derived from platelets and damaged tissue. A few years later, Howell coined the term "thromboplastin," by which he meant a complex with clotting-accelerating activity derived from tissue, with the ability to convert prothrombin to thrombin. The numerous studies on thromboplastin allowed the successive purification of tissue factor (TF) from human and bovine tissue.

One important discovery in enzymology was "limited proteolysis" [1], i.e., the breaking of specific peptide bonds depending on the amino acid sequence of a protein (as opposed to "unlimited proteolysis," which refers to the complete breakdown of a peptide to amino acids). Limited proteolysis is common to those complex biological systems based on highly regulated cascades, such as the complement system, apoptosis pathways, and blood coagulation.

P. Pradella (✉)
Hemostasis Laboratory, Transfusion Medicine Department,
University Hospital (AOUTS), Trieste,
Trieste, Italy
e-mail: paola.pradella@aots.sanita.fvg.it

G. Berlot (ed.), *Hemocoagulative Problems in the Critically Ill Patient*,
DOI: 10.1007/978-88-470-2448-9_1, © Springer-Verlag Italia 2012

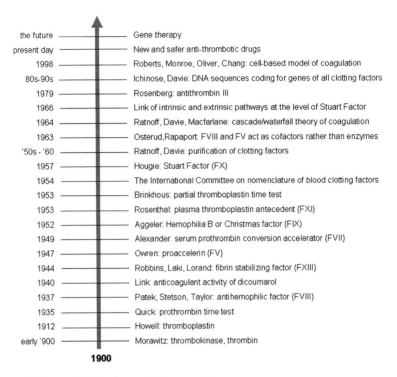

Fig. 1.1 Milestones in blood coagulation research

The understanding of blood coagulation in humans is closely linked to the study of patients with blood coagulation disorders. In the years from the mid-1930s to the end of the 1950s, almost all clotting factors were described (Fig. 1.1) and isolated using techniques such as column chromatography. As clotting factors were discovered, they were given names (sometimes more than one) in an unorganized manner, generating confusion; in 1954 the International Committee on Nomenclature of Blood Clotting Factors was established and has met several times since [2].

Given that a number of coagulation factors were described, the problem was to understand in which way they interacted to form the blood clot. What seemed to be relatively certain quite early on was that clotting factors were present in plasma as precursors (inactive form) and became activated by enzymes in a stepwise manner, probably by the mechanism of limited proteolysis. Another important observation was that calcium ions played a major role in the activation of some clotting factors.

At the beginning of the 1960s, the idea of an intrinsic as opposed to an extrinsic pathway of blood coagulation started to emerge; whereas the former can be initiated in a test tube, the latter needs tissue extracts to be triggered.

In 1964 two seminal articles were published, one in *Science* [3] and one in *Nature* [4]. Davie and Ratnoff [3] claimed the following: "A simple waterfall sequence is proposed to explain the function of the various protein clotting factors during the formation of the fibrin clot. When clotting is initiated, each clotting factor except fibrinogen is converted to a form that has enzymatic activity. This activation occurs in a stepwise sequence with each newly formed enzyme reacting with its specific substrate, converting it to an active enzyme." It is interesting to note that the article by MacFarlane [4] used a term very similar to that employed by Davie and Ratnoff, "coagulation cascade."

So by the mid-1960s, a good model of blood coagulation was available. It was duly refined in successive years, mainly clarifying the role of Stuart factor (factor X, FX), which is the link between the intrinsic and extrinsic pathways. Other major advancements in coagulation were the recognition of the more prominent role played by the extrinsic rather than the intrinsic pathway in blood coagulation as a consequence of vascular injury, and that some coagulation factors (factor VIII, FVIII, and factor V, FV) acted as cofactors and did not display enzymatic activity.

In the 1970s, the plasma inhibitor antithrombin (AT) III was discovered and intensive research on regulatory pathways of coagulation allowed the identification of protein C and protein S.

The 1980s marked the beginning of the molecular era, with the cloning and sequencing of all the clotting factors. This was a very significant advancement in coagulation since it allowed mutations in clotting factors of patients with bleeding disorders to be determined. It also paved the way for the production of recombinant clotting factors for patients with hemorrhagic diseases.

In 1998, a novel coagulation theory was proposed by Roberts et al. [5], termed the cell-based model of coagulation. Currently, this is the accepted model and will be discussed at length in the following sections of this chapter.

1.2   Evolution of Blood Coagulation Systems

Comparative biology is a branch of biological science which applies a multidisciplinary approach to the study of biodiversity and complexity of biological systems, including coagulation.

One of the more primitive and well known coagulation systems is that of the horseshoe crab, or *Limulus*, an invertebrate of the Arthropoda phylum which has lived on Earth for more than 350 million years and is therefore also known as a living fossil [6]. These organisms have an open circulation and their blood (hemolymph) contains a protein called hemocyanin which transports oxygen. Amebocytes, also known as hemocytes, are the only circulating cells and have two main functions: that of killing pathogenic bacteria by means of bactericides and that of releasing coagulation zymogen proteins (proteases) which convert coagulogen (a clottable protein) to coagulin (a monomer), which in turn is polymerized by a transglutaminase. It is clear that this "ancient" and very basic coagulation system has many similarities to the more sophisticated coagulation systems of mammals.

The question that comparative biologists and coagulation experts asked themselves was why in vertebrates did the coagulation system evolve into such a complicated pathway composed of so many factors which, apparently, achieve the same result (blood clotting) as the more simple systems of invertebrates?

The reasonable explanation is that in *Limulus* the open circulation has a low pressure and the rather simple coagulation system suffices. On the other hand, vertebrates have high-pressure vascular systems and therefore evolution has "selected" a more sophisticated coagulation system able to produce localized clotting at the vascular injury level.

The availability of molecular biology tools such as degenerate PCR, reverse transcription techniques, cloning, and sequencing has allowed further insights into the evolution of coagulation systems of different species. Davidson et al. [7] investigated the coagulation systems of chickens (*Gallus gallus*) and the teleost puffer fish (*Fugu rubripes*); whereas the common ancestor of the former and humans dates to some 350 million years ago, the latter shared an ancestor with humans 430 million years ago. The authors were able to demonstrate that domains common to the proteases factor VII (FVII), factor IX (FIX), FX, and protein C (Gla-EGF1-EGF2-SP) and domains common to FV and FVIII (A1-A2-B-A3-C1-C2) were indeed present in both chicken and bony fish, proving that blood coagulation systems evolved over 430 million years ago.

1.3 Models of Coagulation: Cascade Versus Cell-Based

As mentioned previously, a "waterfall" or "cascade" model was proposed in 1964 [3, 4] and was subsequently refined, elucidating the identity and function of the single procoagulant proteins in a sequential series of proteolytic reactions. Each clotting factor is believed to be a proenzyme that cleaves and activates the next in the series, leading to a burst of thrombin generation. Successively, this model was corrected with the observation that some procoagulant molecules are cofactors and do not possess proteolytic activity. It is recognized that thrombin and other coagulation factors are serine proteases and that their activity requires calcium, phosphatidylserine, and other anionic phospholipids. The coagulation process is depicted as a Y-shaped scheme, with factor XII and FVII initiating, respectively, "intrinsic" and "extrinsic" pathways, merging at the level of activated FX (FXa)/activated FV (FVa) (prothrombinase complex) on a "common" pathway (Fig. 1.2). The intrinsic pathway is triggered by a negatively charged surface (contact phase) and all the components are present in blood, whereas the extrinsic pathway, primed by a trauma in a vessel wall, requires TF, a protein mostly present on subendothelial cells, as described in the specific section. In this model, coagulation factors direct and control the overall process and cells merely provide a surface containing phospholipids, on which procoagulant complexes are assembled.

Eventually this model was found to be inconsistent with some clinical observations, for example the TF/activated FVII (FVIIa)-initiated activation of FX cannot compensate for FVIII or FIX deficiency in hemophiliacs, and the reduction of single coagulation factors, mostly of the intrinsic pathway, is associated with different risks of hemorrhage. Subsequently, the hypothesis that intrinsic and extrinsic pathways are linked in vivo and the TF/FVIIa complex is the major initiator of hemostasis was proposed, as a consequence of the observation

1 Physiology of Hemostasis

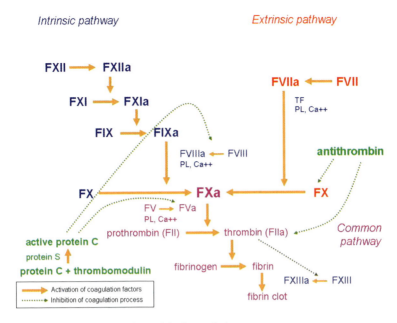

Fig. 1.2 The waterfall or cascade model of coagulation

that TF/FVIIa can activate FIX as well as FX, and thrombin is a physiologic "activator" of factor XI (FXI) on activated platelets. Moreover, in the last decades different receptors for many components of hemostasis and procoagulant or anticoagulant proteins on different cells have been detected, thus suggesting that cell surfaces have a central role in the coagulation process. Therefore, at the end of the 1990s, a cell-based model of coagulation was proposed, consisting of three stepwise and partially overlapping phases [5, 8]:

1. Initiation of coagulation on TF-bearing cells, during which FX and FIX are activated and a small amount of thrombin is produced to promote the coagulation process and platelet activation.
2. Amplification of the response, which implies that coagulation is shifted from TF-bearing cells to the nearby platelets; platelets adhere to subendothelial structures, undergo activation, and collect activated proteins on their membranes. The fact that the TF/FVIIa complex is close to activated platelets represents a crucial step for priming the hemostatic process or thrombosis.
3. Propagation phase, when platelets are recruited to the site of injury, and activated coagulation factors meet their cofactors to compose the procoagulant complexes necessary for the burst of thrombin generation and the fibrin polymerization.

In this model the extrinsic and intrinsic pathways are viewed as not independent. The role of the cell-based extrinsic pathway is to generate, on the TF-bearing cells, the small amount of thrombin needed to initiate and amplify the coagulation process, and that of the cell-based intrinsic pathway is to produce, on the platelet

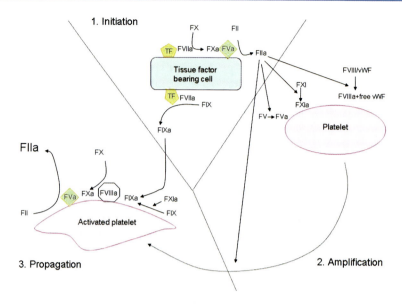

Fig. 1.3 The cell-based model of hemostasis

surface, the burst of thrombin to form a stable fibrin clot. Platelets adhere to the site of injury, become activated, and provide the surface on which clotting factors are collected and coagulation response may take place [8] (Fig. 1.3).

Further studies in genetically modified mice and using intravital imaging techniques have suggested that platelet activation may occur both by thrombin generated by the TF/FVIIa complex on the TF-bearing cells and through interactions with subendothelial exposed collagen. These two distinct pathways for platelet activation can work separately or in parallel, depending on the injury or the disease, but the final effect is the same, as shown in Fig. 1.4 [9, 10]. In this way initiation and amplification phases should be considered as a continuum of events.

The cell-based model for thrombus formation may be summarized as follows.

Initiation phase. When the vessel wall is injured or endothelium is disrupted, TF and collagen have a crucial role in sealing the breach. TF-bearing cells, such as fibroblasts and smooth muscle cells encircling the endothelium, are exposed to flowing blood and initiate the production of thrombin needed for platelet activation. TF acts as a receptor and activator of coagulation FVII and the resulting TF/FVIIa complex converts FX and FIX to FXa and activated FIX (FIXa), respectively. FXa activates its cofactor FV to FVa to form the prothrombinase complex; thus, a small amount of thrombin is generated directly on the TF-bearing cells to stimulate platelets. The functions of FXa are limited to TF-bearing cells, because dissociated FXa is rapidly inactivated in blood by antithrombin (AT) or by a specific inhibitor (TF pathway inhibitor), which is synthesized in endothelial cells and attenuates the TF-initiated coagulation. This pathway ensures that a small procoagulant stimulus does not trigger an uncontrolled and excessive burst of

1 Physiology of Hemostasis

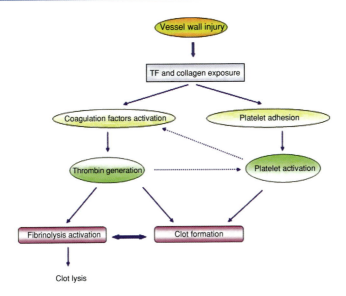

Fig. 1.4 Overview of clot formation

thrombin. In contrast, FIXa is not involved in this phase, but it can diffuse to the membrane of nearby activated platelets, binding to a specific receptor. In this way FIXa plays an important role in the subsequent propagation of thrombus.

Upon vascular injury, also the exposure of subendothelial collagen can initiate platelet activation.

The early contact between platelets and the extracellular matrix is influenced by flux: in veins and larger arteries, where circulation is characterized by a low shear rate, tethering of platelets to subendothelium depends on their interactions with collagen by means of specific receptors, glycoprotein VI and integrin $\alpha_2\beta_1$, whereas in vessels with a high shear rate, platelets adhere to von Willebrand factor (vWF) [11]. vWF is a constitutive component of subendothelium, where it is associated with collagen and is able to support platelet adhesion directly. Furthermore, also plasma-derived vWF can become immobilized onto subendothelial surfaces, binding either extracellular matrix components, mainly collagen, or other vWF molecules. Although many collagen types are present in the subendothelium, the association of vWF with fibrillar collagen type I, III, and VI has been shown and is considered a key step in supporting platelet docking to the injured vessel wall. In conditions of high shear stress, the interaction between vWF and the glycoprotein Ib-IX-V complex on the platelet membrane mediates the initial platelet tethering with short-lived contacts; the consequent deceleration supports platelet rolling on the exposed subendothelial structures [12]. This slow movement allows the interactions of collagen with glycoprotein VI and integrin $\alpha_2\beta_1$ on platelets and the subsequent interactions of vWF with integrin $\alpha_{IIb}\beta_3$. Other receptors on platelets, mostly but not only integrins, create additional bonds with subendothelial matrix molecules to form stable interactions, leading to the definitive arrest of single platelets in the next steps of thrombus formation [12]. Binding to extracellular matrix proteins partially activates platelets and localizes them close to TF-bearing cells, where a small amount of thrombin is generated and binds to the glycoprotein Ib-IX-V complex on the platelet surface, enhancing adhesion. Thrombin fully activates platelets, cleaving the membrane protease-activated receptors (PARs), and is responsible also for activation of FV, FVIII, and FXI [8]. Now the clotting system is set for the large-scale thrombin generation.

Propagation phase. In a monolayer on the exposed vWF and collagen, adherent and activated platelets form a reactive surface for the recruitment of circulating platelets and further platelet deposition. They stick to each other in a process named aggregation, and release or produce soluble agonists, such as ADP, thrombin, thromboxane A2 (TXA$_2$), and epinephrine [13]. These agonists interact with specific receptors on the membrane, producing a wide range of activation events, such as cytosolic calcium concentration elevation, protein phosphorylation, cytoskeleton reorganization, shape change, and granule secretion, which lead to a consequent "inside-out" signaling pathway. This signaling mechanism induces the ligand-binding function of integrin $\alpha_{IIb}\beta_3$, allowing this receptor to bind fibrinogen and vWF and form stable bridging between platelets [14]. In a growing thrombus, just a subgroup of recruited platelets undergo activation, and others are only transiently associated with and ultimately separate from the thrombus, which may be considered a dynamic structure in which some platelets adhere and others disengage [10, 15].

Moreover, platelets constitute the major tool for localizing clotting factors at the site of vascular damage, and in this phase the "tenase" (FIXa plus FVIIIa) and "prothrombinase" (FXa plus FVa) complexes are assembled on the surface of activated platelets [8]. The tenase complex is formed because FIXa diffuses from the TF-bearing cells to its specific receptor on platelets and activates FX in plasma. Also, FXI can bind to platelets to be activated by thrombin, generating further FIXa; the resulting FXa promptly associates with FVa in the prothrombinase complex and generates a large amount of thrombin, which transforms soluble fibrinogen into fibrin and activates FXIII. In this way fibrin monomers are cross-linked and a stable hemostatic fibrin clot is formed in the last step for thrombus stabilization (Fig. 1.5).

Undesired widespread activation of coagulation is prevented by several mechanisms of control, involving endogenous inhibitors of plasma proteases and platelet functions, as described later.

1.4 The Endothelium and Hemostasis

The hemostatic process involves both the coagulation system and fibrinolysis, with the aim of avoiding excessive blood loss, restoring the integrity of the vascular wall, and obtaining a vascular surface with no imperfections in order to allow proper blood circulation.

1 Physiology of Hemostasis

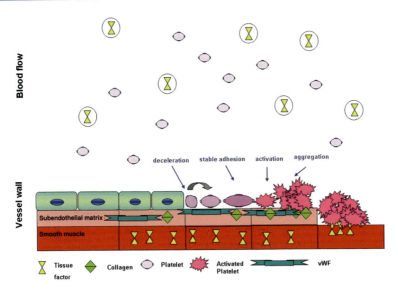

Fig. 1.5 Interactions between platelets and the vessel wall

Endothelium, on one hand, allows the interaction between platelets and coagulation factors, favoring the clotting process and, on the other hand, plays a key role in fibrinolytic events, and thus usually procoagulant and anticoagulant forces are in equilibrium. When under pathological conditions the regulatory mechanisms of hemostasis are overwhelmed, an excessive amount of thrombin is produced and thrombosis takes place. In the view of Virchow, changes in the vessel wall, in the blood composition, and in blood flow are the three major causes contributing in different ways to venous and arterial thrombosis. In the venous district, thrombosis is thought to be due mainly to changes in the composition of the blood, whereas in the arterial circulation, where the high flow rate prevents the accumulation of procoagulation factors, the changes in the vessel wall have a pivotal role in developing thrombus. Venous thrombosis and arterial thrombosis have long been viewed as different and separate disorders because of anatomical differences and distinct clinical presentations, but recent evidence suggests a potential link between these two diseases [16].

The endothelium is present throughout the vascular system, which is composed of three broad categories of vessels: arteries, veins, and capillaries. In each of these, a different structure of the vessel wall is observed, resulting in diverse reactions to vascular injury. The artery wall consists of three concentric layers whose thickness and structure varies according to vessel size. They are (1) the tunica intima, covered by endothelium, (2) the tunica media, composed mainly of elastic fibers (large-caliber arteries) or smooth muscle cells (arteries of medium and small size), and (3) the tunica adventitia, consisting of connective tissue and containing small blood vessels (vasa vasorum) and nerve filaments (nervi vasorum). The three layers described in the arteries are also present in veins, although in general the vein walls are thinner than those of arteries. The capillary wall is made of endothelium, which rests on a thin basement membrane, often reinforced by a delicate sheath of reticular fibers.

The endothelium is represented by a single layer of cells lining the inner part of the vascular bed. Endothelial cells have elongated or polygonal shapes and have pinocytotic vesicles, which are the main mode of transfer of nutrients from the luminal to the abluminal side. They contain Weibel–Palade granules, surrounded by membrane structures that are storage organelles for vWF [17].

The vascular endothelium is considered an organ displaying various activities:

1. Modulation of vascular tone and blood flow.
2. Modification of lipoproteins deposited on artery walls, through the release of toxic oxygen radicals.
3. Regulation of the passage of molecules through the vascular wall.
4. Regulation of immune and inflammatory responses.
5. Production of growth factors that regulate proliferation and differentiation of smooth muscle cells of the tunica media.
6. Regulation of the hemostatic mechanisms to maintain blood fluidity [18].

Vascular endothelium has both anticoagulant and prothrombotic features, which act through a variety of factors, depending on the circumstances.

1.4.1 Anticoagulant Activity

1. Inhibition of platelet aggregation. The electronegative charge of the surface of the endothelium prevents spontaneous deposition and adhesion of platelets. The vascular endothelium controls platelet reactivity through different pathways:
   - Nitric oxide (NO) in platelets regulates cGMP-dependent protein kinases, inducing a decrease of intracellular calcium flux and the consequent affinity of integrin $\alpha_{IIb}\beta_3$ for fibrinogen [19].
   - Prostacyclin is produced from arachidonic acid by means of cyclooxygenase 1 or 2 and increases cyclic AMP (cAMP) levels, inhibiting platelet functions.
   - A component of the endothelial membrane, CD39, is ADPase and limits the plasma levels of ATP and ADP, interfering with platelet reactivity [20].
2. Inhibition of blood coagulation:
   - When thrombin binds to thrombomodulin, a specific receptor on the endothelial surface, it changes its affinity for the substrate and activates protein C, triggering the anticoagulation pathway [21].
   - TF pathway inhibitor binds FXa when complexed with TF/FVIIa, damping the procoagulant stimulus in a similar way as plasmatic AT [6].
3. Promotion of fibrinolysis. The blood drag force on the endothelium triggers the release of tissue-type plasminogen activator (tPA) as well as urokinase-type plasminogen activator (uPA) [22].

1.4.2 Prothrombotic Activity

1. Induction of platelet aggregation and adhesion [23]. Endothelial cells are a major source of platelet-activating factor, a key inflammatory mediator with multiple functions, among which is that of being a potent agonist of platelet aggregation. In addition, the endothelium produces vWF, the main "glue" of platelet adhesion.
2. Activation of blood coagulation. Mechanical damage induces exposure of subendothelial TF on the luminal surface, which triggers the initial phase of coagulation [24].
3. Inhibition of fibrinolysis. In response to tissue injury, deceleration of blood flow, or inflammatory cytokines from endothelial cells, plasminogen activator inhibitor is also released, as described later.

Other Regulatory Mechanisms

In addition to endothelial specific anticoagulants, the clotting system is also balanced by other factors:

- Plasmatic AT is a plasma serine protease and is the major inhibitor of many coagulation factors, such as thrombin, FXa, and FIXa. Heparan sulfate, a glycosaminoglycan secreted by endothelial cells, binds circulating AT and catalyzes its anticoagulant function.
- Other regulatory mechanisms control single steps in the overall process, such as ADAMTS-13, a metalloproteinase that cleaves the largest and most prothrombotic vWF multimers when vWF is secreted from the cellular storage granules. The physiologic function of this protease is thought to reduce the activity of vWF to the site of release and to limit the propagation of platelet aggregates near a site of vessel injury [6].

The first event that occurs as a result of vascular trauma is primary hemostasis. It is characterized by vessel contraction in the injured area and platelet activation with adhesion and aggregation, which lead to the formation of a soft plug [25].

The mechanisms of vasoconstriction are more efficient in the larger vessels with vascular smooth muscle cells (tunica media), but also occur in capillaries owing to the contractile proteins of endothelial cells.

Two mechanisms underlie vasoconstriction:

1. Trauma causes stretching of the smooth muscle cells, triggering an autonomic vasomotor reflex.
2. Trauma induces endothelial cells to release vasoconstrictive agents such as endothelin and platelet-activating factor.

This process would be ineffectual if platelets did not intervene in the later stage. They can adhere to the site of injury, aggregate with each other, and release serotonin from δ-granules. Platelets can prime the coagulation system and cause a sequence of events referred to as "secondary hemostasis," as described in the previous section. The contribution of platelets to thrombus development is dependent on the location of the thrombus and rheologic conditions: in the venous district, thrombi are rich in red blood cells and fibrin, whereas in arterial thrombi, platelets are more represented [12].

1.5 Tissue Factor

This is an integral membrane protein which has an essential role in the extrinsic pathway of blood coagulation. Synthesized as an inactive precursor, TF consists of a signal peptide linked to the mature chain.

Three domains are important for its biochemical function:
1. The first extracellular N-terminal binds with high affinity to FVIIa.
2. The second transmembrane domain binds it to the cell membrane.
3. The third cytoplasmic carboxyl is required for signal transduction.

TF is present in interstitial tissue fibroblasts of the extraendothelial matrix of tunica media and tunica adventitia, where it can bind to FVIIa only after the loss of blood vessel integrity. Through biochemical stimuli, monocytes and endothelial cells can be induced to express TF under pathological conditions.

In normal conditions, TF is separated from circulating FVIIa by the layer of endothelial cells to prevent the inappropriate activation of the coagulation cascade [9]. However, there also exists a certain amount of inactive TF in the circulating blood, transported within vesicles derived from cells such as leukocytes, platelets, monocytes, endothelial cells, and smooth muscle [26]. During the hemostatic process, platelets are activated and express P-selectin, a receptor for vesicles containing TF; this binding allows the propagation of coagulation, even when the damage is limited to the endothelium. In fact, circulating blood TF is present in two forms: a latent one without immediate coagulation capacity and an active one that promotes thrombus formation [9]. The inactive form, after a conformational change, is able to form a complex with FVIIa and bind FX. This binding increases the enzymatic efficiency of serine protease FVIIa with regard to FX, which is activated to FXa, with the consequences referred to earlier. The continuous release of FXa, thrombin, and soluble fibrin into the circulation leads to the activation of the fibrinolytic system, which is described later.

1.6 Platelets and Hemostasis

Platelets are fragments of the bone marrow megakaryocytes and circulate as discoid anucleated cells with a critical function in hemostasis, by acting in concert with coagulation factors and other cells. They contain mitochondria, glycogen particles, lysosomes, and different secretory granules, which are essential for normal platelet function:
- The α-granules containing large polypeptides that contribute to hemostasis, such as vWF and fibrinogen, and platelet factor 4, FV, and other factors.

- The δ-granules (dense granules) rich in low molecular weight compounds that potentiate platelet activation, such as ADP, ATP, GTP, serotonin, and calcium [27].

The cytoskeleton, containing tubulin, actin, and filamin, is responsible for the shape of the resting platelets and for the contractile events, such as the secretion of granules and clot retraction. Despite the lack of genomic DNA, platelets contain more than traces of messenger RNA and the translational machinery necessary for protein synthesis [28]. A wide variety of mobile transmembrane receptors are displayed on the surface and work synergistically in platelet adhesion, activation, and aggregation. The subendothelial components involved in the interactions with platelets include vWF, different types of collagen, fibronectin, thrombospondin, and laminin. Fibrin and fibrinogen, which are not produced by endothelial cells, are immobilized onto extracellular matrix at the site of vascular damage and also bind to platelets. Although several tissue components are able to interact with platelets, only a few may have an essential role in initiating thrombus formation.

Table 1.1 summarizes the characteristics of the main platelet receptors, whose functions are extensively described in the review published by Rivera et al. [13].

Under normal conditions, platelets circulate in a nonadherent resting state, but after vascular injury they interact with exposed proteins in the subendothelium, mainly collagen and vWF, become activated, and undergo a transformation from a smooth discoid to a spherical shape with long dendritic extension. During this process the content of α-granules and δ-granules is released from within the platelets to the surrounding milieu, enhancing activation and promoting adhesion with subendothelium and other platelets. To develop a hemostatic thrombus over this activated monolayer, the recruitment of additional platelets from the flowing blood is mediated by increased local concentrations of soluble and diffusible agonists. They are secreted from dense granules (ADP, ATP, serotonin), synthesized in the platelets (TXA_2), or produced by the coagulation process (thrombin). These agonists interact with specific G-protein-coupled receptors on the platelet membrane and induce signaling events downstream, involving several molecules and second messengers. The resulting rise in cytosolic calcium levels and reorganization of cytoskeleton is referred to as the "inside-out" pathway and is thought to enable the high-affinity state of integrin $\alpha_{IIb}\beta_3$. Binding of vWF and fibrinogen to the active integrin $\alpha_{IIb}\beta_3$ elicits an "outside-in" signaling pathway, which leads to platelet spreading, additional release of granule content, further adhesion and aggregation, and clot retraction. Therefore, platelet activation can be considered a dynamic process involving multiple feedback loops and cross talk between different pathways, as extensively described by Li et al. [14]. Platelet activation can be dampened, increasing the internal concentrations of nitric oxide and cyclic AMP or decreasing the local concentration of platelet agonists, with the consequent reduction of cytoplasmic calcium levels, blockade of TXA_2 receptor, reorganization of cytoskeleton, inhibition of granule release, and downregulation of integrin $\alpha_{IIb}\beta_3$ [20]. These multiple mechanisms contributing to the negative regulation of platelet activity have the role of preventing undesirable platelet accumulation and pathological thrombosis (Fig. 1.6).

Table 1.1 Platelet receptors

Receptor	Ligands/agonists	Functions	References
GPIb-IX-V	vWF, thrombin, FXI, FXII, P-selectin, Mac-1, HMWK, thrombospondin	Adhesion to subendothelium, binding to leukocytes and macrophages, concentration of active factors	[13, 31, 32]
$\alpha_{IIb}\beta_3$	Fibrinogen, vWF, vitronectin, fibronectin, thrombospondin	Firm adhesion, aggregation, spreading on ECM, clot reaction, etc., outside-in signaling	[13, 32, 33]
GPVI	Collagen, laminin	Platelet adhesion and activation by outside-in signaling	[13, 33, 34]
$\alpha_2\beta_1$	Collagen	Platelet adhesion and activation by outside-in signaling	[13, 33, 34]
$\alpha_5\beta_1$	Fibronectin	Adhesion promoting engagement of other integrins	[32]
$\alpha_6\beta_1$	Laminin	Adhesion by outside-in signaling	[32]
$\alpha_V\beta_3$	Vitronectin	Adhesion strengthening	[32]
PARs	Thrombin	Activation of aggregation	[13, 35]
P2Y1, P2Y12	ADP	Amplifying activation of aggregation	[13, 36]
TPα, TPβ	Thromboxane A_2	Amplifying activation of aggregation	[13, 37]
α_2-Adrenergic receptors	Epinephrine	Amplifying activation of aggregation	[13]
PECAM-1	Tyrosine/serine/lipid phosphatases	Signaling inhibition	[13]

GP glycoprotein, *PARs* protease-activated receptors, *PECAM-1* platelet–endothelial cell adhesion molecule 1, *vWF* von Willebrand factor, *FXI* factor XI, *FXII* factor XII, *HMWK* high molecular weight kininogen, *ECM* extracellular matrix

1.7 Fibrinolysis and Hemostasis

Fibrinolysis is a process closely linked to coagulation and its aim is the destruction of the fibrin clot to restore the original tissue integrity, and the restraint of the clotting process to prevent undesired widespread coagulation.

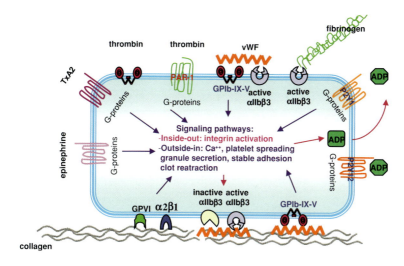

Fig. 1.6 Platelet signaling pathways

Fibrinolysis begins immediately after clot formation on fibrin molecules settled at the site of thrombus development, and it is composed of two major reactions:
1. Activation of plasminogen to plasmin.
2. Degradation and solubilization of fibrin molecules by plasmin.

These two processes involve several activators and inhibitors in different stages.

Fibrinolytic enzymes are produced as inactive precursors (zymogens), with the exception of tPA. Through a proteolytic function on their substrates, they can activate the target enzyme.

All inhibitors of fibrinolysis belong to the SERPIN (serine protease inhibitor) family and have a reactive center that is very similar to a portion of the target physiological substrate. This tool improves the affinity of enzymes for their substrates, leading to a greater efficiency of action [29].

Table 1.2 summarizes the characteristics of the enzymes involved in fibrinolysis.

1.7.1 Fibrinolytic Process

Fibrin acts as a cofactor for the conversion of Glu-plasminogen to Glu-plasmin. Glu-plasminogen starts to catalyze the digestion of fibrin molecules by cleavage of specific residues, subsequently completed by Glu-plasmin. Then fibrin changes its shape, promoting a bond with tPA and Glu-plasminogen. Thus, the modified fibrin is able to induce upregulation of the overall process with high efficiency [30].

Fibrin also serves as a cofactor for the proteolytic conversion of Glu-plasminogen and Glu-plasmin to Lys-plasminogen and Lys-plasmin, respectively.

Table 1.2 Factors involved in fibrinolysis

Fibrinolytic enzyme	Site of production	Function	Activated by	References
Activators of fibrinolysis				
Plasminogen/plasmin	Liver	Degradation of fibrin	tPA	[38]
tPA	Principally endothelial cells	Activation of plasminogen	Plasmin	[39]
uPA	Monocytes, macrophages, fibroblasts, and endothelial cells	Activation of plasminogen	Plasmin	[39]
Inhibitors of fibrinolysis				
Plasminogen activators inhibitor type 1	Several cell types such as hepatocytes, endothelial cells, and platelet α-granules	Inhibition of tPA and uPA	Numerous stimuli such as hormones, growth factors, inflammatory mediators, and clotting factors	[40]
Plasminogen activators inhibitor type 2	Placenta	Inhibition of tPA and uPA	Numerous stimuli such as hormones, growth factors, inflammatory mediators, and clotting factors	[41]
α_2-Antiplasmin	Liver and in a smaller amount in platelets	Inhibition of plasmin	Plasmin	[42]
Thrombin-activated fibrinolysis inhibitor	Liver	Inhibition of plasmin	Thrombin/thrombomodulin	[30]
Metalloproteinases	Liver	Digestion of plasminogen	Plasmin	[43, 44]

tPA tissue-type plasminogen activator, *uPA* urokinase-type plasminogen activator

Lys-plasminogen is more efficient than Glu-plasminogen as a substrate for tPA, which catalyzes the formation of Lys-plasmin. Thus, the modified fibrin formation represents a positive feedback in the fibrinolytic process. At this point in the response to thrombin, particularly thrombin bound to thrombomodulin, thrombin-activated fibrinolysis inhibitor (TAFI) is transformed to activated TAFI (TAFIa).

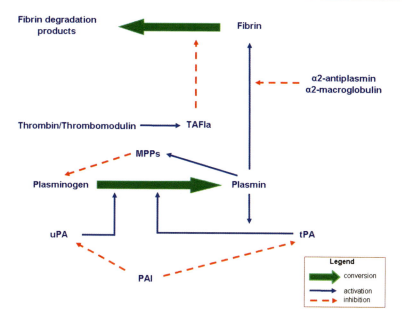

Fig. 1.7 Fibrinolysis

This enzyme catalyzes the removal of C-terminal residues of lysine and arginine on fibrin, producing a further modified molecule, with a low cofactor activity. TAFIa, therefore, does not stop the activation of plasminogen, but reduces its positive feedback, attenuating the fibrinolytic process [30].

The fibrinolysis is also subjected to downregulation of two fast-acting serpins:
1. Plasminogen activator inhibitor type 1, which targets tPA.
2. α_2-Antiplasmin, which acts against Glu-plasmin and Lys-plasmin.

The fibrinolytic process reaches the final step of fibrin digestion and the formation of fibrin degradation products (Fig. 1.7).

References

1. Davie EW (2003) A brief historical review of the waterfall/cascade of blood coagulation. J Biol Chem 278(51):50819–50832
2. Monroe DM, Hoffman M, Roberts HR (2007) Fathers of modern coagulation. Thromb Haemost 98:3–5
3. Davie EW, Ratnoff OD (1964) Waterfall sequence for intrinsic blood clotting. Science 145:1310–1312
4. MacFarlane RG (1964) An enzyme cascade in the blood clotting mechanism, and its function as a biochemical amplifier. Nature 202:498–499
5. Roberts HR, Monroe DM, Oliver JA et al (1998) Newer concepts of blood coagulation. Haemophilia 4:331–334

6. Tanaka KA, Key NS, Levy JH (2009) Blood coagulation: hemostasis and thrombin regulation. Anesth Analg 108:1433–1446
7. Davidson CJ, Hirt RP, Lal K et al (2003) Molecular evolution of the vertebrate blood coagulation network. Thromb Haemost 89:420–428
8. Hoffman M, Monroe DM (2001) A cell-based model of hemostasis. Thromb Haemost 85:958–965
9. Furie B, Furie BC (2008) Mechanisms of thrombus formation. N Engl J Med 359:938–949
10. Bellido-Martin L, Chen V, Furie B, Furie BC (2011) Imaging fibrin formation and platelet and endothelial cell activation in vivo. Thromb Haemost 105:776–782
11. Savage B, Almus-Jacob F, Ruggeri ZM (1998) Specific synergy of multiple substrate-receptor interactions in platelet thrombus formation under flow. Cell 94:657–666
12. Ruggeri ZM (2009) Platelet adhesion under flow. Microcirculation 16(1):58–83
13. Rivera J, Lozano ML, Navarro-Núñez L, Vicente V (2009) Platelet receptors and signaling in the dynamics of thrombus formation. Haematologica 94(5):700–711
14. Li Z, Delaney MK, O'Brien KA, Du X (2010) Signaling during platelet adhesion and activation. Arter Thromb Vasc Biol 30:2341–2349
15. Dubois C, Panicot-Dubois L, Gainor JF, Furie BC, Furie B (2007) Thrombin-initiated platelet activation in vivo is vWF independent during thrombus formation in a laser injury model. J Clin Invest 117(4):953–960
16. Prandoni P (2007) Links between arterial and venous disease. J Intern Med 262(3):341–350
17. Roberts HR, Monroe DM, Escobar MA (2004) Current concepts of hemostasis. Anesthesiology 100:722–730
18. Ignarro LJ, Buga GM, Wood KS, Byrns RE, Chaudhuri G (1987) Endothelium-derived relaxing factor produced and released from artery and vein is nitric oxide. Proc Natl Acad Sci USA 84:9265–9269
19. Palmer RM, Ferrige AG, Moncada S (1987) Nitric oxide release accounts for the biological activity of endothelium-derived relaxing factor. Nature 327:524–526
20. Jin RC, Voetsch B, Loscalzo J (2005) Endogenous mechanisms of inhibition of platelet function. Microcirculation 12:247–258
21. Esmon CT (2000) Regulation of blood coagulation. Biochim Biophys Acta 1477:349–360
22. Mann KG, Bovill EG, Krishnaswamy S (1991) Surface-dependent reactions in the propagation phase of blood coagulation. Ann N Y Acad Sci 614:63–75
23. Löwenberg EC, Meijers JCM, Levi M (2010) Platelet-vessel wall interaction in health and disease. Neth J Med 68:242–251
24. Davie EW, Fujikawa K, Kisiel W (1991) The coagulation cascade: initiation, maintenance, and regulation. Biochemistry 30:10363–10370
25. Lippi G, Favaloro EJ, Franchini M, Guidi GC (2009) Milestones and perspectives in coagulation and hemostasis. Thromb Hemost 35:9–22
26. Butenas S, Bouchard BA, Brummel-Ziedins KE, Parhami-Seren B, Mann KG (2005) Tissue factor activity in whole blood. Blood 105:2764–2770
27. George JN (2000) Platelets. Lancet 355:1531–1539
28. Healy AM, Pickard MD, Pradhan AD, Wang Y, Chen Z, Croce K, Sakuma M, Shi C, Zago AC, Garasic J, Damokosh AI, Dowie TL, Poisson L, Lillie J, Libby P, Ridker PM, Simon DI (2006) Platelet expression profiling and clinical validation of myeloid-related protein 14 as a novel determinant of cardiovascular events. Circulation 113:2278–2284
29. Colucci M, Semeraro N (2006) Il sistema fibrinolitico. In: Burlina A (ed) Trattato italiano di medicina e laboratorio, vol 6. Piccin Nuova Libraria, Padua, pp 1–12
30. Nesheim M (2003) Thrombin and fibrinolysis. Chest 124:33S–39S
31. Clemetson KJ, Clemetson JM (2008) Platelet GPIb complex as a target for anti-thrombotic drug development. Thromb Haemost 99:473–479
32. Kasirer-Friede A, Kahn ML, Shattil SJ (2007) Platelet integrins and immunoreceptors. Immunol Rev 218:247–264

33. Bennet JS (2005) Structure and function of the platelet integrin alphaIIbbeta3. J Clin Invest 115(12):3363–3369
34. Clemetson KJ, Clemetson JM (2001) Platelet collagen receptors. Thromb Haemost 86:189–197
35. Coughlin SR (2005) Protease-activated receptors in hemostasis, thrombosis and vascular biology. J Thromb Haemost 3:1800–1814
36. Gachet C (2008) P2 receptors, platelet functions and pharmacological implications. Thromb Haemost 99:466–472
37. Smyth EM (2010) Thromboxane and the thromboxane receptor in cardiovascular disease. Clin Lipidol 5(2):209–219
38. Collen D, de Maeyer L (1975) Molecular biology of human plasminogen I. Physiochemical properties and microheterogeneity. Thromb Diath Haemorrh 34:396–402
39. Lin Z, Jiang L, Yuan C, Jensen JK, Zhang X, Luo Z, Furie BC, Furie B, Andreasen PA, Huang M (2011) Structural basis for recognition of urokinase-type plasminogen activator by plasminogen activator inhibitor-1. J Biol Chem 286:7027–7032
40. Wind T, Hansen M, Jensen JK, Andreasen PA (2002) The molecular basis for anti-proteolytic and non-proteolytic functions of plasminogen activator inhibitor type-1: roles of the reactive centre loop, the shutter region, the flexible joint region and the small serpin fragment. Biol Chem 383(1):21–36
41. Brenner B (2004) Haemostatic changes in pregnancy. Thromb Res 114(5–6):409–414
42. Shaller J, Gerber SS (2011) The plasminplasmin-antiplasmin system: structural and functional aspects. Cell Mol Life Sci 68:785–801
43. Lijnen HR (2002) Matrix metalloproteinases and cellular fibrinolytic activity. Biochemistry 67:92–98
44. Tsurupa G, Yakovlev S, McKee P, Medved L (2010) Noncovalent interaction of alpha(2)-antiplasmin with fibrin(ogen): localization of alpha(2)-antiplasmin-binding sites. Biochemistry 49(35):7643–7651

Monitoring of Hemostasis

2

Carlo Giansante and Nicola Fiotti

2.1 Introduction

Critically ill patients (CIP) are patients who, because of dysfunction or failure of one or more organs/systems depend on advanced instruments for monitoring and therapy for their survival. Coagulation abnormalities are common in CIP. The most common (35–44%) is thrombocytopenia (platelet count less than 150,000/µl), due to sepsis, disseminated intravascular coagulation (DIC), thrombotic microangiopathy, or induced by drugs, such as heparin. Prolonged global coagulation times, beyond antithrombotic therapy, are also found, and are a result of quantitative defects of coagulation factors, caused by synthesis defects (liver insufficiency), excessive loss (massive hemorrhage), or consumption (DIC), low levels of one or more coagulation factors due to antibodies, antiphospholipid antibodies, or the presence of inhibitors [1–3]. This chapter will provide information on the principles, clinical significance, technology and open problems in laboratory assessment of hemostasis in critically ill patients.

2.2 Principles and Limitations of Laboratory Assessment

Healing a macroscopic or microscopic injury represents a great biologic advantage for every living being. It requires a complex sequence of cellular and extracellular events, partly unknown, aiming at rebuilding the scaffold and, eventually, structure of an organ or tissue. Hemostasis, the earliest and quickest mechanism of tissue

---

C. Giansante (✉)
Unità Clinica Operativa di Clinica Medica Generale e Terapia Medica,
University of Trieste, Trieste, Italy
email: giansant@units.it

G. Berlot (ed.), *Hemocoagulative Problems in the Critically Ill Patient*,
DOI: 10.1007/978-88-470-2448-9_2, © Springer-Verlag Italia 2012

repair, prevents excessive loss of blood, a liquid connective tissue. This process has evolved during evolution to become highly efficient in mammals, in which high blood pressure poses an important challenge to hemostasis.

There is not an ideal model to study in vitro hemostasis, and vast majority of tests revolve around the concept of triggering a biochemical pathway to highlight a deficiency of the system rather than evaluating excessive in vivo efficiency of the system maybe leading to thrombosis. The tests designed to match specific requirements (drug monitoring, or detection of specific coagulation abnormalities) are mainly oriented to reproduce in vitro—rather than to assess in vivo—a specific condition or drug effect. This leaves almost completely unexplored the actual state of the patient, in favor of the analysis of very few reactions. Only recently, in vivo coagulation markers have been introduced in hemostasis laboratory equipment, but cost, sampling peculiarities, and lack of studies are still limiting their use.

Another limitation is in the method which is used for the common test. Armand James Quick developed the test which has his name with laboratory equipment worth around US \$100, according to George Collentine, one of his students. With such a tiny budget, poor technology, and very limited knowledge of the complex coagulation enzyme network and kinetics, the observation of the coagulation phenomena relied on measuring the time to (visually) observe the formation of the first fibrin filaments. Such observation constituted the paradigm for all the coagulation tests developed thereafter. For decades, the method for the tests used in clinics to evaluate the global efficiency of hemostasis relied on the time to reach a certain clot size. Indeed, clot formation in vitro requires the generation of 50 nM thrombin, which represents only about 1% of the whole potential of thrombin generation in vivo, and is therefore poorly predictive of the in vivo process. Assessment of the whole potential of thrombin generation holds great promise in the study of hemostasis, but has been introduced only recently and, notably, describes the in vitro potential of blood, not the actual in vivo state. Therefore, for clinical purposes, such assessment of hemostasis based on coagulation times is widely accepted and actual evaluation of hemostasis defects or monitoring of some old drugs is based on such a technique.

As a consequence, the pathophysiological significance, i.e., correlation of an in vitro test with in vivo activity as well as interlaboratory standardization, has always been a critical point in hemostasis. The prothrombin time, activated partial thromboplastin time (aPTT), and specific assays of platelet function and fibrinolysis were invented in the 1930s and 1940s and led to more sophisticated laboratory tests based on the very same method and inspired by the same approach.

A peculiar problem in emergency medicine, perioperative, and critical care areas, and for CIP in general, is the turnaround time. The importance of a precise diagnosis is obvious for every patient, but in an emergency environment this has to be obtained in a short time, often within the turnaround time of a common laboratory test. Therefore, in recent years, micronization and the development of new technologies have allowed the development of a rapid hemostasis test which can be done at the bedside, by generic personnel, providing a test and diagnosis within minutes instead of some hours.

2.3 Blood Collection Guidelines for Monitoring Hemostasis

Blood sampling is the first, unavoidable, step in order to obtain a hemostasis test. Blood can provide different results according to the source (venous, capillary, or arterial), but also according to the quality of the preanalytical management, i.e., sampling. Surprisingly, the most common cause of an abnormal clotting test is not a pathology-related issue, but rather an improperly obtained sample.

The standard approach in hemostasis is to collect blood and stop coagulation reactions by chelating the plasma calcium with sodium citrate. This blocks the coagulation reactions, except for minimal calcium-independent thrombin activity. Samples can be kept at room temperature. When platelet in vivo activation markers (β-thromboglobulin, βTG, platelet factor 4, PF4) or coagulation activity (fibrinopeptide A, FPA) is being evaluated, calcium chelation is not sufficient, since serious ex vivo platelet aggregation and coagulation could produce false-positive results. For these markers, either blockers of platelet activities (adenosine, citrate, theophylline) or broad spectrum protease inhibitors (namely, aprotinin) for coagulation factors together with immediate cooling (4°C) have to be used.

The personnel conducting the sampling are responsible for adhering to collection and processing guidelines.

Specimen requirements for coagulation assays (described in Ref. [4]) are summarized below.

2.3.1 Before Collection

Patient Identification and Conditions

- Prior to a blood specimen being obtained from any patient, the personal or documental identification of the patient must be verified by checking the patient's wristband for the name and the hospital number.
- Hyperlipemia (and hyperbilirubinemia) can interfere with the test results and their accuracy. For the former condition, if possible, the test should be planned for fastening patients or far from meals.
- Check if the patient has a hematocrit between 20 and 55. If not, see below for special directions.

Identification of the Blood Collection Site

The best samples are obtained with a *peripheral stick* with evacuated tube system. Vascular access devices are not suitable for many routine assessments and definitely *not* for measurement of in vivo activity markers.

Identification and Preparation of Consumables for the Collection

Vacutainer collection tubes (light blue) should be used together with another vial to take out the first milliliters of blood and a 19G to 22G needle. Smaller needles could cause hemolysis; larger are probably unnecessary, unless a platelet aggregation test is conducted. If Vacutainer collection tubes are not available or such a type of sampling is not possible, then a syringe draw is an alternative, using a small (less than 20 ml) syringe and adding blood to the anticoagulant in less than 1 min.

If a sample is drawn from pediatric patients, a pediatric size tube may be used (2.7 ml blood to 0.3 ml of citrate is necessary).

Special Case: Anemia and Polycythemia

To perform a functional test (aPTT, international normalized ratio, INR, and others), plasma samples are collected with calcium-chelating sodium citrate and are then recalcified with calcium chloride in the reaction cuvettes to restore the plasma calcium concentration and the coagulation potential. A sodium citrate concentration of 3.6% provides adequate calcium chelation when the volume of plasma (determined by the red blood cell count of the blood) is within physiological ranges.

In the usual mixing proportions, 10% of the final volume of the anticoagulant solution combines with 90% of blood, which is 60% plasma. In a 5-ml vial, 4.5 ml blood has 2.7 ml of plasma (4.5 × 0.6), which combines with 0.5 ml of 3.6% sodium citrate in a ratio of approximately 5:1, or 0.2 ml of anticoagulant solution for each milliliter of plasma.

The amount of plasma in blood samples varies as the result of changes in the hematocrit, like in anemia and polycythemia. If a standard volume of anticoagulant is used, as in Vacutainer tubes, large amounts of plasma, typical of anemia, can result in a higher amount of available calcium and insufficient neutralization; in contrast, in polycythemia, with less plasma calcium available in the vials, residual chelating activity could interfere with calcium chloride and falsely lengthen functional tests.

These conditions require either modification of the filling of the tube or a different amount of anticoagulant. Keeping in mind the ratio above, we can assume that a sample with a hematocrit of 20 (i.e., around 4 ml of plasma) requires 0.8 ml of sodium citrate (4 ml of blood × 0.2).

If the amount of blood is the target of the correction, then for a standard amount of anticoagulant (0.5 ml) the volume has to be (0.5/0.2) 2.5 ml of plasma. With a hematocrit of 20, the whole volume of blood is approximately 3.1 ml (2.5/0.8). The same principles apply to calculations for polycythemia.

2.3.2   During Collection

From a Peripheral Vein

Clean venipuncture is essential; therefore, trauma should be avoided. Prolonged tourniquet use should be avoided as should "digging" to find the vein since it can cause activation of clotting factors, which can result in a clotted sample. Contamination with tissue factor, activation of clotting factors and platelets, and hemolysis can occur from use of multiple sticks, slapping the vein, excessive pumping of the

2 Monitoring of Hemostasis

hand, air bubbles in the syringes, or placing the tourniquet on too tightly or for too long a period of time.

From a peripheral vein, draw 2–3 ml of blood (which can be rich in cell debris and tissue factor) into a vial and discard it or use it for other purposes. Then use a 5-ml blue-top tube containing the anticoagulant.

The tubes must be properly filled to achieve the proper ratio of blood to citrate (9:1, i.e., nine parts blood to one part anticoagulant). Vials less than 90% full are unacceptable for many routine laboratories, but never combine the contents of two underfilled tubes to make one filled tube.

Mix the anticoagulant with whole blood promptly and thoroughly by gently inverting (do not shake) the vial.

From a Vascular Access Device

If one is drawing from central line, flush the line with 5 ml saline and discard the first 5 ml or six dead space volumes. If one is drawing from a saline lock, discard two dead space volumes.

Use a discard tube (around 3–5 ml) before using light-blue-stoppered tubes (the discard will fill the "dead space" of winged collection set tubing). If this is not done, an underfilled tube or diluted sample/analyte could result.

2.3.3 Afterward

Mix the contents thoroughly by gentle inversion. Do not shake the vials. The samples should be labeled in the patient's presence. Deliver the samples by hand (never by a pneumatic tube) as soon as possible to the laboratory, or conduce the test in a point-of-care setting within the appropriate time. Usually, samples should be stored at *room temperature* (ice will activate leukocytes in the sample, resulting in shortened clotting times), unless special tests are to be run (β-TG, PF4, FPA).

2.4 The Particular Approach for CIP

Some critical aspects of the treatment of CIP need to be considered in the choice, performance, and interpretation of the hemostasis test. The extension of the time of care, the turnaround time for the laboratory test, and deployment are the main issues in treating CIP.

Time extension. CIP require special monitoring as long as they remain in such state. This means that the hemostasis test should be repeated every 24 h using, for comparison purposes, the same instrument and assuming the same (possibly high) grade of reliability.

Turnaround time. The time needed to conduct a test is critical in those patients with intense anticoagulation such as in cardiothoracic surgery, bleeding, or simply who are at risk of bleeding. Sometimes, even the analytic phase of standard coagulation tests (30–60 min) is often too long an interval to wait for reliable guidance on the use of blood products for a massively bleeding patient. As a result, many clinicians have turned their attention toward point-of-care coagulation testing, which is able to provide a less precise result in 15 min, rather than a perfect result in 30–60 min, as long as most of the time the result they obtain is close to the "true" value or at least is sufficiently accurate to prevent the inappropriate transfusion of blood products.

Settings. CIP may be in different settings (some within and some beyond the reach of a hemostasis laboratory). Among the many are: surgery rooms and emergency areas, but also in war settings, tragedy settings (in mobile clinics), and also the patient's house. Different locations also drive different prognoses: military patients with trauma have a 31–38% chance of coagulopathy, associated with a fivefold increase in mortality when compared with civilian trauma patients [5]. Prompt diagnostic support is essential for these patients. Two strategies have been developed to manage this problem. The first, which can be offered only to patients with reach of a laboratory, is to create an array of tests which can be conducted in the routine central laboratory and in a short time. In a study omitting some steps of the laboratory workbench and speeding up others, some hemostasis tests maintained sufficient/good quality and the results were ready after around 20 min [6]. Such a strategy is not suitable when a patient is far from a laboratory facility.

The most relevant advance in this context is the development of point-of-care testing (POCT), a bedside set of coagulation tests. Even considering the many limitations in reproducibility and comparability, POCT can provide information on hemostasis in real time and drive diagnosis and therapy of some CIP.

2.5 Evaluation and Use of Coagulometers

Automation in coagulation laboratories has greatly improved accuracy, precision, and standardization, and has facilitated tests requiring specific training and special conditions. In the 1990s, a number of manufacturers successfully included multiple detection methods, which now give a single laboratory the possibility of applying different methods using the same equipment, and fully automated instruments are today quite common in hemostasis laboratories. They provide efficiency, comparability, repeatability, and reproducibility. Today, instruments can perform clotting, chromogenic, and immunological tests.

2.5.1 Principles of Operation

Mechanical tests. These rely on the increased viscosity of the plasma when fibrin is formed. A steel ball within the plasma sample is subjected to a magnetic field, resulting in a swinging movement of the ball. The increased viscosity from coagulation hinders movement and when a predetermined level of oscillation is not reached, the chronometer stops. The time relates to the speed of fibrin formation.

Photo-optical test. Fibrin clot formation induces a change in the optical density of the specimen: therefore, the time to reach certain a degree of change, assessed with a light beam, is related to the coagulation efficacy.

Nephelometric principle. Laser dispersion can be an alternative way to assess fibrin formation. Light is scattered when it encounters a fibrin clot and measurements are related to a certain level of dispersion (90° or 180°) lateral or backward with respect to the vial.

Chromogenic principle. A color-specific generating substance known as a chromophore (*para*-nitroaniline is the most common) can be linked to synthetic substrates (chromogenic substrate) of proteins involved in coagulation. The analyte protease cleaves the chromogenic substrate, generating a yellow color (*para*-nitroaniline is measured at 405 nm) proportional to the amount/activity.

Immunological principle. Specific antibodies can be bound to latex microparticles, and reaction with the specific antigen will cause agglutination of many particles into a larger agglomerate of particles. This method assesses the amount of an analyte/antigen using the property of microparticles absorbing light when their size approaches the wavelength of (monochromatic) light. Such an increase in light absorbance is proportional to the agglutination, which, in turn, is proportional to the amount of the antigen present in the sample.

2.6 Primary Hemostasis Tests

A test able to screen primary hemostasis is not available in clinical settings. So far the only test, the Ivy skin test, is expressed as the time required to observe the primary hemostasis after a standardized incision in the volar surface of the forearm. Platelet adhesion and aggregation (intrinsic defects, von Willebrand disease, drugs), vascular tone, and integrity, as well as skin resistance, determine the bleeding time, but the thickness and vascularization of the skin, the site and depth of the incision, the skin temperature, and patient anxiety can affect the results, making the Ivy test imprecise, inaccurate, and irreproducible. These limitations make the bleeding time not suitable for any clinical use.

2.6.1 Platelet Function

Platelet Count

A low platelet count is the most common hemostasis defect in CIP. The accuracy of hematology analyzers, based on electrical impedance or light scattering techniques, is ±5% in the range between 1,000 and 3,000,000 platelets per microliter. The mean platelet volume is also provided by the same instruments, together with a platelet size distribution curve.

Spontaneous platelet aggregates, cold agglutinins, or use of EDTA as an anticoagulant can spuriously reduce the platelet count, inducing so-called pseudothrombocytopenia. In contrast, particulate debris, i.e., red or white cell fragments, can account for spurious thrombocytosis.

Since thrombocytopenia can induce an overestimate of the platelet count, low platelet counts need manual inspection of a peripheral smear [7].

Platelet Aggregation

Platelet aggregation is measured by either conventional or whole blood platelet aggregometry. The former uses a modified spectrophotometer using light transmission variation to measure formation of the platelet, whereas the latter is based on changes of electrical impedance due to the cell–cell (platelets and leukocytes) contact in whole blood. Platelets in platelet-rich plasma are triggered in vitro by an agonist to diagnose inherited and acquired platelet disorders, for the assay for von Willebrand factor activity (ristocetin cofactor assay), and for the diagnosis of heparin-induced thrombocytopenia.

The type of agonist is chosen to diagnose specific platelet defects. Whole-blood aggregometers have a faster turnaround time. Also, lumiaggregometers measure aggregation and ATP release at once, to provide a more accurate diagnosis of platelet function defects. Routinely, the platelet agonists used to differentiate various platelet function defects are ADP, adrenaline, collagen, ristocetin, and arachidonic acid, whereas thrombin, vasopressin, serotonin, thromboxane A_2, platelet-activating factor, and other agents are mainly used for research.

The main utilization is in the diagnosis of platelet defects. The most relevant is *Glantzman* thromboasthenia, consisting in the aberration of the activatable fibrinogen-binding glycoprotein (GP) IIb/IIIa. In this condition, all fibrinogen-dependent aggregation is defective, i.e., that to ADP, epinephrine, arachidonic acid, and collagen, whereas passive aggregation ristocetin-mediated aggregation is maintained. *Bernard–Soulier* disease is characterized by lack of GPIb/IX, thrombocytopenia, and large platelets. In these patients, fibrinogen-mediated aggregation is efficient, whereas binding to thrombin, ristocetin, and von Willebrand factor (i.e., GPIb/IX-mediated aggregation) is poor.

A more sophisticated use of aggregometry relies on mixing studies, i.e., tests where either the patient's platelets or plasma is mixed with control components and triggered with specific agonists. In *heparin-induced thrombocytopenia*, plasma (containing antibodies against the PF4–heparin complex) can induce control platelet aggregation in the presence of heparin as an agonist. The complex binds to CD32 (FcγRIIA), resulting in platelet aggregation. The relatively low sensitivity and turnaround time make enzyme immunoassay and flow cytometry preferable in the initial diagnosis of heparin-induced thrombocytopenia, and the platelet aggregation test should only be used as a confirmatory test in antibody-positive patients.

Von Willebrand disease is another condition requiring platelet aggregation. Ristocetin aggregability is impaired when plasma from these patients, lacking von

Willebrand factor, is used, but not when the patient's platelets are matched with control plasma.

In conclusion, although very precise, platelet aggregometry is a complex, time-consuming, expensive test, the utility of which, in CIP, is limited to confirmation of inherited diseases, but with few consequences for acute treatment of the patient.

2.7 Clot-Based Assays

Although some guidelines state that the INR can be conducted even after 24 h, no matter whether the sample is centrifuged or not, or is taken from thawed plasma stored at $-70°C$ for 6 months, fresh clean plasma should be the only option for CIP.

2.7.1 Activated Partial Thromboplastin Time

The aPTT is a functional evaluation of the intrinsic pathway of coagulation (involving fibrinogen, prothrombin, factors V, VIII, IX, XI and XII, prekallikrein, high molecular weight kininogen). In the aPTT, an aliquot of undiluted, platelet-poor plasma is incubated with a particulate factor XII activator (e.g., silica, Celite, kaolin, micronized silica, ellagic acid, etc.) and a reagent containing phospholipid (partial thromboplastin) at 37°C. After 5 min, i.e., after generation of a sufficient amount of activated factor XI, the sample is recalcified with $CaCl_2$ and the chronometer starts. A cascade reaction takes place and results in fibrin production, which stops the chronometer. The normal value is between 24 and 37 s [3]. Statistically, the aPTT is slightly lengthened in young individuals and slightly shortened in older populations. Premature infants have prolonged aPTT values, which return to normal by 6 months of age. However, age-specific normal ranges are not utilized in patient care at this time.

The sensitivity of the assay to factor deficiencies, inhibitors, and heparin varies with the reagents used in the assay. Lipemia and hyperbilirubinemia interfere with the detection of clot formation by photo-optical methods.

Clinical Use
The aPTT is a fundamental assay of the intrinsic pathway of the coagulation system. The principal clinical uses of the aPTT include:
1. The detection of hereditary or acquired deficiencies or defects of the intrinsic and common pathway coagulation factors and monitoring their eventual correction, such as coagulation factor replacement therapy in patients with hemophilia. The time increases beyond the upper limit when a single factor is below 40% of activity.
2. Monitoring intravenous unfractionated heparin anticoagulant therapy.

3. Detection of coagulation inhibitors (i.e., lupus anticoagulant, antibodies against coagulation factors), and of resistance to activated protein C (i.e., genetic defects of factor V).

Liver disease, disseminated intravascular coagulation (DIC), intense oral anticoagulant therapy, and improper specimen collection (i.e., traumatic phlebotomy or hemolyzed specimen) are other causes of inaccurate aPTT.

For some uses, variants of the test have been developed. These include reptilase time, protein C and protein S activity, tests for lupus anticoagulant diagnosis (dilute Russell's viper venom time, dRVVT), and activated C protein resistance test.

2.7.2 Prothrombin Time and INR

Test methodology. In the prothrombin time, an aliquot of plasma is incubated at 37°C with a reagent containing a phospholipid–protein tissue extract mix (complete thromboplastin). $CaCl_2$ is then added and the time required for clot formation is measured by one of a variety of techniques (photo-optical, electromechanical, etc.). The result is reported in seconds (prothrombin time), or as a ratio compared with the laboratory mean normal control (prothrombin ratio). Indeed, the prothrombin time is critically dependent on the characteristics of the thromboplastin used in the assay and in particular on tissue factor content. This receptor (CD142), a transmembrane protein widely expressed on cells of nonvascular origin, activates factor VII during the initiation of the extrinsic coagulation pathway. It is commercially taken from the uterus and brain of animals (and only recently has been obtained by recombinant technology) and its amount differs critically according to the type of organ and the age and strain of the animal. Thus, potentially, different laboratories might provide different and sometimes opposite results, leading to different clinical decisions. For this reason, the WHO requires that the activity of each batch of thromboplastin from manufacturers of INR kits is matched with a reference sample from the WHO. The result of such a comparison is the international sensitivity index (ISI), a power factor to be assigned to the ratio of the times (patient/reference) to obtain the INR. Nowadays, only the INR should be considered for monitoring the extrinsic pathway.

What the prothrombin time measures. The prothrombin time is a functional determination of the extrinsic (tissue factor) pathway of coagulation (prothrombin, factors V, VII, and X, fibrinogen) and is extremely sensitive to the vitamin K dependent clotting factors (prothrombin, factor VII and X). The prothrombin time is used for the detection of inherited or acquired coagulation defects related to the extrinsic pathway of coagulation and for monitoring oral anticoagulation maintained with vitamin K antagonists. Its normal values are in the range 8.8–11.6 s and the INR should be between 0.8–1.2 [7].

2.7.3 Fibrinogen Assay

Fibrinogen is a large asymmetrical clotting protein in the plasma, with a normal level ranging from 200 to 350 mg/dl and a half-life of 4 days. Its plasma concentration is essential in the diagnosis and management of many coagulopathies. In addition, it is also an acute phase reactant, and high levels represent a risk index in some patients who will develop myocardial infarction and stroke.

The methods for its measurement are numerous and many of them provide significantly different results. The washed clot assay (dry weight of the total clottable fibrinogen, or the protein content in a washed and dissolved clot), proposed by the WHO, is a time-consuming reference technique but is definitely not suitable for CIP and emergency settings.

The von Clauss technique is the standard method used in clinical laboratories, and provides the best results in terms of interlaboratory and intralaboratory accuracy and precision [8]. In this technique, a high concentration of thrombin is added to buffer-diluted (1:5 or 1:10) plasma. Dilution reduces the effect of clotting inhibitors and the clotting time is, therefore, directly proportional to the level of clottable fibrinogen. The times are then converted into fibrinogen concentration on a standard curve made with purified fibrinogen of known concentration. Accuracy is good in the range of approximately 50–800 mg/dl.

Interference in such a measurement can come from high (beyond therapeutic) levels of heparin or hirudin, hyperfibrinolytic activity (which will require a special tube containing aprotinin or another plasmin inhibitor), and fibrin degradation products (FDPs). All these can result in underestimation by the Clauss or coagulation-based technique.

2.8 Plasma Mixing Studies

A high INR value or a prolonged aPTT indicate either a factor deficiency or the presence of an inhibitor of coagulation. The plasma mixing study is the initial step in the evaluation of a prolonged clotting time, provided that 50% of any coagulation factor is sufficient to restore a normal value of the test, but the presence of an inhibitor requires a more important dilution and is able to prolong coagulation times of normal pooled plasma. So, even the 1% factor VIII level encountered in severe hemophilia can be corrected to the normal range by mixing with normal pooled plasma, whereas an inhibitor requires a higher plasma dilution and 1:1 mixing will not completely restore the coagulation time. The single deficient clotting factor will be then identified by "factor assays": in principle, mixing the plasma of the patient with plasmas known to be deficient in a different coagulation factor will identify the defective protein (the level in the mix in one of the vials will not be above 50%, resulting in a prolonged time). The failure of a mixing study to correct a prolonged clotting test indicates an "inhibitory" substance retarding coagulation.

Precise identification of the inhibitor requires cooperation with the clinicians and further laboratory tests. Inhibitors can be considered "specific," such as antibodies directed against phospholipids (like in lupus anticoagulant) or a specific coagulation factor (factor inhibitor), or "global", i.e., FDPs, monoclonal paraproteins, and drugs such as heparin. The former group is not corrected by the mixing studies, and the latter is corrected only in part, but not completely. Clinical and other laboratory clues are necessary to identify the inhibitor. For example, lupus anticoagulant is not associated with clinical bleeding, whereas specific factor inhibitors frequently induce bleeding. The diagnosis can be confirmed by a phospholipid-sensitive test such as the dRVVT.

Heparin and other global inhibitors (paraproteins and FDPs) can be confirmed by other coagulation tests, such as the thrombin clotting time and the reptilase time, which are insensitive to these inhibitors.

The incubation time can provide further information on the activity of the inhibitor. Fast-reacting inhibitors prolong the coagulation time immediately after the mixing (most factor inhibitors, except factor VIII, and most lupus anticoagulants), whereas slow-reacting inhibitors (most factor VIII inhibiting factors and 15% of lupus anticoagulants) require 1–2 h of incubation at 37°C to inhibit the test.

In the case of hereditary prekallikrein deficiency, inducing a markedly prolonged aPTT, a prolonged preincubation (i.e., 10 min) of the plasma with aPTT reagent before the assay is performed normalizes the time.

2.8.1 Reptilase Time

Reptilase replaces thrombin and is not affected by heparin, hirudin, and antithrombin antibodies, but is still sensitive to the presence of myeloma proteins and FDPs. Prolongation of both the thrombin time and the reptilase time suggests myeloma, FDPs, hypofibrinogenemia, or dysfibrinogenemia. A prolonged aPTT and a normal reptilase time indicates that, beyond the aforementioned causes, heparin, hirudin, or other antithrombins are the cause of the prolonged aPTT. If these drugs, FDPs or myeloma can be ruled out, then the cause of the prolonged reptilase time may be hypodysfibrinogenemia.

2.8.2 Dilute Russell's Viper Venom Assay

Lupus anticoagulants are IgG and IgM autoantibodies that interfere with the function of anionic phospholipids found in patients with antiphospholipid antibody syndrome. The effect on coagulation is to prolong phospholipid-dependent clotting tests such as the aPTT and particularly the dRVVT. Russell's viper venom contains a serine protease that directly activates factor X. The activated factor X then activates prothrombin (factor II) in the presence of factor V and phospholipid. In the dRVVT test, the phospholipid content (of plant origin) is lowered to make the test more sensitive to the presence of substances blocking the availability of the phospholipid surface. Starting by activation of factor X, moreover, the test is not influenced by deficiencies of the contact or intrinsic pathway factors or antibodies against factors VIII, IX, or XI, as can be the case for aPTT.

2.9 POCT Technologies

POCT refers to testing that is performed near or at the site of the patient, with the result leading to a possible change in the care of patient. The development of devices incorporating microchemistry, miniaturization, and microcomputerization has led us to a point where many of the hemostasis tests can be performed in real time at the bedside or at the point of patient interaction.

Hemostasis tests currently available in POCT are:

- International normalized ratio (INR)
- Activated partial thromboplastin time (aPTT)
- Activated clotting time (ACT)
- Modifications of the thrombin time
- Thromboelastography
- Platelet function
- D-dimer

They can be performed in venous (whole or centrifuged) as well as in capillary blood. Some further difficulties can be encountered with POCT devices compared with standard devices: insufficient volume of blood sample (usually 3–50 µl), coordination between warm up of the strip and capillary blood sampling, access to the test strip (when inserted in the device), unavailable heparin neutralizing reagent in some kits, high INR (above 4.5), high viscosity, hematocrit extremes (below 25 or above 55), hyperbilirubinemia, and hypertriglyceridemia.

The technologies used in POCT are quite different and the main problems are standardization of the results and comparability among different POCT devices and coagulometers. Conflicting reports exist on comparability with regular coagulometers. External quality assessment programs do exist but, at the moment, they are very few. The tests described below are those peculiar to or better performed with POCT technologies [9].

2.9.1 Thromboelastography

Native blood is put in the cuvette and left to coagulate with a 45° swinging movement. A pin is immersed in the vial and suspended by a torsion wire—a transductor attached to the wire records the strength of the forming clot. This allows one to record the formation/dissolution speed, and the amplitude of the clot. Thromboelastography is mainly used in monitoring blood replacement products in perioperative patients.

Thromboelastography has been adopted into the resuscitation protocols of some centers. However, although the turnaround time for rapid thromboelastography (19 + 3.1 min) may seem advantageous compared with that of routine laboratory tests, in most centers this time is spent by the clinician performing laboratory testing, instead of direct treatment of the patient, which could negatively affect the delivery of health care.

2.9.2 Platelet Test

Recently, POCT platelet tests have been used in CIP treatment. One type of assessment studies aggregability and is based on impedance platelet counting. The principle is that a thrombocytopenia (low platelet count) is expected in a blood sample aggregated by an agonist and such a reduction in platelet count is directly proportional to the aggregation potential. Two separate samples are taken, one containing a prefixed dose of angonist (ADP and collagen), and the difference in the platelet counts between the two samples expressed as a percentage reflects the effect of antiplatelet drugs (clopidogrel, NSAIDs, or GPIIb/IIIa antagonists) in patients with different cardiovascular disease undergoing procedures.

Another method (PFA-100) is to study aggregation under flow conditions. Blood mixed with a platelet agonist is forced through a narrow pore (150 μm) at a high shear rate corresponding to that of a small artery. Platelets undergo platelet adherence, activation aggregation, and finally occlusion of the pore. The time to occlusion (closure time) is the final result of the assay. This test is versatile and can provide information also on inherited platelet dysfunction, aspirin resistance or antiplatelet compliance, monitoring desmopressin acetate in von Willebrand disease patients (types 1 and 2).

The limitations of this test are the insensitivity to low levels of fibrinogen or other coagulation factors and some platelet defects, requiring a strict clinical cooperation in order to evaluate the results. Moreover, the test is affected by preanalytical conditions such as hematocrit, platelet count, and the collection technique.

Alternatively, in the platelet test, blood is forced into a slit at constant pressure. The bleeding time is the time that elapses between the start of the flow and the blood clotting in the slit. Phase I studies suggest that such a test is able to diagnose dysfunctional platelets and thrombotic thrombocytopenic purpura and to monitor the effects of plasma exchange.

Recently, microbead agglutination technology has been used in the evaluation of platelet function (VerifyNow system). Anticoagulated blood is put into contact with fibrinogen-coated microbeads, which, after agglutination, change the optical absorbance of the sample.

All these POCT devices/techniques have a shorter turnaround time but none are comparable in terms of sensibility or sensitivity with classic platelet aggregometry.

2.9.3 Activated Clotting Time

The ACT is useful in monitoring coagulation status and high-level heparinization in immediate-need situations such as cardiac surgery. The ACT uses tubes containing a negatively charged particulate activator of coagulation, such as kaolin, Celite, or diatomaceous earth. When whole blood is drawn into the tube, the contact system is activated and clotting occurs. The manual ACT device has been replaced in recent years by an increasingly sophisticated variety of microprocessor-controlled instruments. The assay is useful at high levels of heparin, when the aPTT assay would provide an unclottable sample, but is also affected by platelets. For this reason, some manufacturers also provide ACT reagents containing heparinase so that a patient's baseline value can be established in the presence of heparin. These instruments are increasingly being applied to the near-patient monitoring of direct thrombin inhibitors and low molecular weight heparins in critical situations.

2.9.4 D-dimer

D-dimer is a marker of fibrin turnover, its level being increased as a result of both increased formation and increased degradation of fibrin. Although this marker is hardly used in emergency situations, it still retains its utility in the treatments of CIP to rule out deep vein thrombosis. This semiquantitative test has reached sufficient reliability for clinical settings and is considered negative when values are below 500 ng/ml. Different antibody-related techniques are employed in the analysis of this marker.

References

1. Levi M, Opal SM (2006) Coagulation abnormalities in critically ill patients. Crit Care 10:222
2. Perry DJ, Fitzmaurice DA, Kitchen S, Mackie IJ, Mallett S (2010) Point-of-care testing in haemostasis. Br J Haematol 150:501–514
3. Wheeler AP, Rice TW (2010) Coagulopathy in critically ill patients—part 2. Chest 137:185–194
4. NCCLS (1998) Collection, transport and processing of blood specimens for coagulation testing and general performance of coagulation assays, approved guideline 3rd edn, H21-A3. Wayne, PA
5. Borgman MA, Spinella PC, Perkins JG, Grathwohl KW, Repine T, Beekley AC, Sebesta J, Jenkins D, Wade CE, Holcomb JB (2007) The ratio of blood products transfused affects mortality in patients receiving massive transfusions at a combat support hospital. J Trauma 63:805–813
6. Chandler WL, Ferrel C, Trimble S, Moody S (2010) Development of a rapid emergency hemorrhage panel. Transfusion 50:2547–2552
7. Jordan CD, Flood JG, Laposata M, Lewandrowski KB (1992) Normal reference laboratory values. N Engl J Med 327:718–724

8. Palareti G, Maccaferri M, Manotti C, Tripodi A, Chantarangkul V, Rodeghiero F, Ruggeri M, Mannucci PM (1991) Fibrinogen assays: a collaborative study of six different methods. C.I.S.M.E.L. Comitato Italiano per la Standardizzazione dei Metodi in Ematologia e Laboratorio. Clin Chem 37:714–719
9. Louie RF, Tang Z, Shelby DG, Kost GJ (2000) Point of care testing: millennium technology for critical care. Lab Med 31:402–408

Anticoagulation Therapy in ICU Patients

3

Emanuele Marras, Luigi Lo Nigro and Giorgio Berlot

3.1 Introduction

Most patients admitted to a critical care unit have multiple risk factors for thromboembolic complications, which are very present in the guise of deep venous thrombosis (DVT) and/or pulmonary thromboembolism (PTE) [1]. Risks factors may be present before the ICU admission (i.e., advanced age, malignancy, major surgery, and major trauma), or may be related to the ICU stay (such as mechanical ventilation and central venous catheters [2–5]). In such settings, there are strong indications for prolonged thromboprophylaxis and/or treatment of thrombotic complications [6, 7]. This is achieved by a number of pharmacological and nonpharmacological provisions, each having specific advantages and shortcomings. To date, heparin and vitamin K antagonists (VKAs) are the two most widely used measures for both prevention and treatment of DVT and PTE.

3.2 Biological Actions of Unfractioned Heparin and Low Molecular Weight Heparin

Unfractioned heparin (UFH) is a heterogeneous mixture of glycosaminoglycans with molecular masses between 3,000 and 30,000 Da, which act by binding to antithrombin III (ATIII) and accelerating the inhibitory activity against thrombin. The heparin–ATIII complex can also inhibit factor X. The best activities are obtained using heparin administered by continuous infusion intravenously (10–20 UI/kg/h)

E. Marras (✉)
Anesthesia and Intensive Care, Cattinara Hospital,
University of Trieste, Trieste, Italy
e-mail: dottorsulcis@gmail.com

G. Berlot (ed.), *Hemocoagulative Problems in the Critically Ill Patient*,
DOI: 10.1007/978-88-470-2448-9_3, © Springer-Verlag Italia 2012

after a bolus (5,000 U intravenously), which will ensure the proper achievement of the steady-state drug concentration. The pharmacological effect should be monitored with the tissue thromboplastin time (activated partial thromboplastin time, aPTT), and checks should be performed every 6 h until the desired level of anticoagulation is achieved. Heparin has a half-life of about 90 min, so its action is over after 2–4 h from its discontinuation. To modulate the pharmacological effect of heparin, if needed, protamine can be administered at a dose of 1 mg/100 U of heparin administered. The dose of protamine that should be administered to neutralize a bolus of heparin decreases in proportion to the time elapsed since the bolus (immediately after the bolus, 100% of the dose, after 1 h 50%, after 2 h 25%).

In critically ill patients heparin resistance may occur, likely either because of binding of heparin to some acute phase proteins or because of low levels of ATIII. In the former case, the heparin dose must be increased, whereas in the latter case, ATIII levels of 70% or greater must be obtained.

UFH may also be administered subcutaneously at low doses, primarily for prophylaxis of DVT [8]. The common dosage is approximately 5,000 U every 12 h, and it usually does not require monitoring through the aPTT.

The low molecular weight heparins (LMWH) are derived from the fractionation of UFH. These molecules inhibit the coagulation cascade by blocking activated factor X (factor Xa). The LMWH have been shown to be superior to UFH in the prophylaxis of DVT [9].

Moreover, the dose–effect response is more predictable, and bleeding complications and heparin-induced thrombocytopenia (HIT) are more uncommon. The half-life of LMWH is longer than that of UFH (about 4 h) and their effect is only partially reverted by protamine. The elimination of LMWH is primarily renal, and their effect can be prolonged in patients with acute kidney injury [10]. The route of administration of LMWH is usually subcutaneous. The DVT prophylaxis dose and the interval of administration differ depending on the type of molecule.

The efficacy of heparin anticoagulation during the first few days of therapy after the DVT diagnosis is relevant for the long-term risk of late recurrent thromboembolism. The absence of an initial heparin treatment is associated with unacceptable high relapse rates of DVT in the long term [11].

3.3   Prevention of DVT and PTE

According to the American College of Chest Physicians, actions to prevent DVT and PTE are recommended for several surgical procedures [2]. All major trauma [4] and all spinal cord injury patients should receive thromboprophylaxis (grade of recommendation 1A), whereas in patients admitted to hospital with an acute medical illness [12], thromboprophylaxis with LMWH, low-dose UFH, or fondaparinux is recommended (each grade 1A). Finally, the venous thromboembolism (VTE) risk of all patients admitted to the ICU should be assessed, and most should receive thromboprophylaxis (grade of recommendation 1A) [11, 13].

3.4 Treatment of DVT

The goals of treatment of DVT are (1) to stop local extension of the thrombus and the detachment of emboli, (2) to prevent lysis of the clot, and (3) to prevent long-term complications (postthrombotic syndrome) [14, 15]. These aims are commonly achieved by using anticoagulants (heparins and oral anticoagulants), fibrinolytic agents, and vena cava filters.

3.4.1 Unfractioned Heparin

The evidence proving the efficacy of UFH in the treatment of DVT of the lower limbs [16] was provided in the 1990s. There was a remarkable reduction of thromboembolic events, 6 months after the episode, combined with an even more significant reduction of asymptomatic thrombosis extensions [8].

High doses of UFH are required to inhibit the growth of a thrombus. To prevent PTE and the extension/recurrence of DVT, it is vital to achieve the desired anticoagulant effect in a short time.

When patients are admitted to hospital, UHF is administered by a continuous intravenous infusion. This approach provides a more effective level of anticoagulation compared with the one achieved by administering multiple doses. Moreover, it also reduces the risk of bleeding caused by intermittent hypocoagulability associated with administration of multiple doses. On the basis of the drug administration guidelines, the loading dose should be 50–100 IU/kg intravenously, followed by a continuous intravenous infusion of 1,250–1,500 IU/h, titrated according to the aPTT, with a maintenance ratio of 1.5–2.5 times the control value. In the first 48 h, the heparin required may be substantially higher than that required successively (60,000 IU/day or more), especially in patients with extended thrombosis.

The optimal therapeutic aPTT range, reported in baseline studies, corresponds to plasma heparin levels between 0.2 and 0.4 IU/ml (measured by protamine titration), or between 0.35 and 0.7 (measured as the level of anti-factor Xa activity).

Over the past years, treatment and prophylaxis of VTE, long done with UFH, has been gradually complemented and partly replaced by use of LMWH, which have a greater bioavailability, a longer half-life, and a more predictable anticoagulant action [9], although evidence of moderate quality (Chest, February 24, 2011) suggests that subcutaneous UFH twice daily and UFH thrice daily do not differ in their effect on DVT, pulmonary embolism, major bleeding, and mortality. Either of the two dosing regimens of UFH or LMWH appears to be a reasonable strategy for thromboprophylaxis in patients [13, 17].

3.4.2 Low Molecular Weight Heparins

It has been shown that subcutaneous LMWH is effective in the acute phase of DVT and is a good alternative to the intravenous method. A meta-analysis of studies comparing the two routes of administration showed a substantial balance, in terms of both efficacy and bleeding risk [18]. The rate of hospitalization was reduced and a more rapid mobilization was observed with subcutaneous administration. Compared with the intravenous route, therapeutic concentrations are reached more slowly (1–2 h after injection). The initial cumulative daily dose should not be less than 35,000 U, divided into two or three doses. Monitoring of the aPTT is essential and should be performed on venous samples taken 4–6 h after the administration of each dose.

3.4.3 Vitamin K Antagonists

VKAs, or coumarins, have been the mainstay of oral anticoagulant therapy for more than 60 years. Despite their proven effectiveness and wide use in clinical practice, their optimal management may be challenging. In fact, effective treatment greatly depends on the time within the therapeutic window; this range is actually rather narrow for all currently used coumarins.

Pharmacodynamics
VKAs produce their anticoagulant effect by interfering with the cyclic interconversion of vitamin K and its 2,3-epoxide (vitamin K epoxide), thereby modulating the γ-carboxylation of glutamate residues on the N-terminal regions of vitamin K dependent proteins [19]. The vitamin K dependent coagulation factors prothrombin, VII, IX, and X require γ-carboxylation for their procoagulant activity, and treatment with VKAs results in the hepatic production of partially carboxylated and decarboxylated proteins with reduced coagulant activity. Moreover, the VKAs inhibit carboxylation of the regulatory anticoagulant proteins C, S, and Z, thus having a procoagulant potential.

Pharmacokinetics
The two most widespread VKAs, warfarin and acenocoumarol, are a racemic mixture of two optically isomers, the R and S enantiomers. Both drugs are taken orally. Warfarin is highly water soluble and rapidly absorbed, has high bioavailability, and reaches maximal blood concentrations about 90 min after oral administration. Racemic warfarin has a half-life of 36–42 h, circulates bound to plasma proteins (mainly albumin), and accumulates in the liver, where the two enantiomers are transformed by different pathways (the S enantiomer is metabolized by the CYP2C9 enzyme of the cytochrome P450 system, whereas the R enantiomer is metabolized by CYP1A2 and CYP3A4). (R)-Acenocoumarol has an elimination half-life of 9 h, whereas (S)-acenocoumarol has an elimination half-life of 0.5 h. The former is primarily metabolized by CYP2C9 and CYP2C19 and is more potent than the latter, which is primarily metabolized by CYP2C9.

Clinical Uses

VKAs have a broad spectrum of uses in clinical practice:

- Primary and secondary prevention of VTE
- Prevention of systemic embolism in patients with prosthetic heart valves or atrial fibrillation (AF)
- Adjunct in the prophylaxis of systemic embolism after myocardial infarction (MI)
- Reducing the risk of recurrent MI

In a healthy adult, the initial amount of warfarin is about 10 mg/day for 2 days. In the case of increased prothrombin time, heart failure, abnormalities in transaminases, or when the patient is subjected to parenteral nutrition or is underweight, the induction dose should be less than 10 mg/day. The subsequent maintenance dose is chosen based on the international normalized ratio (INR) of the person and is about 3–9 mg/day.

During warfarin treatment [20], it is essential to periodically check the INR, to change the administered dose, should this prove necessary, and to maintain an INR within the therapeutic range. The British Society for Haematology recommended an INR to achieve optimal values in different situations (Table 3.1)

When replacement of VKAs with heparin is needed, current recommendations propose initial coadministration of heparin and VKAs and discontinuation of heparin after obtaining an adequate prothrombin time expressed in seconds or as a ratio with a control value (INR).

3.4.4 Complications of Heparin Treatment

Bleeding

The main complication of heparin therapy is bleeding, whose incidence and severity is highly variable: minor complications are reported with a frequency from 10 to 15%; major complications (defined as fatal bleeding, or vital organ bleeding, resulting in a decrease in hemoglobin below 2 g/dl, and therapeutic transfusion) have a frequency of 2–7%.

Risk factors for bleeding during heparin treatment are age above 60 years (especially women), severe intercurrent diseases, recent surgery, history of alcohol abuse, history of peptic ulcer, and platelet count below 150,000/mL, and renal injury [21].

Heparin-Induced Thrombocytopenia

The most common adverse drug effects associated with heparin administration are bleeding and HIT [22]. HIT is an immune-mediated disorder typically occurring between the fifth and the 15th day of treatment. However, it can develop much earlier (first and second days) in patients who have previously received the drug [23, 24]. HIT is caused by an IgG that activate platelets through their Fc receptors (RII).

Table 3.1 International randomized ratio (INR) recommended by the British Society for Haematology

Indication	Therapeutic range (INR)	Duration
Treatment and secondary prevention of pulmonary embolism		
Without persistent thromboembolic risk	2–3	3–6 months
Presence of thrombophilic conditions or recurrent events	2–3	According to case-by-case assessment
Treatment and secondary prevention of distal vein thrombosis		
Without persistent thromboembolic risk	2–3	3–6 months
Presence of thrombophilic conditions or recurrent events	2–3	According to case-by-case assessment
Prevention of DVT in high-risk patients (i.e., orthopedic surgery), as an alternative to LMWH	1.5–2.5	7–10 days
Arterial thromboembolism	3–4.5	Indefinite
Chronic atrial fibrillation		
Cardioversion in recent-onset AF	2–3	Start at least 2 weeks before cardioversion Continue at least 3 weeks after cardioversion
Valvular prosthesis		
Mechanical	3–4.5	Indefinite
Biological	2–3	3 months
Intracardiac mural thrombosis	2–3	Until all thrombi have disappeared
Myocardial infarction:		
Prevention of thromboembolic risk	2–3	3 months
Prevention of reinfarction	3–4.5	At least 3 years

DVT deep venous thrombosis, *LMWH* low molecular weight heparins, *AF* atrial fibrillation, *INR* international normalized ratio

The incidence of HIT ranges from 0.3 to 4%, according to various reports [25–27] and, as far as the risk of inducing HIT is concerned, there is no substantial difference between therapeutic and prophylactic administration of heparin.

HIT is frequently associated with arterial or venous thrombosis, including MI, ischemic stroke, acute arterial occlusion of the lower extremities, disseminated intravascular coagulation (DIC), DVT and PTE, with an incidence from 25 to 89% [28]. In addition, myocardial necrosis and bilateral adrenal hemorrhage have also been observed in 1–2% of patients with HIT [28, 29]. Therefore, HIT should be suspected in patients with thrombocytopenia and receiving heparin who are experiencing abdominal pain and/or hypotension. Platelet counts should be monitored in all patients treated with heparin owing to the severity of thrombotic events that may be HIT-related. For hospitalized patients receiving a therapeutic dose of heparin, a baseline control is recommended, and platelet counts should be monitored at least every 2–3 days from the fourth day to the 14th day, whereas in patients treated at home, monitoring should be done at least once on the seventh or eighth day together with the baseline control. In the case of low platelet count, and in the absence of a convincing alternative cause, heparin administration should be ceased immediately and alternative options should be implemented. Different medications can be used to replace heparin, including:

- Danaparoid, which has a 10–40% in vitro cross-reactivity rate, but it is not associated with adverse clinical outcomes. The initial bolus is 2,250 IU, followed by 400 IU/h every 4 h, then 300 IU/h every 4 h, followed by a maintenance dose.
- Recombinant hirudin, which has been successfully used in many cases [30]. It has no cross-reactivity, and this medication has already been approved in different countries. The most common initial bolus is 0.4 mg/kg, followed by an infusion of 0.15 mg/kg/h, with laboratory monitoring to maintain the aPTT at 1.5–3 times the baseline value. The use of hirudin may be associated with thrombolytic therapy of vascular occlusion.
- Other direct antithrombin inhibitors, such as argatroban (Novostan), have been successfully used in patients with HIT who required extracorporeal circulation [31] and in patients who underwent carotid stenting [32].

Pentasaccharide can also be effective in these kind of diseases, as no cross-reactivity was observed in vitro [33].

3.4.5 Antiplatelet Therapy

Direct Inhibitors of Thrombin

The two reference new antiplatelet medications are tirofiban and eptifibatide [34, 35], whose mechanism of action is similar to that of abciximab. They prevent platelet aggregation by antagonizing the platelet glycoprotein IIb/IIIa receptor, and, as a consequence, the bond between fibrinogen and von Willebrand factor (vWF) [36].

Their effect lasts for about 4 h versus 24–48 h for abciximab. They are administered by intravenous infusion: for tirofiban, the loading dose is 400 ng/kg/min for 30 min followed by a maintenance infusion of 100 ng/kg/min for at least 48 h; eptifibatide infusion is 2 μg/kg/min for up to 72 h, preceded by an initial bolus dose of 180 μg/kg. However, the efficacy of these antiplatelet agents in acute coronary syndromes and non-Q-wave MI therapy is less clear, and their precise role is yet to be defined [34, 36–38].

Several studies revealed that patients with instable angina using glycoprotein IIb/IIIa inhibitors showed greater clinical benefits when they had at least one of the following factors: troponin positive levels, recurrent ischemia, hemodynamic instability, severe arrhythmia disorders, early post-MI angina, and previous coronary artery bypass surgery. Tirofiban and eptifibatide have not been directly compared in clinical trials. Presently, studies are being conducted to establish the efficacy of tirofiban combined with fibrinolitic therapy in acute MI in order to improve coronary reperfusion [34, 35].

Finally, glycoprotein IIa/IIIb inhibitors may increase the risk of excessive bleeding [39–41].

3.5 VTE in Nonsurgical Patients

3.5.1 Preliminary Considerations

Necropsy studies have shown that among all fatal pulmonary embolisms, only 25% were subsequent to a recent surgery. The remaining 75% occurred in bed-ridden patients with medical illnesses. The incidence of DVT observed in some categories of patients (i.e., stroke patients) is similar to that of orthopedic patients. This is not surprising since both groups have the same risk factors, such as age, immobilization, and tissue damage. The incidence of DVT in other categories of medical patients (i.e., acute MI [38], heart failure, pulmonary infections, ICU stay) is similar to that in surgical patients (25%).

The overall mortality in hospitalized patients is approximately 10% (1% of all admissions) [42–45]. Randomized controlled trials have shown that mortality is lower in surgical patients (4%), moderate in general medical patients, including patients with acute MI (10%, SCATI Group 1989), and high in stroke patients [46, 47].

The available data suggest that prophylaxis with anticoagulants (usually low-dose UFH—Collins 1996—and LMWH) or with antiplatelet inhibitors (usually acetylsalicylic acid) relatively reduces the risk of DVT in medical patients and in acute ischemic stroke [48] and equalizes the risk in surgical patients [38].

No clinical studies have been conducted in medical patients on the efficacy of mechanical prophylaxis with graduated compression stockings or with intermittent pneumatic compression devices [49]. However, there are reasons to believe that these methods are less effective than in surgical patients; further studies are therefore required to give a proper recommendation.

All patients in general practice should be classified according to the thromboembolic risk, and prophylaxis should be implemented in patients at moderate and high risk (International Consensus Statement of the International Union of Angiology—IUA—1997).

3.5.2 Acute Ischemic Stroke

Patients with acute stroke and paraplegia have high risk of developing DVT (more frequent in hemiplegic patients) and are at high risk of mortality, where fatal pulmonary embolism represents the most common cause of death. A review of ten

3 Anticoagulation Therapy in ICU Patients

studies has confirmed that prophylaxis with UFH, LMWH, or heparinoids is effective in reducing the incidence of DVT in patients with suspected or proven stroke [13, 46]. Each of those treatments is recommended for patients with stroke and paraplegia (level of evidence I, grade of recommendation A) [47].

However, results of other studies recommend a cautious attitude in the administration of heparin, where low doses (5,000 U twice daily) are generally preferred in the acute phase of stroke. Nevertheless, it is necessary to exclude intracranial hemorrhage, usually via early CT scans, before starting heparin prophylaxis [50, 51]. In patients with stroke, as demonstrated from studies of other antiplatelet general medical patients at high risk (Antiplatelet Trialists' Collaboration 1994), aspirin has proven effective in reducing DVT (level of evidence III) [47, 48].

3.5.3 Hemorrhagic Stroke

The prevention of VTE in stroke bleeding is even more problematic. In fact the incidence of DVT is comparable to that of ischemic stroke. A clear recommendation for the use of mechanical devices (intermittent pneumatic compression and graduated compression stockings) [49, 52] was given by the NIH Consensus Conference in 1986 and confirmed by the International Consensus Statement of the International Union of Angiology (1997).

In patients with suspected or proven hemorrhagic stroke and in patients at high risk of bleeding, mechanical prophylaxes such as intermittent pneumatic compression or graduated compression stockings are recommended [49, 52, 53] (grade of recommendation C) on the basis of studies on general surgery and neurosurgery patients.

3.6 Atrial Fibrillation

AF is one of the most common rhythms seen in critical patients. This is consistent with its association with many acute, cardiac and noncardiac, illnesses. ICU physicians mostly encounter acute AF, defined as AF of less than 48 h duration. This definition covers both paroxysmal AF (which may be a consequence, or the cause, of the critical status) and the first symptomatic presentation of persistent AF. The acute onset involves high risk of embolic complications, mostly as ischemic stroke or systemic embolism; moreover, strokes frequently occur in clusters. For these reasons, thromboprophylaxis has paramount importance in the management of this disturbance [54–56].

Current recommendations for antithrombotic therapy in the prevention of thromboembolism in AF are listed below:

- Preventing thromboembolism (for recommendations regarding antithrombotic therapy in patients with AF undergoing cardioversion)

Class I

1. Antithrombotic therapy to prevent thromboembolism is recommended for all patients with AF, except those with lone AF or contraindications (level of evidence A).
2. The selection of the antithrombotic agent should be based upon the absolute risks of stroke and bleeding [41] and the relative risk and benefit for a given patient (level of evidence A).
3. For patients without mechanical heart valves at high risk of stroke, chronic oral anticoagulant therapy with a VKA is recommended in a dose adjusted to achieve the target INR of 2.0–3.0, unless contraindicated. Factors associated with the highest risk of stroke in patients with AF are prior thromboembolism [stroke, transient ischemic attack (TIA), or systemic embolism] and rheumatic mitral stenosis (level of evidence A).
4. Anticoagulation with a VKA is recommended for patients with more than one moderate risk factor. Such factors include age of 75 years or greater, hypertension, heart failure, impaired left ventricular systolic function (ejection fraction 35% or less or fractional shortening less than 25%), and diabetes mellitus (level of evidence A).
5. The INR should be determined at least weekly during initiation of therapy and monthly when anticoagulation is stable (level of evidence A).
6. Aspirin, 81–325 mg daily, is recommended as an alternative to VKAs in low-risk patients or in those with contraindications to oral anticoagulation (level of evidence A).
7. For patients with AF who have mechanical heart valves, the target intensity of anticoagulation should be based on the type of prosthesis, maintaining an INR of at least 2.5 (level of evidence B).
8. Antithrombotic therapy is recommended for patients with atrial flutter as for those with AF (level of evidence C).

Class IIa

9. For primary prevention of thromboembolism in patients with nonvalvular AF who have just one of the following validated risk factors, antithrombotic therapy with either aspirin or a VKA is reasonable, based upon an assessment of the risk of bleeding complications, the ability to safely sustain adjusted chronic anticoagulation, and patient preferences: age greater than or equal to 75 years (especially in female patients), hypertension, heart failure, impaired left ventricular function, or diabetes mellitus (level of evidence A).
10. For patients with nonvalvular AF who have one or more of the following less well validated risk factors, antithrombotic therapy with either aspirin or a VKA is reasonable for prevention of thromboembolism: age 65–74 years, female gender, or coronary artery disease. The choice of the agent should be based

3 Anticoagulation Therapy in ICU Patients

upon the risk of bleeding complications, the ability to safely sustain adjusted chronic anticoagulation, and patient preferences (level of evidence B).

11. It is reasonable to select antithrombotic therapy using the same criteria irrespective of the pattern (i.e., paroxysmal, persistent, or permanent) of AF (level of evidence B).

12. In patients with AF who do not have mechanical prosthetic heart valves, it is reasonable to interrupt anticoagulation for up to 1 week without substituting heparin for surgical or diagnostic procedures that carry a risk of bleeding (level of evidence C).

13. It is reasonable to reevaluate the need for anticoagulation at regular intervals (level of evidence C).

Class IIb

14. In patients 75 years of age and older at increased risk of bleeding but without frank contraindications to oral anticoagulant therapy, and in other patients with moderate risk factors for thromboembolism who are unable to safely tolerate anticoagulation at the standard intensity of INR 2.0–3.0, a lower INR target of 2.0 (range 1.6–2.5) may be considered for primary prevention of ischemic stroke and systemic embolism (level of evidence C).

15. In patients with AF younger than 60 years without heart disease or risk factors for thromboembolism, the risk of thromboembolism is low without treatment and the effectiveness of aspirin for primary prevention of stroke relative to the risk of bleeding has not been established (level of evidence C).

16. In patients with AF who sustain ischemic stroke or systemic embolism during treatment with low-intensity anticoagulation (INR 2.0–3.0), rather than add an antiplatelet agent, it may be reasonable to raise the intensity of the anticoagulation to a maximum target INR of 3.0–3.5 (level of evidence C).

Class III

Long-term anticoagulation with a VKA is not recommended for primary prevention of stroke in patients below the age of 60 years without heart disease (lone AF) or any risk factors for thromboembolism (level of evidence C).

- Prevention of thromboembolism in patients with AF undergoing cardioversion

Class I

17. For patients with AF of 48 h duration or longer, or when the duration of AF is unknown, anticoagulation (INR 2.0–3.0) is recommended for at least 3 weeks prior to and 4 weeks after cardioversion, regardless of the method (electrical or pharmacological) used to restore sinus rhythm (level of evidence B).

18. For patients with AF of more than 48 h duration requiring immediate cardioversion because of hemodynamic instability, heparin should be administered concurrently (unless contraindicated) by an initial intravenous bolus injection followed by a continuous infusion in a dose adjusted to prolong the

aPTT to 1.5–2 times the reference control value. Thereafter, oral anticoagulation (INR 2.0–3.0) should be provided for at least 4 weeks, as for patients undergoing elective cardioversion. Limited data support subcutaneous administration of LMWH in this indication (level of evidence C).

19. For patients with AF of less than 48 h duration associated with hemodynamic instability (angina pectoris, MI, shock, or pulmonary edema), cardioversion should be performed immediately without delay for prior initiation of anticoagulation (level of evidence C).

Class IIa

20. During the 48 h after onset of AF, the need for anticoagulation before and after cardioversion may be based on the patient's risk of thromboembolism (level of evidence C).

21. As an alternative to anticoagulation prior to cardioversion of AF, it is reasonable to perform transesophageal echocardiography in search of thrombus in the left atrium or left atrial appendage (level of evidence B).

22. For patients with no identifiable thrombus, cardioversion is reasonable immediately after anticoagulation with UFH (e.g., initiated by intravenous bolus injection and an infusion continued at a dose adjusted to prolong the aPTT to 1.5–2 times the control value until oral anticoagulation has been established with an oral VKA (e.g., warfarin) as evidenced by an INR equal to or greater than 2.0) (level of evidence B). Thereafter, continuation of oral anticoagulation (INR 2.0–3.0) is reasonable for a total anticoagulation period of at least 4 weeks, as for patients undergoing elective cardioversion (level of evidence B). Limited data are available to support the subcutaneous administration of a LMWH in this indication (level of evidence C).

23. For patients in whom thrombus is identified by transesophageal echocardiography, oral anticoagulation (INR 2.0–3.0) is reasonable for at least 3 weeks prior to and 4 weeks after restoration of sinus rhythm, and a longer period of anticoagulation may be appropriate even after apparently successful cardioversion, because the risk of thromboembolism often remains elevated in such cases (level of evidence C).

24. For patients with atrial flutter undergoing cardioversion, anticoagulation can be beneficial according to the recommendations as for patients with AF (level of evidence C).

Oral anticoagulation therapy with VKAs has been shown to be highly efficacious for preventing stroke in most patients with AF. However, there is increasing evidence that oral anticoagulation therapy is underused in this population. This underutilization may have many reasons: the presence of contraindications, the inconvenience associated with prolonged monitoring of the INR, patient compliance, fear of major bleeding. Moreover, even when oral anticoagulant therapy is used, the INR value is not maintained within its therapeutic margin, eventually making the treatment ineffective. Several studies have evaluated the effectiveness of drugs that do not require a continuous monitoring of coagulation

3 Anticoagulation Therapy in ICU Patients

factors, including the direct thrombin inhibitors [39–41]. Moreover, even when oral anticoagulant therapy is used, the therapeutic INR value is not maintained consistently between 2 and 3, thus making the treatment ineffective. Given the concrete need for improvement, new classes of medications have been developed which do not require periodic monitoring. The first class to undergo clinical testing is the direct thrombin inhibitors.

Dabigatran etexilate, an orally administered competitive and reversible direct thrombin inhibitor, has been evaluated as an alternative to warfarin in the Randomized Evaluation of Long-Term Anticoagulation Therapy (RE-LY) trial [39]. The study randomized 18,133 patients with a nonvalvular cause of AF who were at risk of ischemic stroke to open-label adjusted-dose warfarin or blinded dabigatran at a fixed dose of 110 or 150 mg twice daily; 3,623 patients had a history of stroke or TIA. The dabigatran 150-mg dose was superior to warfarin at preventing stroke or systemic emboli, with a decreased risk of hemorrhagic stroke and similar rates of major hemorrhage, but with an increased risk of MI and gastrointestinal hemorrhage. Dabigatran dosed at 110 mg twice daily is equivalent to warfarin in efficacy but is associated with lower rates of major hemorrhage (2.7 vs. 3.4% per year).

Presently, the results do not actually demonstrate whether it is possible to differentiate the dose in subgroups of patients characterized by different basal thromboembolic and/or hemorrhagic risk [57]. From the results, 150 mg dabigatran twice daily appears to be safer than 110 mg twice daily in the prevention of hemorrhagic events, whereas it is inferior in preventing ischemic complications. Considering its simple dosing regimen with no requirements for follow-up testing, the drug appears promising. The FDA has approved the drug for prevention of stroke or systemic embolism in moderate- to high-risk patients (age around 75 years, hypertension, history of stroke or TIA, systemic embolism, or ventricular fraction below 45%, peripheral arterial disease, or age between 55 and 74 years associated with diabetes mellitus or coronary artery disease) with AF.

Another new oral anticoagulant class evaluated for prevention in AF is factor Xa inhibitors (e.g., rivaroxaban, apixaban). The Rivaroxaban, Once Daily, Oral, Direct Factor Xa Inhibition Compared with Vitamin K Antagonism for Prevention of Stroke and Embolism Trial in Atrial Fibrillation (ROCKET-AF) study is a randomized, double-blind, double-dummy, event-driven trial, which aims to establish the noninferiority of rivaroxaban compared with dose-adjusted warfarin in patients with nonvalvular AF who have a history of stroke or at least two additional independent risk factors for future stroke [58]. The primary objective is to compare the efficacy of rivaroxaban with that of dose-adjusted warfarin titrated to a target INR of 2.5 (range 2.0–3.0) for the prevention of thromboembolic events in patients with nonvalvular AF. The primary end point comprises stroke (ischemic and hemorrhagic) and noncentral nervous system systemic embolism; secondary end points include all causes of death, vascular death, and MI. Patient population qualifying criteria include prior stroke, TIA, or systemic embolism, or two or more of the following risk factors: clinical heart failure and/or left ventricular ejection fraction of 35% or below, hypertension, age 75 years or greater, or diabetes mellitus (CHADS2). In addition, the patients with only two risk factors will be capped at 10% of the overall trial population, with the remaining patients requiring three of more risk factors (CHADS2 ≥ 3) or a prior stroke, TIA, or systemic embolism.

Patients with AF and hemodynamically significant mitral stenosis or any valve prostheses are excluded, as are those with transient AF caused by a reversible disorder, excessive hemorrhagic risk, and planned cardioversion.

Rivaroxaban was found to be noninferior to warfarin [40, 41] for the prevention of stroke or systemic embolism; the risk of major bleeding between different groups was not significant, although the rivaroxaban group had a lower frequency of intracranial and fatal bleeding (New Engl J Med Sept 2011).

The ACTIVE-W trial assessed whether clopidogrel plus aspirin is noninferior to oral anticoagulation therapy for prevention of vascular events in patients with nonvalvular AF and one or more risk factor for stroke. A population of 6,706 patients were randomly allocated to receive oral anticoagulation therapy (target INR of 2.0–3.0; $n = 3{,}371$) or clopidogrel (75 mg per day) plus aspirin (75–100 mg per day recommended; $n = 3{,}335$). Clear evidence of the superiority of oral anticoagulation therapy versus clopidogrel plus acetylsalicylic acid in prevention of primary events emerged early during the course of the study (annual risk of 3.93 vs. 5.60%, rate ratio 1.44, 95% confidence interval 1.18–1.76, $P = 0.0003$), which was stopped.

3.6.1 Disorders of Coagulation Associated with Drug Therapy in the ICU

Disorders of coagulation are common adverse drug effects in critically ill patients [59–61].

Critically ill patients are peculiar in having altered pharmacokinetic and pharmacodynamic variability. This variability can lead to unpredictable drug effects, greater toxicity, and increased potential for adverse drug effects associated with disorders of coagulation. ICU patients can receive simultaneously several different medications throughout their admission, increasing the potential for drug interactions or a synergistic/enhanced response [62].

3.6.2 Other Clinical Conditions

A considerable proportion of acutely ill medical patients are at high risk of developing VTE, especially in the absence of adequate thromboprophylaxis [63]. To date, there is still uncertainty about appropriate risk stratification in patients hospitalized for acute medical conditions. In any case, it is acknowledged that a complete risk assessment includes consideration of both predisposing factors, inherited or acquired, and all transient ones associated with the hospitalization [64]. An acute medical condition such as acute stroke or acute MI, or exacerbation of heart failure or pulmonary failure, or infectious disease may create the need for elective or

3 Anticoagulation Therapy in ICU Patients

emergency surgery, apart from being a major independent risk factor for VTE and a possible cause of prolonged immobilization (another independent risk factor).

Common conditions that may be risk factors for VTE in critical patients are heart failure, pulmonary failure, acute limb plegia, diabetic ketoacidosis or coma, nephrotic syndrome, history of previous DVT or pulmonary embolism, and primary or acquired thrombophilia. Many other important risk factors are listed as follows [63]:

- Acute medical illness: stroke, MI, illness requiring ICU admission ,other acute illnesses requiring immobilization for at least 3 days
- Clinical risk factors: previous pulmonary embolism or DVT, collagen vascular disorders, cancer, an internal cardiac defibrillator, congestive heart failure, stroke with limb paresis, chronic obstructive pulmonary disease, diabetes mellitus, varicose veins, inflammatory bowel disease, hormone replacement therapy, antipsychotic drug use, obesity, chronic in-dwelling central venous catheter, cancer chemotherapy, permanent pacemaker
- Thrombophilia: factor V Leiden mutation, prothrombin gene mutation, hyperhomocysteinemia (including mutation in methylene tetrahydrofolate reductase), antiphospholipid antibody syndrome, deficiency of ATIII, protein C, or protein S, high concentrations of factors VIII, IX, or XI, increased level of lipoprotein(a)

The degree of risk of VTE, according to the relevant medical conditions, is generally categorized as (IUA 1997):

- High: major medical illness with thrombophilia or a history of VTE, lower limb plegia (paraplegia, hemiplegic stroke)
- Moderate: major medical illnesses such as heart or lung disease, cancer, and inflammatory bowel disease
- Low: minor medical illnesses associated with thrombophilia or a history of thromboembolism

Prophylaxis with LMWH is recommended in patients with heart failure [65], bronchopneumonic processes [66, 67], and patients in intensive care [62] (grade A recommendation). It is also recommended in patients with additional risk factors. (grade C recommendation). Patients with cancer are often hospitalized if they present with an acute medical illness. Current evidence supports the use of thromboprophylaxis in this patient population, guided by a case-by-case risk assessment. So, acute patients with a history of cancer such as pancreatic, prostate, lung, breast, stomach, or colon cancer are considered to be at significant risk of VTE and may benefit from receiving thromboprophylaxis, whereas patients with a history of minor skin cancer or Hodgkin's disease, for example, may not.

LMWH and heparinoid showed efficacy and safety equal to those of UFH. One study has demonstrated the prophylactic efficacy of a high dose of LMWH (4,000 U enoxaparin) in patients with acute medical conditions [38, 65].

Although age does increase the risk of VTE, age over 65 years alone does not justify routine prophylaxis.

The treatment of patients with congestive heart failure has shown a relatively low incidence of clinically relevant thromboembolic events (2–3% of patients per year). On the basis of this observation, there is a reasonable indication for chronic anticoagulant therapy, burdened with a risk of major bleeding events of 2–3% per year [65].

Secondary thrombocytosis is apparently not associated with an increased risk of thromboembolism, which is instead expected with essential thrombocythemia and other myeloproliferative diseases. Anyway, in these diseases there is no clear correlation between thromboembolic risk and platelet count.

3.6.3 Recommendations

1. Acute ischemic stroke. Administration of heparin in the acute phase of stroke should be cautious: ruling out intracranial hemorrhage before commencing pharmacological prophylaxis is mandatory. In stroke patients, aspirin was effective in reducing DVT (level III evidence).
2. Hemorrhagic stroke. Prevention of VTE is still problematic. In patients with suspected or proven hemorrhagic stroke, recommended thromboprophylaxis methods are intermittent pneumatic compression and/or graduated compression stockings.
3. Acute MI. Oral anticoagulation is effective in the prevention of VTE [68]. Aspirin is also effective in the prevention of DVT/pulmonary embolism in patients at high risk [38]. Intermittent pneumatic compression and graduated compression stockings are recommended in patients with contraindication to anticoagulation.
4. Trombofilia and contraceptives. Oral contraceptives should be discontinued at least 1 month before elective surgery and prophylaxis should be considered in the case of major trauma, prolonged hypomobility, or an emergency surgical procedure. A general screening for all women considering oral contraceptive use is not feasible. Screening for major congenital thrombophilic conditions is recommended in women with a personal or family history of VTE.

3.6.4 Colloids

Excessive hemodilution after volume expansion may increase the risk of bleeding by decreasing the concentration of platelets and coagulation factors, and some colloids may have other properties that can increase the risk of bleeding. Colloids are used because of their ability to maintain intravascular volume and regional tissue perfusion more efficiently than crystalloids [69–71]

Several mechanisms have been suggested by which colloids impair blood coagulation [72].

Large molecules of colloids interfere with fibrinogen, coagulation factor VIII, and vWF more than predicted from hemodilution alone [73, 74].

Hydroxyethyl starch (HES) and gelatin promote platelet dysfunction [75], disturb the reticular fibrin mesh, decrease clot firmness, and reduce functional clot quality [76–79]. In such conditions, the resulting thrombus may be less stable and more susceptible to lysis. Also, hemodilution might reduce thrombin generation and fibrin clot formation independently of each other [80].

Gelatins may decrease clot strength and decrease platelet aggregation through binding to and decreasing the concentration of vWF. Dextrans are known to

3 Anticoagulation Therapy in ICU Patients

decrease the levels of vWF and factor VIII and increase fibrinolysis, and they have been shown to be effective in preventing thrombosis and pulmonary embolism. Therefore, the dextrans are utilized more as an anticoagulant than as a plasma expander. HES-based compounds have also been found to decrease the levels of vWF and factor VIII as well as to increase fibrinolysis.

However, the exact mechanism remains unclear. Reduced fibrinogen concentration could impair fibrin polymerization in conditions of hemodilution [81].

3.6.5 Dextrans

Dextrans are polydisperse glucose polymers produced by bacteria growing in sucrose-containing media. Commercially available dextran-based plasma substitutes have an average molecular mass of 40–70 kDa. Besides their plasma-expanding properties, they also exert an anticoagulant effect. Indeed, dextrans have been shown to be effective in preventing postoperative venous thrombosis and pulmonary embolism [82–84].

Dextran infusion induces a "von Willebrand syndrome," with decreased levels of vWF and associated factor VIII (VIII:c) [85, 86]. The fall in the levels of vWF and factor VIII:c after dextran administration is more than can be explained by its dilutional effects. vWF is the ligand between the platelet surface receptor protein glycoprotein Ib and subendothelial collagen, thereby causing platelet adhesion to the vessel wall. Decreased levels of vWF, therefore, may lead to an impaired primary hemostasis.

3.6.6 Gelatins

Gelatins are polydisperse polypeptides produced by degradation of bovine collagen.

There is now increasing evidence that gelatins influence platelet function and blood coagulation. Clots produced in the presence of gelatin had decreased weight and strength and loss of the normal reticular network of fibrin strands [87]. It was suggested that vWF binds to gelatin by means of its collagen binding site. Also, a decrease in thrombin generation, as measured by thrombin–antithrombin complexes and prothrombin fragment F1 [88], was observed after gelatin administration, probably caused by hemodilution [89]. The clinical relevance of the impairment of hemostasis after gelatin infusion is uncertain. Studies comparing gelatin with HES [90] or HES and albumin [91] found no difference or, in some cases, even an improvement [92] in postoperative blood loss when gelatin was given.

3.6.7 Hydroxyethyl Starch

HES is generally considered as an effective and safe plasma substitute. However, bleeding complications have been reported after administration of HES in various clinical settings. High molecular weight HES (Hetastarch, average molecular mass 480,000 Da) has been associated with increased postoperative bleeding after neurosurgery [93] and in patients undergoing cardiac surgery [91, 94, 95]. It has been suggested that not all HES solutions have negative effects on blood coagulation, but that these effects depend on the average molecular weight of the HES molecules and the kinetics of elimination.

HES solutions modify blood coagulation in vivo and in vitro by prolonging the coagulation time and decreasing clot strength [76, 77].

3.6.8 Pharmacokinetics of HES

Natural starches cannot be used as plasma substitutes because they are rapidly degraded by circulating amylase and they are insoluble at neutral pH. HES are polymers of glucose units derived from amylopectin and modified by substituting hydroxyethyl for hydroxyl groups on glucose molecules. The substitution results in slower degradation and highly increased solubility. HES are very polydisperse solutions of molecules with a broad range of molecular masses from very low to several hundred thousand daltons. After administration of HES, the low molecular weight fraction is rapidly lost by renal elimination and the large molecules are progressively hydrolyzed, resulting in an average in vivo molecular weight that is significantly lower than the average molecular weight of the infused fluid. The rate at which degradation of HES molecules occurs depends on the degree of substitution, that is, the proportion of glucose units having a hydroxyethyl group substituted for a hydroxyl group. There are three possible sites for substitution, leading to a maximum degree of substitution of 3. Currently available HES solutions have a degree of substitution of 0.5–0.7. The rate of degradation and elimination is highest with low values of the degree of substitution [96]. Because substitution is possible at positions 2, 3, or 6 of the glucose unit, different patterns of substitution are possible. The substitution pattern is characterized by the C2/C6 hydroxyethylation ratio. Clearance of HES is slowest with high C2/C6 ratios [97]. The characteristics of HES solutions are given by their initial molecular weight, the degree of substitution, and the C2/C6 ratio. Thus, HES 200/0.5/6 has an initial average molecular mass of 200,000 Da, with 50% of glucose units having a hydroxyethyl group and with a C2/C6 ratio of 6 (i.e., six times more substitutions at the C2 position as compared with the C6 position).

3.6.9 Albumin

Albumin is generally considered not to influence blood coagulation and is often used as control fluid in studies evaluating the effects of other colloids. It has been reported that albumin induces an impairment of platelet aggregation and

3 Anticoagulation Therapy in ICU Patients

prolongation of the bleeding time [98, 99]. The mechanism by which platelet function is impaired is uncertain.

3.6.10 Desmopressin

Desmopressin is used in a variety of conditions, including hemophilia A, von Willebrand disease type I, diabetes insipidus, and primary nocturnal enuresis [100]. Desmopressin stimulation of extrarenal V2 receptors increases the levels of factor VIII and vWF, and has been used in an attempt to control bleeding in patients with and without normal coagulation physiologic behavior.

3.7 Conclusions

Patients in ICUs are at high risk of VTE, which is one of the most common challenges for critical care physicians. In fact, many patients are at high risk of thromboembolism and bleeding simultaneously. Current guidelines recommend that all patients who have sustained major trauma and/or spinal cord injury receive prophylaxis with LMWH as soon as possible after hemostasis has been ascertained. For patients in the ICU at risk of thrombosis, heparin or LMWH is recommended at low doses. For those with a very high risk of bleeding, mechanical prophylaxis should be started as soon as possible and continued until the pharmacological prophylaxis may be initiated. The prophylactic use of inferior vena cava filters is no longer recommended, as the risks outweigh the benefit in most cases. Despite its large evidence base, thromboprophylaxis is often poorly implemented. This gap between evidence-based recommendations and clinical practice may be a result of many factors, i.e., poor education, costs, and fear of severe bleeding. Finally, thromboprophylaxis is a definite priority in patient safety, especially in critical settings, where most patients have multiple risk factors. For these reasons, thromboprophylaxis should be one of the cornerstones of any local continuous quality improvement program.

References

1. Illingworth C, Timmons S (2007) An audit of intermittent pneumatic compression (IPC) in the prophylaxis of asymptomatic deep vein thrombosis (DVT). J Perioper Pract 17(11): 522–524, 526–528
2. Harris LM, Curl GR, Booth FV, Hassett JM Jr, Leney G, Ricotta JJ (1997) Screening for asymptomatic deep vein thrombosis in surgical intensive care patients. J Vasc Surg 26(5): 764–769
3. Ibrahim EH, Iregui M, Prentice D, Sherman G, Kollef MH, Shannon W (2002) Deep vein thrombosis during prolonged mechanical ventilation despite prophylaxis. Crit Care Med 30(4):771–774
4. Geerts WH, Code KI, Jay RM, Chen E, Szalai JP (1994) A prospective study of venous thromboembolism after major trauma. N Engl J Med 331(24):1601–1606

5. Joynt GM, Kew J, Gomersall CD, Leung VY, Liu EK (2000) Deep venous thrombosis caused by femoral venous catheters in critically ill adult patients. Chest 117(1):178–183
6. Geerts WH, Pineo GF, Heit JA, Bergqvist D, Lassen MR, Colwell CW, Ray JG (2004) Prevention of venous thromboembolism: the Seventh ACCP conference on antithrombotic and thrombolytic therapy. Chest 126(Suppl 3):338S–400S
7. Geerts WH, Bergqvist D, Pineo GF, Heit JA, Samama CM, Lassen MR, Colwell CW, American college of Chest Physicians (2008) Prevention of venous thromboembolism: American College of chest physicians evidence-based clinical practice guidelines, 8th edn. Chest 133(Suppl 6):381S-453S
8. Vardi M, Zittan E, Bitterman H (2009) Subcutaneous unfractionated heparin for the initial treatment of venous thromboembolism. Cochrane Database Syst Rev 7(4):CD006771
9. McGarry LJ, Stokes ME, Thompson D (2006) Outcomes of thromboprophylaxis with enoxaparin versus unfractionated heparin in medical inpatients. Thromb J 27(4):17
10. Bauersachs R, Schellong SM, Haas S, Tebbe U, Gerlach HE, Abletshauser C, Sieder C, Melzer N, Bramlage P, Riess H (2011) Prophylaxis of venous thromboembolism in patients with severe renal insufficiency. Thromb Haemost 105(6):981–988 [Epub 2011 Apr 20]
11. Antithrombotic therapy for venous thromboembolic disease: American college of Chest Physicians Evidence-Based Clinical Practice Guidelines (8th Edn.)
12. Hirsch DR, Ingenito EP, Goldhaber SZ (1995) Prevalence of deep venous thrombosis among patients in medical intensive care. JAMA 274(4):335–337
13. Cook D, Meade M, Guyatt G, Walter SD, Heels-Ansdell D, Geerts W, Warkentin TE, Cooper DJ, Zytaruk N, Vallance S, Berwanger O, Rocha M, Qushmaq I, Crowther M (2011) Prophylaxis for thromboembolism in critical care trial protocol and analysis plan. J Crit Care 26(2):223.e1–9
14. Hirsh J, Gordon G, Gregory WA, Robert H, Holger JS (2008) American college of chest physicians evidence-based clinical practice guidelines (8th edn.) Chest 134(4):892
15. Hirsh J, Guyatt G, Gregory WA, Robert H, Holger JS (2008) Antithrombotic and thrombolytic therapy: American college of chest physicians evidence-based clinical practice guidelines (8th edn.) Chest 133:110S–112S. doi:10.1378/chest.08-0652
16. Hillis C, Warkentin TE, Taha K, Eikelboom JW (2011) Chills and limb pain following administration of low-molecular-weight heparin for treatment of acute venous thromboembolism. Am J Hematol 86(7):603–606. doi:10.1002/ajh.22043
17. Phung OJ, Kahn SR, Cook DJ, Murad MH (2011) Dosing frequency of unfractionated heparin thromboprophylaxis: a meta-analysis. Chest [Epub ahead of print]
18. Quinlan DJ, McQuillan A, Eikelboom JW (2004) Low-molecular-weight heparin compared with intravenous unfractionated heparin for treatment of pulmonary embolism: a meta-analysis of randomized, controlled trials. Ann Intern Med 140(3):175–183
19. Ansell J, Hirsh J, Hylek E, Jacobson A, Crowther M, Palareti G, American College of Chest Physicians (2008) Pharmacology and management of the vitamin K antagonists: American college of chest physicians evidence-based clinical practice guidelines (8th edn.). Chest 133(Suppl 6):160S–198S
20. Ansell J, Hirsh J, Hylek E, Jacobson A, Crowther M, Palareti G (2008) Pharmacology and management of the vitamin K antagonists: American college of chest physicians evidence-based clinical practice guidelines (8th edn.) Chest 133:160S–198S. doi:10.1378/chest.08-0670
21. Tafur AJ, McBane R, Wysokinski WE, Litin S, Daniels P, Slusser J, Hodge D, Beckman MG, Heit JA (2012) Predictors of major bleeding in peri-procedural anticoagulation management. J Thromb Haemost 10(2):261–267. doi:10.1111/j.1538-7836.2011.04572.x
22. Falvo N, Bonithon-Kopp C, Rivron Guillot K, Todolí JA, Jiménez-Gil M, Di Micco P, Monreal M, The RIETE investigators (2011) Heparin-associated thrombocytopenia in 24,401 patients with venous thromboembolism. Findings from the RIETE registry. J Thromb Haemost doi:10.1111/j.1538-7836.2011.04402.x
23. Cuker AJ (2011) Heparin-induced thrombocytopenia: present and future. Emerg Trauma Shock 4(1):97–102

3 Anticoagulation Therapy in ICU Patients 57

24. Kato S, Takahashi K, Ayabe K, Samad R, Fukaya E, Friedmann P, Varma M, Bergmann SR (2011) Heparin-induced thrombocytopenia: analysis of risk factors in medical inpatients. J Thromb Thrombolysis 31(3):353-66. doi:10.1111/j.1365-2141.2011.08746.x
25. Greinacher A, Juhl D, Strobel U, Wessel A, Lubenow N, Selleng K, Eichler P, Warkentin TE (2007) Heparin-induced thrombocytopenia: a prospective study on the incidence, platelet-activating capacity and clinical significance of antiplatelet factor 4/heparin antibodies of the IgG, IgM, and IgA classes. J Thromb Haemost 5(8):1666-1673 [Epub 2007 May 7]
26. Kappers-Klunne MC, Boon DM, Hop WC, Michiels JJ, Stibbe J, van der Zwaan C, Koudstaal PJ, van Vliet HH (1997) Heparin-induced thrombocytopenia and thrombosis: a prospective analysis of the incidence in patients with heart and cerebrovascular diseases. Br J Haematol. 96(3):442–446
27. Kahl K, Heidrich H (1998) The incidence of heparin-induced thrombocytopenias. Int J Angiol 7(3):255–257
28. Hirsh J, Warkentin TE, Raschke R, Granger C, Ohman EM, Dalen JE (1998) Heparin and low-molecular-weight heparin: mechanisms of action, pharmacokinetics, dosing considerations, monitoring, efficacy, and safety. Chest. 114(Suppl 5):489S–510S
29. Kurtz LE, Yang S (2007) Bilateral adrenal hemorrhage associated with heparin induced thrombocytopenia. Am J Hematol 82(6):493–494
30. Schmidt OH, Lang W (1997) Heparin-induced thrombocytopenia with thromboembolic arterial occlusion treated with recombinant hirudin. N Engl J Med 337(19):1389
31. Matsuo T, Koide M, Kario K (1997) Application of argatroban, direct thrombin inhibitor, in heparin-intolerant patients requiring extracorporeal circulation. Artif Organs 21(9):1035–1038
32. Lewis BE, Rangel Y, Fareed J (1998) The first report of successful carotid stent implant using argatroban anticoagulation in a patient with heparin-induced thrombocytopenia and thrombosis syndrome: a case report. Angiology 49(1):61–67
33. Amiral J, Lormeau JC, Marfaing-Koka A, Vissac AM, Wolf M, Boyer-Neumann C, Tardy B, Herbert JM, Meyer D (1997) Absence of cross-reactivity of SR90107A/ORG31540 pentasaccharide with antibodies to heparin-PF4 complexes developed in heparin-induced thrombocytopenia. Blood Coagul Fibrinolysis 8(2):114–117
34. Brown DL et al (2001) Meta-analysis of effectiveness and safety of abciximab versus eptafibatide or tirofiban in percutaneous coronary intervention. Am J Cardiol 87:537–541
35. Topol EJ et al (2001) Comparison of two platelet glycoprotein IIb/IIIa inhibitors, tirofiban and abciximab for the prevention of ischemic events with percutaneous coronary revascularization. N Engl J Med 344:1888–1894
36. Coller BS (2001) Anti-GPIIb/IIIa: current strategies and future directions. Thromb Haemost 86:427–443
37. Bosh X, Marrugat J. Platelet glycoprotein IIb/IIIa blockers for percutaneous coronary revascularization, and unstable angina and non-ST-segment elevation myocardial infarction
38. Ferro M, Crivello R, Rizzotti M (2000) Comparison of subcutaneous calcium heparin and acetylsalicylic acid in the prevention of ischemic events and death after myocardial infarction: a randomized trial in a consecutive series of 90 patients. Heart Dis 2(4):278–281
39. Sawaya FJ, Musallam KM, Arnaout S, Rabah A (2011) To RE-LY or not to rely. In: Sawaya J (ed) Int J Cardiol, Switching patients from warfarin to dabigatran therapy
40. Connolly SJ, Ezekowitz MD, Yusuf S, Eikelboom J, Oldgren J, Parekh A, Pogue J, Reilly PA, Themeles E, Varrone J, Wang S, Alings M, Xavier D, Zhu J, Diaz R, Lewis BS, Darius H, Diener HC, Joyner CD, Wallentin L (2009) RE-LY steering committee and investigators. Dabigatran versus warfarin in patients with atrial fibrillation. N Engl J Med 361(12): 1139–1151 [Epub 2009 Aug 30]
41. Connolly S, Pogue J, Hart R, Pfeffer M, Hohnloser S, Chrolavicius S, Pfeffer M, Hohnloser S, Yusuf S (2006) ACTIVE writing group of the ACTIVE investigators. Clopidogrel plus aspirin versus oral anticoagulation for atrial fibrillation in the atrial fibrillation clopidogrel trial with irbesartan for prevention of vascular events (ACTIVE W): a randomised controlled trial. Lancet 367(9526):1903–1912

42. Lindblad B, Sternby NH, Bergqvist D (1991) Incidence of venous thromboembolism verified by necropsy over 30 years. BMJ 302(6778):709–711

43. Anderson FA Jr, Wheeler HB, Goldberg RJ, Hosmer DW, Forcier A (1992) The prevalence of risk factors for venous thromboembolism among hospital patients. Arch Intern Med 152(8):1660–1664

44. Lindblad B, Bergqvist D, Nordström M, Kjellström T, Björgell O, Nylander G, Sternby NH, Anderson H (1992) A survey in Malmö. The frequency of venous thromboembolism has not changed during the last 30 years. Lakartidningen. 89(37):2941–2942, 2947

45. Sandler DA, Martin JF (1989) Autopsy proven pulmonary embolism in hospital patients: are we detecting enough deep vein thrombosis? J R Soc Med 82(4):203–205

46. The SCATI (Studio sulla Calciparina nell'Angina e nella Trombosi Ventricolare nell'Infarto) Group (1989) Randomised controlled trial of subcutaneous calcium-heparin in acute myocardial infarction. Lancet 2(8656):182–186

47. Kase CS, Albers GW, Bladin C, Fieschi C, Gabbai AA, O'Riordan W, Pineo GF, PREVAIL Investigators (2009) Neurological outcomes in patients with ischemic stroke receiving enoxaparin or heparin for venous thromboembolism prophylaxis: subanalysis of the prevention of VTE after acute ischemic stroke with LMWH (PREVAIL) study. Stroke 40(11):3532–3540. [Epub 2009 Aug 20]

48. Sandercock PA, Counsell C, Gubitz GJ, Tseng MC (2008) Antiplatelet therapy for acute ischaemic stroke. Kochrane Database Syst Rev 16;(3):CD000029

49. Morris RJ, Woodcock JP (2010) Intermittent pneumatic compression or graduated compression stockings for deep vein thrombosis prophylaxis? A systematic review of direct clinical comparisons. Ann Surg 251(3):393–396

50. Cohen A (1997) Interpretation of IST and CAST stroke trials. International stroke trial. Chinese acute stroke trial. Comment on: Lancet. 349(9065):1569–1581, 350(9075):440, author reply 443–444

51. Low molecular weight heparinoid ORG 10172 (danaparoid), and outcome after acute ischemic stroke: a randomized controlled trial. The Publications Committee for the trial of ORG 10172 in acute stroke treatment (TOAST) Investigators. JAMA. 279(16):1265–1272

52. Goldstein JN, Gilson AJ (2011) Critical care management of acute intracerebral hemorrhage. Curr Treat Options Neurol 13(2):204–216

53. Paciaroni M, Agnelli G, Venti M, Alberti A, Acciarresi M, Caso V (2011) Efficacy and safety of anticoagulants in the prevention of venous thromboembolism in patients with acute cerebral hemorrhage: a meta-analysis of controlled studies. J Thromb Haemost 9(5):893–898. doi:10.1111/j.1538-7836.2011.04241.x

54. Fuster V, Rydén LE, Cannom DS, Harry CJ, Anne CB, Kenneth EA, Jonathan HL, Kay NG, Jean-Yves LH, James LE, Olsson BS, Eric PN, Luis JT, Samuel WL, Smith SC, Silvia GP (2011) ACCF/AHA/HRS focused updates incorporated Into the ACC/AHA/ESC 2006 guidelines for the management of patients with atrial fibrillation: a report of the American college of cardiology foundation/American heart association task force on practice guidelines. Circulation 123:e269–e367

55. Daniel ES, Albers GW, Dalen JE, Fang MC, Alan SG, Jonathan LH, Gregory YHL, Warren JM (2008) Antithrombotic therapy in atrial fibrillation: American college of chest physicians evidence-based clinical practice guidelines (8th edn.). Chest 133;546S-592S. doi:10.1378/chest.08-0678

56. Antonio R, Marcello D, Alboni P, Bertaglia E, Botto G, Brignole M, Cappato R, Capucci A, Del Greco M, de Ponti R, Di Biase M, Di Pasquale G, Michele G, Lombardi F, Sakis T, Tritto M (2011) AIAC 2010 guidelines for the management and treatment of atrial fibrillation. G Ital Cardiol 12(Suppl 1):7–69

57. Ezekowitz MD, Connolly S, Parekh A, Reilly PA, Varrone J, Wang S, Oldgren J, Themeles E, Wallentin L, Yusuf S (2009) Rationale and design of RE-LY: randomized evaluation of long-term anticoagulant therapy, warfarin, compared with dabigatran. Am Heart J 157(5):805–810, 810.e1-2

3 Anticoagulation Therapy in ICU Patients 59

58. Rivaroxaban once daily, oral, direct factor Xa inhibition compared with vitamin K antagonism for prevention of stroke and embolism trial in atrial fibrillation: rationale and design of the ROCKET AF study. Am Heart J 159(3):340–347.e1

59. Bates DW, Cullen DJ, Laird N et al (1995) Incidence of adverse drug events and potential adverse drug events. Implications for prevention. ADE Prevention Study Group. JAMA 274:29–34

60. Kopp BJ, Erstad BL, Allen ME et al (2006) Medication errors and adverse drug events in an intensive care unit: direct observation approach for detection. Crit Care Med 34:415–425

61. Leape LL, Brennan TA, Laird N et al (1991) The nature of adverse events in hospitalized patients. Results of the Harvard Medical practice study II. N Engl J Med 324:377–384

62. Cullen DJ, Sweitzer BJ, Bates DW et al (1997) Preventable adverse drug events in hospitalized patients: a comparative study of intensive care and general care units. Crit Care Med 25:1289–1297

63. Cohen AT, Alikhan R (2005) Assessment of venous thromboembolism risk and the benefits of thromboprophylaxis in medical patients. Thromb Haemost 94(4):750–759

64. Leizorovicz A, Mismetti P (2004) Preventing venous thromboembolism in medical patients. Circulation 110:IV-13-IV-19

65. Bechtold H, Janssen D (2004) Anticoagulation with low-molecular-weight heparin in patients with heart diseases. Eur J Med Res 9(4):186–198

66. Baum GL, Fisher FD (1960) The relationship of fatal pulmonary insufficiency with cor pulmonale, rightsided mural thrombi and pulmonary emboli: a preliminary report. Am J Med Sci 240:609–612

67. Greene R, Zapol WM, Snider MT, Reid L, Snow R, O'Connell RS, Novelline RA (1981) Early bedside detection of pulmonary vascular occlusion during acute respiratory failure. Am Rev Respir Dis 124(5):593–601

68. Lip GY, Lane DA (2010) Does warfarin for stroke thromboprophylaxis protect against MI in atrial fibrillation patients? Am J Med 123(9):785–789. [Epub 2010 Jul 23]

69. Gallandat Huet RC, Siemons AW, Baus D, et al (2000) A novel hydroxyethyl starch (Voluven) for effective perioperative plasma volume substitution in cardiac surgery. Can J Anaesth 47:1207–1215

70. Karanko MS, Klossner JA, Laaksonen VO (1987) Restoration of volume by crystalloid versus colloid after coronary artery bypass: hemo- dynamics, lung water, oxygenation, and outcome. Crit Care Med 15:559–566

71. Verheij J, van Lingen A, Beishuizen A et al (2006) Cardiac response is greater for colloid than saline fluid loading after cardiac or vascular surgery. Intensive Care Med 32:1030–1038

72. Boldt J, Haisch G, Suttner S, Kumle B, Schellhaass A (2002) Effects of a new modified, balanced hydroxyethyl starch preparation (Hextend) on measures of coagulation. Br J Anaesth 89:72

73. Nielsen VG (2006) Effects of Hextend hemodilution on plasma coagulation kinetics in the rabbit: role of factor XIII-mediated fibrin polymer crosslinking. J Surg Res 132:17–22

74. Niemi TT, Kuitunen AH (2005) Artificial colloids impair haemostasis. An in vitro study using thromboelastometry coagulation analysis. Acta Anaesthesiol Scand 49:373–378

75. Boldt J, Knothe C, Zickmann B, Andres P, Dapper F, Hempelmann G (1993) Influence of different volume therapies on platelet function in patients undergoing cardiopulmonary bypass. Anesth Analg 76:1185–1190

76. Niemi TT, Kuitunen AH (1998) Hydroxyethyl starch impairs in vitro coagulation. Acta Anaesthesiol Scand 42:1104–1109

77. Niemi TT, Suojaranta-Ylinen RT, Kukkonen SI, Kuitunen AH (2006) Gelatin and hydroxyethyl starch, but not albumin, impair hemostasis after cardiac surgery. Anesth Analg 102:998–1006

78. Niemi TT, Kuitunen AH (2005) Artificial colloids impair haemostasis. An in vitro study using thromboelastometry coagulation analysis. Acta Anaesthesiol Scand 49:373–378

79. Boldt J, Wolf M, Mengistu A (2007) A new plasma adapted hydroxyethylstarch preparation: in vitro coagulation studies using thrombelastography and whole blood aggregometry. Anesth Analg 104:425–430
80. Schols SE, Lance MD, Feijge MA (2010) Impaired thrombin generation and fibrin clot formation in patients with dilutional coagulopathy during major surgery. Thromb Haemost 103:318–328
81. Van der Linden P, Ickx BE (2006) The effects of colloid solutions on hemostasis. Can J Anaesth 53:30–39
82. Bergqvist D (1998) Modern aspects of prophylaxis and therapy for venous thromboembolic disease. Aust N Z J Surg 68:463–468
83. Clagett GP, Anderson FAJ, Geerts W et al (1998) Prevention of venous thromboembolism. Chest 114:531S–60S
84. Ljungstrom KG (1983) Dextran prophylaxis of fatal pulmonary embolism. World J Surg 7:767–772
85. Aberg M, Hedner U, Bergentz SE (1979) Effect of dextran on factor VIII (antihemophilic factor) and platelet function. Ann Surg 189:243–247
86. Batlle J, del Rio F, Lopez FM et al (1985) Effect of dextran on factor VIII/von Willebrand factor structure and function. Thromb Haemost 54:697–699
87. Mardel SN, Saunders FM, Allen H et al (1998) Reduced quality of clot formation with gelatin-based plasma substitutes. Br J Anaesth 80:204–207
88. Aberg M, Hedner U, Bergentz SE (1979) The antithrombotic effect of dextran. Scand J Haematol Suppl 34:61–68
89. de Jonge E, Levi M, Berends F et al (1998) Impaired haemostasis by intravenous administration of a gelatin-based plasma expander in human subjects. Thromb Haemost 79:286–290
90. Beyer R, Harmening U, Rittmeyer O et al (1997) Use of modified fluid gelatin and hydroxyethyl starch for colloidal volume replacement in major orthopaedic surgery. Br J Anaesth 78:44–50
91. Boldt J, Knothe C, Zickmann B et al (1993) Influence of different intravascular volume therapies on platelet function in patients undergoing cardiopulmonary bypass. Anesth Analg 76:1185–1190
92. Mortelmans YJ, Vermaut G, Verbruggen AM et al (1995) Effects of 6% hydroxyethyl starch and 3% modified fluid gelatin on intravascular volume and coagulation during intraoperative hemodilution. Anesth Analg 81:1235–1242
93. Trumble ER, Muizelaar JP, Myseros JS et al (1995) Coagulopathy with the use of hetastarch in the treatment of vasospasm. J Neurosurg 82:44–47
94. Cope JT, Banks D, Mauney MC et al (1997) Intraoperative hetastarch infusion impairs hemostasis after cardiac operations. Ann Thorac Surg 63:78–82
95. Villarino ME, Gordon SM, Valdon C et al (1992) A cluster of severe postoperative bleeding following open heart surgery. Infect Control Hosp Epidemiol 13:282–287
96. Salmon JB, Mythen MG (1993) Pharmacology and physiology of colloids. Blood Rev 7:114–120
97. Treib J, Haass A, Pindur G (1997) Coagulation disorders caused by hydroxyethyl starch. Thromb Haemost 78:974–983
98. Jorgensen KA, Stoffersen E (1980) On the inhibitory effect of albumin on platelet aggregaion. Thromb Res 17:13–18
99. Kim SB, Chi HS, Park JS et al (1999) Effect of increasing serum albumin on plasma Ddimer, von Willebrand factor, and platelet aggregation in CAPD patients. Am J Kidney Dis 33:312–317
100. Sanofi-Aventis (2007) DDAVP package insert. Bridgewater, NJ

Inborn Prothrombotic States

4

Nicola Fiotti and Carlo Giansante

4.1 Introduction

An efficient hemostatic system limits blood loss and assists tissue repair. This is particularly important in mammals, which rely on high blood pressure (i.e., being at increased risk of hemorrhage after injury) deliver live offspring, and require continuous tissue remodeling. The reactions leading to fibrin mesh deposits, those reactions controlling clot development, and fibrinolytic systems are set in order to reduce hemorrhages or excessive clot formation. A subtle biochemical and physical balance regulates blood coagulation and tissue repair. Critical aspects of these reactions are triggering the reactions only where needed, amplifying them to speed up the process but also controlling their magnitude and localization, and, at the end of hemostasis, starting a repair process.

Congenital or acquired conditions can shift the equilibrium toward either excessive or defective fibrin formation (and sometimes toward both of the extremes). The condition where blood has an increased tendency to clot has long been recognized as the prethrombotic/prothrombotic state, thrombophilia, hypercoagulability, or vulnerable blood. The clinical consequence of this condition is the development (or increased risk) of venous and, sometimes, also arterial thrombosis. Genetic variants are major causes of prothrombotic states and are called inborn prothrombotic states (IPS).

The defects inducing IPS are:
- Prothrombin mutation
- Activated protein C resistance

C. Giansante (✉)
Unità Clinica Operativa di Clinica Medica Generale e Terapia Medica,
University of Trieste, Trieste, Italy
e-mail: giansant@units.it

G. Berlot (ed.), *Hemocoagulative Problems in the Critically Ill Patient*,
DOI: 10.1007/978-88-470-2448-9_4, © Springer-Verlag Italia 2012

- Protein C deficiency
- Antithrombin deficiency
- Protein S deficiency

Prothrombin mutation and protein C resistance can be called either a mutation or a polymorphism according to the populations where it has been studied, the allelic frequency of the former being more than 1% in southern Europe, whereas the same can be observed for protein C resistance in northern Europe.

4.2 Clinical Features of IPS

Venous thromboembolism (VTE) triggered by or associated with the aforementioned genetic variants usually shows some peculiar characteristics which should lead to the investigation of a possible IPS. These clinical abnormalities can be suspected mainly when the age at onset of the thrombosis and the blood vessel site are atypical.

4.2.1 Age at Onset

The most common, first and foremost clinical suspicion of IPS is when the age at presentation of a thromboembolism, either at an arterial or a venous site, is below 50 years. In a broad perspective, age also affects the patient's offspring before their birth. Some genetic defects, namely, type I antithrombin deficiency, have never been found in living individuals, and within the families carrying such a defect, spontaneous abortion is frequent. Therefore, a history of spontaneous abortion needs to be ascertained in the family history of the proband. Also, some other less powerful familial genetic defects combine and increase the risk of abortion.

In keeping with this evidence, homozygous quantitative protein C and protein S deficiencies are associated with abortion in the families and purpura cutanea fulminans in newborns, a rare syndrome caused by progressive thrombosis of the microvasculature inducing widespread cutaneous hemorrhage and tissue death.

The number of genetic defects in a patient has an additive effect on the age at onset: the first VTE episode in patients with two identified genetic defects occurs earlier (17 years on average) than in members of families with VTE either with or without an identified defect (40 years).

The relationship between genetics and age is further corroborated by evidence that a young age at onset of VTE in probands with an ascertained genetic defect is the main determinant of the occurrence of VTE in first-degree relatives [1].

4.2.2 Unusual Sites

Mesenteric vein thrombosis or Budd–Chiari syndrome. This is a rare but characteristic event that should be suspected when abdominal pain becomes worse after eating and with time, and is associated with diarrhea and vomiting.

4 Inborn Prothrombotic States

Upper limb veins. Another site is in the veins of the arm. In a small group of patients, the prevalence of factor V Leiden mutation was around 13%, the prevalence of prothrombin G20210A mutation was 20%, and 5% had protein S deficiency.

Cerebral vein thrombosis. The clinical presentation can be extremely varied, and symptoms evolve within hours to a few weeks. The most frequent signs and symptoms are headache, focal seizures with or without secondary generalization, paresis (unilateral or bilateral), and papilledema, or patients have an impairment of consciousness on presentation. Symptoms of intracranial hypertension (headache, visual disturbance, and papilledema) were found in 20% of patients. Less frequent symptoms include thunderclap headache mimicking subarachnoid hemorrhage. Cortical vein involvement alone, lacking features of raised pressure, is rare and may present with a "stroke-like" episode. Occasionally, cerebellar veins may be involved, usually related to middle-ear infection, and may lead to a slowly evolving syndrome of vertigo, vomiting, and ataxia, often with headache and coma.

In some case–control studies (1,183 cerebral vein thrombosis patients and 5,189 controls), factor V Leiden/G1691A and prothrombin/G20210A increase the risk of cerebral vein thrombosis by 2.40 and 5.48 times, respectively.

Deep vein thrombosis of the lower limbs. The prevalence of VTE in individuals with protein S deficiency is 100%, in individuals with antithrombin deficiency is 90%, in individuals with protein C deficiency is 88%, and in individuals with factor V Leiden is 57%. The probability of developing thrombosis during the lifetime is 8.1 times higher for carriers of antithrombin deficiency than that for noncarriers, 7.3 times higher for carriers of protein C deficiency, 8.5 times higher for carriers of protein S deficiency, and 2.2 times higher for carriers of factor V Leiden. The site of occurrence within the lower limb veins can be guided by genetic factors. Carriers of factor V Leiden have a more distal localization of the thrombus compared with patients without such a mutation [2]. Factor V Leiden carriers have about eightfold lower incidences of deep vein thrombosis in the iliofemoral veins than noncarriers [3]. Together with the observation that deep vein thromboses located in the iliofemoral vein segments, more likely to be associated with pulmonary embolism, this can explain why the prevalence of pulmonary embolism in IPS patients, supposed to parallel the higher prevalence of VTE, is actually not different from that observed in non-IPS VTE [4].

Superficial thrombophlebitis. The prevalence of superficial vein thrombosis in carriers of factor V Leiden is 43%, in carriers of antithrombin deficiency is 10%, in carriers of protein C deficiency is 13%, in carriers of prothrombin G20210 mutation is 3.5%, and in carriers of protein S deficiency is 0%.

Warfarin-induced skin necrosis. This potentially catastrophic complication affects carriers of protein C deficiency at the beginning of warfarin therapy. One day after initiation of the usual doses of warfarin, protein C (and factor VII) activity is reduced by approximately 50%. In normal subjects, such decrease in activity is balanced between procoagulant and anticoagulant sides of fibrin formation reactions because of the short half-life of factor VII. The reduced level of protein C activity, compared with that of the other procoagulant molecules, creates a transient hyper-coagulable state, which generates cutaneous vessel thrombosis, with surrounding interstitial hemorrhage, and ischemic necrosis of the cutaneous tissue. The skin lesions arise on fat-rich regions, such as the bottom and the breast. Around one in three warfarin-induced skin necroses occur in patients with protein C deficiency.

A high prevalence of some mutations/polymorphisms in the population questions the belief that they have a negative impact on survival and health in general. The ascertained risk of a potentially life-threatening condition associated with these variants leads to the hypothesis that IPS were not a disadvantage for ancient populations. Indeed, at least factor V Leiden and prothrombin mutation may offer benefits for reducing blood loss related to menstruation, the postpartum period, or trauma and are associated with a decreased risk of intracranial hemorrhage. In addition, it has been demonstrated that factor V Leiden significantly reduces mortality due to severe infections. Further support for this counterintuitive evidence comes from the statement that aging, prolonged immobility, surgery, and hormonal therapy are thrombosis risk conditions observed only in recent years. It is likely, then, that the risk of thrombosis in the past was lower than now [5].

4.3 Types of Genetic Defects

Five defects have been identified and are recognized on the basis of the risk level and the prevalence in the population, namely, functional antithrombin deficiency, protein C deficiency, protein S deficiency, factor V G1691A, and prothrombin G20210A. The prevalence of the mutations and the odds ratio for development of deep vein thrombosis are reported in Table 4.1.

4.3.1 Prothrombin Mutation G20210A

Biology. Thrombin is a crossroad of many blood coagulation reactions. It catalyzes the conversion of fibrinogen, protein C, protein S, and factors IX and XIII. Prothrombin, the proenzyme of thrombin, is a vitamin K dependent glycoprotein of approximately 70 kDa circulating in human plasma at a concentration of approximately 100 mg/l, and has a half-life of 60 h. Activated by activated factor X (factor Xa) (in the presence of activated factor V, i.e., factor Va, and phospholipids), thrombin converts fibrinogen to fibrin, and activates protein C and protein S (when linked to thrombomodulin) and also factors V, VIII, IX, and XIII.

Gene. A single nucleotide exchange (G $\rightarrow$ A transition) at position 20210 in the 3′-untranslated region of the prothrombin gene (chromosome 11p11), increases the posttranslational 3′ end processing efficiency, thus leading to a higher transcription rate, and is associated with an approximately 25% increase in plasma thrombin activity. Prothrombin 20210A represents the second most frequent prothrombotic polymorphism in humans and the most frequent in southern Europe.

4 Inborn Prothrombotic States

Table 4.1 Inherited thrombophilias: prevalence and relative risk

Thrombophilia	Prevalence in general population (%)	Prevalence in individuals with VTE (%)	Relative VTE risk (OR)
Antithrombin deficiency	0.02–0.04	0.5–4.9	10–20
Protein C deficiency	0.2–0.50	3–9	7–10
Protein S deficiency	0.1–1	1–3	5–10
Factor V Leiden (heterozygous)[a]	3–7	12–20	3–8
Factor V Leiden (homozygous)	0.004–0.065	0.01	9–80
Prothrombin G20210A (heterozygous)[a]	1–3	6–8	2–3
Prothrombin G20210A (homozygous)	0.001–0.012	0.2–4	NA

NA not available, *OR* odds ratio, *VTE* venous thromboembolism
[a] Prevalence varies with the population studied

The mutation is approximately 24,000 years old and a founder effect has been established. Therefore, the prevalence of the prothrombin mutation varies depending on the geographic location and the ethnic background, being as high as 2–4% of healthy individuals in southern Europe, and half that in northern Europe. Its distribution shows, in Europe, a north to south gradient (cutoff at 50°N, prevalence of 0.017 and 0.03, respectively). Similar to FV Leiden, it is rare in Far East Asian populations, in Africa, and in indigenous populations of Australia and the Americas.

In Western societies today, the mutation is found in 6–8% of venous thrombosis patients. The transmission is autosomal dominant. Carriers of the mutation have a threefold to fourfold increased risk of venous thrombosis [5].

Diagnosis. The mutation can be ascertained by DNA amplification and a restriction enzyme (*Hin*dIII).

4.3.2 Activated C Protein Resistance

Biology. Factor V is a regulatory protein allowing (in presence of calcium and phospholipids) the breakdown of prothrombin into thrombin by factor Xa. It needs to be activated to factor Va by thrombin. When thrombin binds to thrombomodulin inside the vessels, it catalyzes the activation of protein C, which, together with protein S, degrades factor Va and activated factor VIII (factor VIIIa) to inactivated factors V and VIII. Thus, thrombin bound to thrombomodulin switches from a procoagulant to an anticoagulant protein. In the 1990s it was discovered that a defect in factor V makes it less susceptible to inactivation by activated protein C. The cleavage of factor V by protein C initially occurs on Arg506, which facilitates subsequent cleavage of Arg306 and Arg679. Failure to degrade factor V increases the amount of prothrombinase complexes, thus predisposing to thrombosis.

Gene. Factor V Leiden (chromosome 1q23) consists of a G1691A nucleotide transition resulting in an R506Q amino acid missense mutation. It accounts for 90–95% of cases of activated C protein resistance, whereas the remaining 5–10% is due to the missense of Arg306 with threonine (factor V Cambridge) or with glycine (factor V Hong Kong). It was thought to have emerged 30,000 years ago, with divergence among Caucasian, Asian, and African populations. Factor V resistance to activated C protein has an incidence of 4.8% in the general population of northern Europe and the USA and is the most common cause of inherited thrombosis, accounting for 40–50% of cases. In these populations, FV Leiden mutation is more frequently found in cases of venous thrombosis than are protein C or protein S deficiency, prothrombin G20210A mutation, and antithrombin deficiency combined. FV Leiden mutation is extremely uncommon in people of African or Asian descent [5].

Diagnosis. The activated protein C resistance is diagnosed by the ratio of two activated partial thromboplastin time (aPTT) tests from the same patient, one following the standard protocol and the other with the addition of activated protein C. In normal subjects, the ratio between the latter and the former is greater than 3, owing to the degradation of factor Va by activated protein C, whereas in carriers of activated C protein resistance, i.e., factor V Leiden, Cambridge, or Hong Kong, the ratio will be lower than 3.

If the aPTT ratio is suggestive of a factor V mutation, then a molecular genetic analysis identifies precisely the defect. This is usually performed by direct sequencing, which allows one to detect all the mutations responsible for activated C protein resistance, i.e., in both the 306 and the 506 amino acid position.

4.3.3 Antithrombin

Biology. The gene encoding antithrombin, *SERPINC1*, is located on the long arm of chromosome 1 (q23–q25.1). Its product, antithrombin (formerly known as antithrombin III) is a 58,200-Da protein synthesized by the liver, and circulates in plasma at a concentration of around 125 mg/l (2.3 μM) with a half-life of around 65 h. The mature form is glycosylated at Asn128, Asn167, Asn187, and Asn224. Around 5–10% of plasma antithrombin is not glycosylated at Asn167 and is termed antithrombin-β, and despite being a minor proportion of antithrombin, it may be physiologically important because it has a higher affinity for heparin than the major form, which is known as antithrombin-α.

When antithrombin binds to specific sulfate groups on the pentasaccharide structure of heparin, the reactive site loop containing the reactive site (Arg425–Ser426) becomes available and antithrombin affinity for serine proteases is

4 Inborn Prothrombotic States

increased by more than 1,000-fold, leading to the formation of a stable inactive 1:1 stoichiometric complex (serine protease–antithrombin) that is removed from circulation. Antithrombin also inhibits factors Xa, IXa, XIa, XIIa and VIIa when in complex with tissue factor, in addition to thrombin. Inhibition of thrombin by antithrombin requires thrombin to bind to heparin and to be close to the heparin-bound antithrombin, and this is only possible with higher molecular weight heparin comprising at least 18 saccharide units. In health, antithrombin is believed to be concentrated on the vascular endothelium, where it is activated by glycosaminoglycans.

Gene. Genetic variants of antithrombin affect around 0.02% of healthy adults, in all ethnic groups, but this prevalence is increased to 1.9% in patients with a personal history of VTE, with an odds ratio of 95. There is also an increased risk of arterial thrombosis, namely, acute myocardial infarction for antithrombin deficiency carriers.

Antithrombin deficiency is a heterogeneous disorder: over 200 distinct *SERPINC1* mutations are known, usually showing an autosomal dominant pattern of inheritance. A database of these mutations can be found at http://www1.imperial. ac.uk/departmentofmedicine/divisions/experimentalmedicine/haematology/coag/antithrombin/.

Such a large number of mutations are categorized into type I and type II antithrombin deficiencies. Type I deficiency refers to the complete quantitative deficiency, usually caused by:

- Nonsense mutations or small insertions and deletions leading to frameshifts and failure in expression of antithrombin.
- Partial or major gene deletions, sometimes induced by the high number of Alu repeats within the gene through the misalignment of DNA strands during replication and the deletion of the intervening sequence.
- Missense mutations such as amino acid substitutions in the signal peptide that result in impaired cotranslational processing and quantitative deficiency of antithrombin have been described.
- Missense mutations causing abnormal glycosylation and intracellular retention of antithrombin or which are associated with reduced conformational stability of antithrombin.

These mutations are scattered throughout the gene; therefore, diagnosis requires complete sequencing of the exons.

Type II deficiency is usually caused by missense mutations affecting residues that are involved in antithrombin function. It can be further classified into three subtypes of mutations:

1. Type II reactive site (most cases of deficiency) affecting the reactive sites Arg425, Ser426, Gly424, Ala414, and Ala416.
2. Type II heparin binding site deficiency involves Pro73, Arg79, Leu131, and Arg161 residues, which are involved in heparin binding.
3. Type II deficiency generating pleiotropic effects is caused by missense mutations affecting amino acids between residues 434 and 441 and between 453 and 462 in the C-terminal region of the protein.

Diagnosis. Timing is very important to obtain a reliable result: sampling should be avoided in the setting of acute thrombosis, because acute thrombosis and heparin therapy may lower antithrombin levels. Also, vitamin K antagonist therapy may increase antithrombin levels owing to coagulation inhibition, thus underestimating antithrombin deficiency.

Causes of acquired antithrombin deficiency can be due to decreased antithrombin synthesis (liver cirrhosis), increased antithrombin losses (nephrotic syndrome, protein-losing enteropathy) enhanced consumption/inactivation of antithrombin (sepsis with disseminated intravascular coagulation, burn injuries, polytrauma, hepatic venoocclusive disease, thrombotic microangiopathies, cardiopulmonary bypass surgery, large hematomas, metastatic tumors, extracorporeal membrane oxygen therapy), or drug-induced antithrombin deficiency (like in L-asparaginase therapy or heparin therapy).

In general, no patient should be diagnosed as having antithrombin deficiency on the basis of a single abnormal test result, although an abnormal test result should lead to repeat testing on a new blood sample.

To determine antithrombin deficiency, the first and foremost test is the determination of antithrombin activity in plasma.

The functional antithrombin assay is an amidolytic (chromogenic) assay. A patient's plasma is incubated in the presence of heparin with excess thrombin (either human or bovine) or factor Xa. The antithrombin in the patient's plasma neutralizes thrombin or factor Xa, and the amount of residual nonneutralized thrombin or factor Xa is inversely proportional to the patient's antithrombin activity level. This remaining thrombin or factor Xa is quantified using an automated chromogenic detection system.

If the results of the functional assays are abnormal, an antithrombin antigen level can be obtained to help differentiate between type I and type II deficiencies. The distinction of antithrombin deficiency subtypes may be clinically relevant, because the type IIb subtype has a much lower risk of thrombosis than the other subtypes.

The antigenic assays are quantitative assays that define the type of antithrombin deficiency. In the absence of secondary causes, and in the appropriate clinical setting, a low antigenic assay result classifies a patient as having a type I (or type IIc) antithrombin deficiency.

Owing to the large number of different mutations underlying antithrombin deficiency, the precise molecular diagnosis will require whole gene sequencing [6].

4.3.4 Protein C

Biology. Protein C is a 62-kDa, vitamin K dependent glycoprotein synthesized in the liver. It circulates in the blood as an inactive zymogen at a concentration of 4 µg/mL and has a half-life of around 6–8 h. Its activation into the serine protease like enzyme, activated protein C, is catalyzed by thrombin when it is bound to the endothelial receptor thrombomodulin. Activated protein C exerts its anticoagulant activity primarily through inactivation of coagulation factors Va and VIIIa.

The catalytic activity of activated protein C is greatly enhanced by the vitamin K dependent cofactor protein S.

Gene. The gene for protein C is located on the long arm of chromosome 2. Around 200 pathogenic heterozygous mutations of this gene have been described, all inherited in an autosomal dominant fashion. These mutations are divided into type I (inducing a quantitative defect) and type II (accounting for a functional defect).

Heterozygous type I protein C deficiency demonstrates protein C antigen and activity levels that are approximately half those of the plasma of a normal patient. The mutation is due to alterations within the promoter, coding, noncoding, and splice areas of protein C leading to defective synthesis of the protein. Protein C deficiency is estimated to be three times higher in Japanese populations. Type I deficiency shows marked phenotypic variation among families, some exhibiting a severe thrombotic tendency, whereas others remain asymptomatic. Interestingly, this variability is seen even among different pedigrees that harbor the same protein C mutation, suggesting that the mutation itself does not fully explain the phenotypic variability.

Type II protein C deficiency is less common than the previous defect, and shows normal immunologic levels of protein C, but decreased functional activity. Here too, a number of point mutations within the protein C gene accounting for this disorder have been reported.

Diagnosis. The functional protein C test is the screening test to assess protein C deficiency. If the value obtained is lower than the reference value, then an immunoenzymatic test is necessary to discriminate between the two types, the value being low in type I deficiency and normal in type II deficiency. Subtypes can then be diagnosed only by sequencing of the gene [7].

4.3.5 Protein S

Biology. Protein S is a vitamin K dependent anticoagulant protein facilitating, as a cofactor, the action of activated protein C on its substrates, factor Va and factor VIIIa. Protein S deficiencies are associated with venous thrombosis but not arterial thrombosis. In blood plasma, protein S exists in both a bound and a free state. A portion of protein S is noncovalently bound with high affinity to the complement regulatory protein C4b binding protein. In healthy individuals, approximately 30–40% of total protein S is in the free state. Only free protein S is capable of acting as a cofactor in the protein C system.

Gene. Two genes for human protein S have been identified and both are linked closely on chromosome 3 (3p11.1–3q11.2). One is the active gene, *PROS*-b (i.e., *PROS1*), and the other, *PROS*-a, is an evolutionarily duplicated nonfunctional gene, which is classified as a pseudogene because it contains multiple coding errors (e.g., frameshifts, stop codons), and has 97% homology compared with the *PROS*-a gene.

Molecular studies into the genetic causes of protein S deficiency are complicated by the presence of the pseudogene, *PROS*-b, and phenotypic variation.

Deletions of large portions of the *PROS*-a gene are associated with protein S deficiency and thrombophilia.

The distinction between free and total protein S levels is important and gives rise to the current terminology regarding the deficiency states:

Type I protein S deficiency is a reduction in the level of free and total protein S.

Type II deficiency is a reduction in the cofactor activity of protein S, with normal antigenic levels.

Type III deficiency is a reduction in the level of free protein S only.

The most common genetic defects in the protein S gene are point mutations rather than gene deletions. Phenotypic variation has been observed in protein S deficiency. Current research indicates that protein S deficiency is five to ten times higher in Japanese populations than in Caucasians.

Diagnosis. Diagnosis is done by determining the total protein S amount by the ELISA method. Functional activity can be determined by precipitating the C4b bound fraction with poly(ethylene glycol) 8000 and measuring the concentration of free protein S in the supernatant. Reduced functional activity is measured with a modified aPTT [7].

4.4   Treatment

Asymptomatic individuals. The risk of VTE is low if the individual's condition was diagnosed because of random screening, but is higher if the individual's conditions was diagnosed because a family member was found to have VTE.

In both cases, the risk of VTE is relatively low and probably does not outweigh the risk of bleeding if long-term oral anticoagulation therapy is given. There is no evidence to support a policy of long-term pharmacological primary thromboprophylaxis of asymptomatic family members found to have thrombophilia, because the risk of serious or fatal hemorrhage considerably outweighs the risk of a fatal VTE event, even for patients with the most severe types of thrombophilia. However, future anticoagulant regimens with a lower risk for bleeding may change this risk–benefit assessment.

Prophylaxis during surgery and immobility. Half of the episodes of VTE in individuals with IPS occur in the setting of transient risk factors. These conditions, therefore, require diligent VTE prophylaxis. The drugs of choice are fondaparinux and subcutaneously administered hirudin. Interestingly, the pentasaccaride seems effective even in antithrombin deficiency.

VTE. The initial management of VTE in patients with IPS is usually not different from that of VTE in any other patient: (1) consideration of thrombolytics; (2) initial therapy with heparin or fondaparinux; and (3) transitioning to a vitamin K antagonist. In individuals with antithrombin deficiency there is, theoretically, a risk of heparin resistance and thrombus progression, no matter whether unfractionated heparin, low molecular weight heparin, or fondaparinux is used, but this does not seem to be a clinical problem in most patients. An international normalized ratio target of 2.0–3.0 appears appropriate. In determining the length of

4 Inborn Prothrombotic States

vitamin K antagonist therapy, the circumstances of the thrombotic event and all the patient's risk factors for recurrence should be weighed, similar to what is done for any other patient who has experienced a VTE. In addition, all risk factors for bleeding and the patient's preference regarding long-term versus time-limited anticoagulation need to be considered in the decision making. The risk of recurrent VTE in patients not treated long term with anticoagulants is high (10% and up to 17% per year). Long-term anticoagulation clearly lowers that risk. It is, therefore, typically recommended that a patient who has had a VTE and IPS should be considered for long-term anticoagulation. It is noteworthy that, despite long-term anticoagulation, a substantial risk of recurrence of 2.7% per year still remains.

Arterial thromboembolism. No data exist as to what the best treatment is for the patient with IPS deficiency who has had an arterial thrombotic event (i.e., whether anticoagulants or antiplatelet agents should be used). If the patient also has significant underlying arteriosclerosis or arteriosclerosis risk factors, which by themselves could explain the thrombotic event, then antiplatelet therapy may be appropriate, because this would be standard therapy in any other patient with a similar arterial event. However, if the thrombotic event occurred in a younger person and in the absence of any obvious arteriosclerosis, the suspicion that hypercoagulability may be the main cause of the thrombotic event is heightened. In this situation, the consideration of longer-term anticoagulation may be appropriate. However, it is important to realize that this approach is derived not from clinical studies, but from the inference that anticoagulants may be more effective than antiplatelet agents in such a specific condition.

Pregnancy. Recommendations for pregnancy management are weak because there are no good quality clinical studies, and reflect only expert committee opinions and/or clinical experience of respected authorities. The uncertainty about the best treatment refers to (1) the pharmacological agents used for VTE prophylaxis and (2) the doses of drugs given.

The recommendations are:
1. In IPS without previous VTE, the American College of Chest Physicians guidelines recommend: antepartum and postpartum prophylaxis.
2. In women with IPS with previous VTE not receiving anticoagulants long term, the American College of Chest Physicians suggests, in addition to postpartum prophylaxis, antepartum prophylactic or intermediate-dose low molecular weight heparin or unfractionated heparin.
3. In women with previous VTE who are receiving long-term vitamin K antagonist therapy, low molecular weight heparin or unfractionated heparin throughout the pregnancy is recommended independent of whether the woman has or does not have antithrombin deficiency.

Moreover, women should wear graduated compression stockings throughout pregnancy and for 6–12 weeks postpartum [8].

References

1. Couturaud F, Leroyer C, Julian JA et al (2009) Factors that predict risk of thrombosis in relatives of patients with unprovoked venous thromboembolism. Chest 136:1537–1545
2. Huisman MV, Klok FA, Djurabi RK et al (2008) Factor V Leiden is associated with more distal location of deep vein thrombosis of the leg. J Thromb Haemost 6:544–545
3. Bjorgell O, Nilsson PE, Nilsson JA, Svensson PJ (2000) Location and extent of deep vein thrombosis in patients with and without FV: R 506Q mutation. Thromb Haemost 83:648–651
4. Hooper WC, de Staercke C (2002) The relationship between FV Leiden and pulmonary embolism. Respir Res 3:8
5. Bauduer F, Lacombe D (2005) Factor V Leiden, prothrombin 20210A, methylenetetrahydrofolate reductase 677T, and population genetics. Mol Genet Metab 86:91–99
6. Patnaik MM, Moll S (2008) Inherited antithrombin deficiency: a review. Haemophilia 14:1229–1239
7. Dahlback B (2008) Advances in understanding pathogenic mechanisms of thrombophilic disorders. Blood 112:19–27
8. Spencer FA, Becker RC (1999) Diagnosis and management of inherited and acquired thrombophilias. J Thrombosis Thrombolysis 7:91–104

Inborn Defects of the Coagulative System

5

Marinella Astuto, Nadia Grasso and Alessandro Trainito

5.1 Introduction

The modern concept of coagulation was presented in 1964 as the waterfall/cascade model, which might overwhelm many nonhematologists with its complexity (Fig. 5.1a) [1]. The model has been further refined as a cell-based model describing a complex networking of various elements of coagulation (Fig. 5.1b) [2].

Over the course of time, blood coagulation has became a highly sophisticated defense mechanism to detect injury to the body and prevent exsanguinations to enhance survival [3–7]. Surveillance and rapid, localized hemostatic actions of the coagulation system are necessary given the multiple number of breaches to vascular integrity that occur over a lifetime.

To understand the evolution of hemostasis, it is useful to examine the primitive coagulation system of invertebrates. Horseshoe crabs (*Limulus*) have lived on Earth for more than 350 million years; in the blood (emolymph) of *Limulus*, oxygen is transported by the copper-containing protein hemocyanin. The only circulating blood cells are amoebocytes (hemocytes), which contain bactericides and coagulation zymogen proteins that are released upon activation. The important evolutionary difference between the vertebral coagulation system and that of invertebrate species is the need to provide localized thrombosis in high-pressure closed networks of blood vessels in contrast to the low-pressure open circulation. Similar to the mechanism by which amoebocytes detect a breach in the horseshoe crab's body armor, in humans, circulating blood reacts quickly to a disruption of the vascular endothelium to limit bleeding.

M. Astuto (✉)
Department of Anesthesia and Intensive Care,
Pediatric Anesthesia and Intensive Care Section,
"Policlinico" University Hospital, Catania, Italy
e-mail: astmar@tiscali.it

G. Berlot (ed.), *Hemocoagulative Problems in the Critically Ill Patient*,
DOI: 10.1007/978-88-470-2448-9_5, © Springer-Verlag Italia 2012

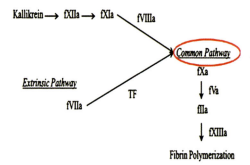

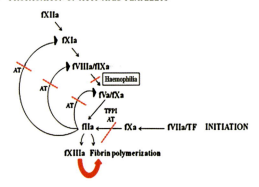

Fig. 5.1 a Intrinsic pathway and b propagation on activated platelets. *AT* antithrombin, *fIIa* activated factor II (thrombin), *fVa* activated factor V, *fVIIa* activated factor VII, *fVIIIa* activated factor VIII, *fIXa* activated factor IX, *fXa* activated factor X, *fXIa* activated factor XI, *fXIIa* activated factor XII, *fXIIIa* activated factor XIII, *TF* tissue factor, *TFPI* tissue factor pathway inhibitor

The coagulation process was understood until a few years ago as a simple "enzyme cascade mechanism." It involves an orderly and sequential activation of various coagulation factors from an inactive form to an enzymatically active form (theory of enzymatic "cascade" from the mid-1960s). According to this theory, there are two pathways (intrinsic and extrinsic) that converge in a common pathway when factor X is activated.

The weak points of this theory are:
- Not all coagulation factors behave as enzymes when activated.
- Many of the reactions of the coagulation process involve the formation of multimolecular complexes rather than the interaction of individual plasma factors.
- The activated factors may exert their enzymatic action on substrates differing from conventional ones.

5 Inborn Defects of the Coagulative System

- Feedback mechanisms and interactions between the various phases and various factors of the hemostatic process are activated.

Currently, it is considered that the two pathways of coagulation activation are not separate, but are interconnected. In fact, factors generated in the extrinsic pathway will activate factors and complexes of the intrinsic pathway. Physiologically, the clotting inside the vessel begins through the extrinsic and not the intrinsic pathway. Then, tissue factor (TF), which is normally expressed on the membrane of fibroblasts and exposed to coagulation factors in response to endothelial damage, activates the coagulation cascade in vivo. TF has affinity for factor VII, leading to the formation of the TF–activated factor VII complex, which activates factor X (extrinsic pathway) or factor IX (intrinsic pathway). The distinction between the two pathways of coagulation activation is still in use but it is important to underline that there are mechanisms of cross-over among the two. The two pathways converge at the final stage, that is, the activation of factor X (common pathway), leading to the transformation of fibrinogen to fibrin.

There are many diseases that can result from abnormalities of one or more of the three compartments. Among these we consider the inherited deficiencies of coagulation factors.

5.2 Congenital Coagulation Defects

5.2.1 Hemophilia

Hemophilia is a group of hereditary genetic disorders that impair the body's ability to control blood clotting or coagulation.

Hemophilia A is the second most common genetic disorder associated with serious bleeding, second only to von Willebrand disease. It is inherited, as an X-linked recessive trait, and thus occurs in males and in homozygous females. However, mild hemophilia A has been described in heterozygous females, presumably owing to extremely unfavorable lyonization (inactivation of the normal X chromosome in most of the cells). The annual incidence of hemophilia A has been estimated at approximately one in 5,000 male births [8, 9].

It is caused by a reduction in the amount or activity of factor VIII: this protein serves as a cofactor for factor IX in the activation of factor X in the coagulation cascade. This disorder results in the formation of fibrin-deficient clots, which makes coagulation much more prolonged, and the clot more unstable. It is classified into three groups:

1. Severe hemophilia: concentration of factor VIII/factor IX below 0.01 IU/ml
2. Moderate hemophilia: concentration of factor VIII/factor IX 0.01–0.05 IU/ml (2–5% of normal activity)
3. Mild hemophilia: concentration of factor VIII/factor IX 0.05–0.4 IU/ml (5–40% of normal activity)

Diagnosis:

- Increased activated partial thromboplastin time (aPTT)

- Normal prothrombin time
- Reduction of activity of factor VIII or factor IX

The one-stage aPTT method is most commonly used because of its reproducibility, simplicity, and low cost. Other laboratory techniques for determination of factor VIII are chromogenic and Nijmegen methods [10]. The values determined by the chromogenic substrate are approximately twice as high as those determined by the one-stage aPTT method [11].

The Nijmegen method [10], a modification of the Bethesda assay, has been recommended as the standard assay by the International Society on Thrombosis and Hemostasis Factor VIII/IX Scientific Subcommittee. This is the recommended method for diagnosis of inhibitors [12]. The result is expressed in Bethesda units (BU) [13]. On the basis of the results of the inhibitor assay, a value less than 5 BU is considered to correspond to a low-titer inhibitor. If the inhibitor titer fails to rise despite repeated challenges with the factor, the patient is termed a low responder. In contrast, a patient in whom the inhibitor titer is greater than 5 BU is considered a high responder [14]. The method has recently been reviewed [15].

Hemophilia B is a blood clotting disorder caused by a mutation of the factor IX gene, leading to a deficiency of factor IX. It is the second most common form of hemophilia, and is rarer than hemophilia A. It is sometimes called Christmas disease after Stephen Christmas, the first patient described as having this disease [16, 17]. It occurs in about one in about 20,000–34,000 male births [18].

Three degrees of clinical severity correspond to the level of plasma coagulant factor activity:

1. Levels less than 1% of normal: severe hemophilia characterized by frequent spontaneous bleeding into joints and soft tissues as well as prolonged bleeding with trauma or surgery.
2. Levels between 1 and 5% of normal level: moderate course characterized by occasional spontaneous bleeding with trauma or surgery.
3. Levels greater than 5% of normal seem to protect against spontaneous bleeding.

The laboratory diagnosis for inhibitors in hemophilia B involves a modification of the Bethesda assay in which plasma deficient in factor IX is used instead of plasma deficient in factor VIII [19].

5.2.2 Von Willebrand Disease

Von Willebrand disease is an inherited hemorrhagic disorder caused by a deficiency or dysfunction of von Willebrand factor, a large adhesive glycoprotein found in plasma, platelets, and endothelial cells. As a result, the interaction of platelets with the vessel wall is defective, and primary hemostasis is impaired. Three major von Willebrand disease types are recognized: type 1 refers to partial quantitative deficiency, type 2 includes qualitative defects, and type 3 refers to virtually complete absence [20]. It affects 35–100 individuals per million individuals (0.0035–0.01%), which is comparable to the prevalence of hemophilia A [21].

5 Inborn Defects of the Coagulative System 77

The *VWF* gene is on human chromosome 12 [22, 23], and von Willebrand disease usually exhibits an autosomal pattern of codominant inheritance: one mutant allele may cause disease (although penetrance and expressivity can be variable), and two mutant alleles usually cause severer disease. Only homozygotes or compound heterozygotes have symptoms.

A typical screening laboratory evaluation for von Willebrand disease, in selected patients, includes assays of plasma von Willebrand factor mediated platelet function, von Willebrand factor antigen level, and factor VIII level [24].

5.2.3 Inherited Thrombophilias

A thrombophilia is defined as a disorder of hemostasis that predisposes a person to both venous and arterial thromboembolic events [25].

Inherited thrombophilias result from deficiencies of components of the coagulation system. They are associated with venous thromboembolism and adverse pregnancy outcomes. Included in the category of inherited thrombophilias are:

1. *Factor V Leiden.* The Leiden mutation is a single-nucleotide substitution in the factor V gene at nucleotide 1691 (G to A) that causes an amino acid substitution (glutamine for arginine) at position 506 in the factor V molecule. In normal clotting, activated protein C inactivates activated factor V and activated factor VIII by cleavage at specific sites. In the presence of the mutation of factor V, the cleavage of this factor is inhibited, leading to enhanced thrombin generation and increased clot formation. The inheritance of the mutation is autosomal dominant. The frequency of the factor V Leiden mutation in whites is 3–8%, and one in 1,000 are homozygous. The factor V Leiden mutation is rare in African-Americans, Asians, and Native Americans. Most patients who are resistant to activated protein C will be heterozygous for factor V Leiden. Acquired activated protein C resistance can be found in pregnancy, with the use of oral contraceptives, and in the presence of antiphospholipid antibodies. The heterozygous condition is associated with a sevenfold increased lifetime risk of thrombosis, whereas the homozygous condition increases the lifetime risk 50-fold to 100-fold. Because the condition is so common, 20–50% of patients diagnosed with a venous thrombosis will have the heterozygous factor V Leiden. Laboratory screening should begin with a test for resistance to activated protein C. If the ratio is less than 2.0, mutation testing for factor V Leiden should follow, with appropriate counseling. Patients should be advised of the increased lifetime risks, counseled to correct any secondary hypercoagulable factors, and advised to have parents, siblings, and perhaps children tested [26].

2. *Prothrombin gene (G20210A) mutation.* In 1996, an additional factor involved in the cause of thrombophilia was discovered: a point mutation, $G{\rightarrow}A$ at nucleotide position 20210 in the $3'$ untranslated region of the prothrombin gene. This mutation is associated with higher plasma prothrombin concentrations, augmented thrombin generation, and increased risk of venous and arterial thrombotic disease. The increased levels of prothrombin are secondary to more

efficient translation or to greater stability of the messenger RNA. Heterozygosity for the mutation is present in 2–3% of the white population. In patients presenting with deep vein thrombosis, approximately 6–18% are positive for the G20210A polymorphism [27].

Polymerase chain reaction methods have been used to detect the G20210A prothrombin gene mutation in genomic DNA [28, 29]. Prothrombin gene mutation is associated with elevated plasma levels of prothrombin, but it should not be used for screening [28–30].

3. *Antithrombin deficiency.* Antithrombin (previously called antithrombin III) is a serine protease inhibitor produced by the liver with naturally occurring anticoagulant properties. It is the major physiologic inhibitor of the coagulation system and inactivates thrombin as well as activated factors IX, X, and XI. Heparin binds to antithrombin and greatly accelerates its activity. Heparin-like molecules in the vessel wall and endothelial cells increase the rate of the antithrombin reaction. Two basic types of antithrombin deficiency have been recognized. Type I deficiencies are quantitative, with decreased levels of antigen and decreased function. These deficiencies are secondary to impaired synthesis, defective secretion, or unstable antithrombin. Type I deficiencies are caused by major gene deletions, nucleotide changes, insertions, or deletions. Type II antithrombin defects are qualitative deficiencies with normal antigen levels but decreased function. These deficiencies are secondary to abnormalities of protease inhibitory activity or abnormalities of the heparin binding site, or both. Type II deficiencies are caused by point mutations with single amino acid changes leading to a dysfunctional protein. More than 80 different mutations have been identified for type I and type II antithrombin deficiency. Acquired deficiencies of antithrombin can be identified in women taking combination oral contraceptives. Other common acquired deficiency states include surgery, liver disease, inflammatory bowel disease, and infection. Clinically, all forms of antithrombin deficiency will have decreased functional test values [26]. The antithrombin deficiency is inherited in an autosomal dominant fashion. Normal plasma activity is 80–120% of normal. Most individuals are heterozygous, with antithrombin levels of 40–60% of normal. The prevalence of heterozygous carriers is estimated at one in 2,000 to one in 5,000 [31]. Type II defects with deficiencies in the heparin-binding function occur in three in 1,000 individuals. It is present in 1% of patients with venous thromboembolism and is the most thrombogenic of the inherited thrombophilias, with a 20–50% lifetime risk of thrombosis [32].

4. *Hyperhomocysteinemia.* Hyperhomocysteinemia can be seen with deficiencies in vitamins B_6 and B_{12}, folic acid, and methylenehydrofolate reductase (MTHFR). Normal circulating plasma levels of homocysteine range from 5 to 16 mmol/l.

Hyperhomocysteinemia can be diagnosed with fasting homocysteine levels and can further be classified as severe (above 100 mmol/l), moderate (25–100 mmol/l), and mild (16–24 mmol/l) [33]. MTHFR can be a cause of mild to severe hyperhomocysteinemia. Frosst et al. [34] explained the

5 Inborn Defects of the Coagulative System

thermolability of MTHFR and how the mechanism was caused by a cytosine to thymine substitution at base pair 677 in the MTHFR gene [35]. Homozygosity for MTHFR is a relatively common cause of mildly elevated plasma homocysteine levels in the general population, often occurring in association with low serum folate levels.

5. *Protein C.* Protein C is a vitamin K dependent serine protease inhibitor synthesized in the liver. Protein C binds to the endothelial cell-surface protein thrombomodulin, is activated by binding to free protein S, and is converted to an active protease by thrombin [36]. Protein C downregulates the coagulation cascade by proteolysis of activated factor V and activated factor VIII. Deficiencies of protein C lead to unregulated fibrin formation secondary to impaired inactivation of activated factors V and VIII. Activated protein C may also stimulate fibrinolysis and accelerate clot lysis. Protein C deficiency is inherited in an autosomal dominant fashion. The gene for protein C is located on chromosome 2 (2q13–14) [37, 38]. More than 160 different mutations have been identified; missense and nonsense mutations are the most common. Two phenotypes of deficiency are recognized. Type I deficiency is the more common and is associated with decreased antigen levels secondary to reduced synthesis or stability of the protein. Activity of protein C is low because of decreased protein. Type II deficiency is characterized by normal antigen levels, but because the protein is defective in some way, function of the protein is low. Thus, clinical screening for protein C deficiency should begin with functional tests. The prevalence of protein C deficiency in the general population is 0.15–0.8%, and is 2.7–4.6% in patients with a history of venous thromboembolism. Normal protein C activity is between 60 and 180% of normal. Deficiency is certain if the protein C level is repeatedly below 55% of normal [36].

6. *Protein S.* Protein S is a vitamin K dependent serine protease inhibitor synthesized in hepatocytes, endothelial cells, megakaryocytes, and in the cells of the human kidney, brain, and testes. Protein S is the principal cofactor of activated protein C, and deficiency states mimic protein C deficiency with increased fibrin formation. Protein S can also bind directly to and inhibit activated factors V, VIII, and X. Protein S exists in two distinct forms in plasma. The free form accounts for 35–40% of total protein S, whereas the remainder is found in a form bound to C4b binding protein. Only the free protein S can serve as a cofactor for protein C. Protein S deficiency is inherited in the autosomal dominant fashion and is identified in 0.1–0.2% of the general population [26]. The gene for protein S is located on chromosome 3 [39, 40]. It is the causative factor in 2–3% of patients with venous thromboembolism. Three types of protein S deficiency have been reported. The most common type I deficiency is associated with a reduction in the level of normal protein S antigen, resulting in lower free protein S level and decreased activity. The uncommon type II deficiency is characterized by low activity but normal free and total protein S levels. Type III deficiency is characterized by a low free protein S level with normal antigen levels but reduced activity. Thus, clinical screening for protein S deficiency should begin with functional tests [26].

5.2.4 Rare Coagulation Factor Deficiencies

Inherited deficiencies of blood clotting proteins distinct from those involved in hemophilia A and hemophilia B are rare, and the clinical presentations, diagnostic options, and treatments differ from those for deficiencies of factor VIII and factor IX. The rare disorders include:

- Deficiencies of fibrinogen
- The plasma protease zymogens prothrombin, factors VII, X, XI, and XII, and prekallikrein
- The cofactors factor V and high molecular weight kininogen.
- The transaminase factor XIII

5.3 Perioperative Changes in Coagulation

Trauma and surgical patients have various degrees of vascular injury and exsanguinations. Massive hemorrhage results in progressive dilution of coagulation factors to 30% of normal after a loss of one blood volume and down to 15% after a loss of two blood volumes. (The calculation of blood volume is based on the Nadler method, which determines the total blood volume in a person on the basis of gender, height, and weight. The average adult body contains between 5.2 and 6 l of blood [41, 42]). In the presence of severe hemodilution, the initiation of thrombin generation is delayed by reduced factor VII, and the propagation is reduced by the gross reduction of procoagulatant serine protease zymogens and accelerators. The efficiency of thrombin generation is further reduced by decreased platelet count, which decreases to 50×10^3 mm^{-3} over the loss of two blood volumes [41].

Prothrombin time and aPTT also indicate a "hypocoagulable state" as they approach more than 1.5 times the normal level. The levels of two important thrombin substrates, fibrinogen and factor XIII, also decrease rapidly during hemodilution; fibrinogen concentration decreases to 100 mg/dl after a loss of 142% of blood volume.

Reduced thrombin generation, a low level of fibrinogen, and low activated factor XIII activity render fibrin clots susceptible to tissue plasminogen activator induced fibrinolysis. Unstable fibrin clot formation because of low levels of fibrinogen and/or factor XIII results in profuse bleeding, but may also represent a problem in localizing procoagulant activity. Polymerized fibrin seems to have a role in containing excess thrombin and activated factor X molecules inside the thrombus [43]. In fact, antithrombin I, which was originally described as an anticoagulant protein, turned out to be fibrin [44]. In severe hemodilution, the levels of anticoagulant proteins, including TF tissue factor pathway inhibitor, antithrombin, protein C, protein S, and endothelium-bound thrombomodulin, are progressively decreased [45, 46]. Thus, thrombin's procoagulant and proinflammatory activities may not be quickly suppressed after thrombin is released (from weak clots at the injury site) into the circulation. The deficiency in either fibrinogen or factor XIII seems to be associated with elevated levels of plasma markers of thrombin generation [44–47]. Current hemostatic therapies for postoperative bleeding consist of allogeneic fresh frozen plasma, cryoprecipitate, and platelet concentrates [48].

More recently, plasma-derived factor concentrates, such as fibrinogen, factor XIII, and recombinant activated factor VII, have been increasingly used in postoperative patients in a empirical manner [49–51]. These components may allow rapid restoration of specific elements of coagulation without the need for a cross-match, while avoiding intravascular volume overload. In addition, the risk of infectious transmission is decreased because they are pasteurized against currently known viruses. However, additional studies are required to prove their safety in the perioperative setting because surgical patients demonstrate multiple deficiencies in procoagulant and anticoagulant proteins [52, 53]. Decreased levels of coagulation factors and inhibitors recover to normal levels after surgery over the course of several days. Acute inflammatory responses associated with vascular injury and wound healing often result in cytokine, platelet count, fibrinogen, von Willebrand factor–factor VIII, and plasminogen activator inhibitor 1 levels over the normal limit [54, 55]. The syntheses of TF pathway inhibitor and antithrombin are not increased, and endothelial thrombomodulin expression is decreased by inflammatory cytokines (e.g., tumor necrosis factor, interleukin-1β). The imbalance of procoagulant and anticoagulant elements may increase the risk of prothrombotic complications in the postoperative period. Prophylactic use of antithrombotic therapy should be considered on the basis of the type of surgery, hematological history, and other patient characteristics (e.g., age, obesity) [56].

References

1. Davie EW (2003) A brief historical review of the waterfall/cascade of blood coagulation. J Biol Chem 278(51):50819–50832
2. Hoffman M, Monroe DM 3rd (2001) A cell-based model of hemostasis. Thromb Haemost 85(6):958–965
3. Patthy L (1985) Evolution of the proteases of blood coagulation and fibrinolysis by assembly from modules. Cell 41(3):657–663
4. Lindqvist PG, Svensson PJ, Dahlback B, Marsal K (1998) Factor V Q506 mutation (activated protein C resistance) associated with reduced intrapartum blood loss–a possible evolutionary selection mechanism. Thromb Haemost 79(1):69–73
5. Krem MM, Di Cera E (2001) Molecular markers of serine protease evolution. EMBO J 20(12):3036–3045
6. Davidson CJ, Tuddenham EG, McVey JH (2003) 450 million years of hemostasis. J Thromb Haemost 1(7):1487–1494
7. Theopold U, Schmidt O, Soderhall K, Dushay MS (2004) Coagulation in arthropods: defence, wound closure and healing. Trends Immunol 25(6):289–294
8. Kar A, Potnis-Lele M (2001) Descriptive epidemiology of haemophilia in Maharashtra, India. Haemophilia 7(6):561–567
9. Fukutake K (2000) Current status of hemophilia patients and recombinant coagulation factor concentrates in Japan. Semin Thromb Hemost 26(1):29–32

10. Verbruggen B, Novakova I, Wessels H, Boezeman J, van den Berg M, Mauser-Bunschoten E (1995) The Nijmegen modification of the Bethesda assay for factor VIII:C inhibitors: improved specificity and reliability. Thromb Haemost 73(2):247–251
11. Kasper CK, Aronson DL, Davignon G, Foster P, Hillman-Wiseman C, Lusher JM et al (1995) Comparison of six commercial plasma references for factor VIII, factor IX and von Willebrand factor. On behalf of the Subcommittee for Factor VIII and IX of the Scientific and Standardization Committee of the ISTH. Thromb Haemost 74(3):987–989
12. Giles AR, Verbruggen B, Rivard GE, Teitel J, Walker I (1998) A detailed comparison of the performance of the standard versus the Nijmegen modification of the Bethesda assay in detecting factor VIII:C inhibitors in the haemophilia A population of Canada. Association of Hemophilia Centre Directors of Canada. Factor VIII/IX Subcommittee of Scientific and Standardization Committee of International Society on Thrombosis and Haemostasis. Thromb Haemost 79(4):872–875
13. Kasper CK, Aledort L, Aronson D, Counts R, Edson JR, van Eys J et al (1975) Proceedings: A more uniform measurement of factor VIII inhibitors. Thromb Diath Haemorrh 34(2):612
14. White GC, Rosendaal F, Aledort LM, Lusher JM, Rothschild C, Ingerslev J (2001) Definitions in hemophilia. Recommendation of the Scientific Subcommittee on factor VIII and factor IX of the Scientific and Standardization committee of the International Society on Thrombosis and Haemostasis. Thromb Haemost 85(3):560
15. Verbruggen B, van Heerde WL, Laros-van Gorkom BA (2009) Improvements in factor VIII inhibitor detection: From Bethesda to Nijmegen. Semin Thromb Hemost 35(8):752–759
16. Biggs R, Douglas AS, Macfarlane RG, Dacie JV, Pitney WR (1952) Merskey. Christmas disease: a condition previously mistaken for haemophilia. Br Med J 2(4799):1378–1382
17. Aggeler PM, White SG, Glendening MB, Page EW, Leake TB, Bates G (1952) Plasma thromboplastin component (PTC) deficiency; a new disease resembling hemophilia. Proc Soc Exp Biol Med 79(4):692–694
18. Giannelli F, Green PM, Sommer SS, Poon M, Ludwig M, Schwaab R et al (1998) Haemophilia B: database of point mutations and short additions and deletions–eighth edition. Nucleic Acids Res 26(1):265–268
19. Hay CR, Baglin TP, Collins PW, Hill FG, Keeling DM (2000) The diagnosis and management of factor VIII and IX inhibitors: a guideline from the UK Haemophilia Centre Doctors' Organization (UKHCDO). Br J Haematol 111(1):78–90
20. Sadler JE, Budde U, Eikenboom JC, Favaloro EJ, Hill FG, Holmberg L et al (2006) Update on the pathophysiology and classification of von Willebrand disease: a report of the Subcommittee on von Willebrand Factor. J Thromb Haemost 4(10):2103–2114
21. Sadler JE, Mannucci PM, Berntorp E, Bochkov N, Boulyjenkov V, Ginsburg D et al (2000) Impact, diagnosis and treatment of von Willebrand disease. Thromb Haemost 84(2):160–174
22. Ginsburg D, Handin RI, Bonthron DT, Donlon TA, Bruns GA, Latt SA et al (1985) Human von Willebrand factor (vWF): isolation of complementary DNA (cDNA) clones and chromosomal localization. Science 228(4706):1401–1406
23. Verweij CL, de Vries CJ, Distel B, van Zonneveld AJ, van Kessel AG, van Mourik JA et al (1985) Construction of cDNA coding for human von Willebrand factor using antibody probes for colony-screening and mapping of the chromosomal gene. Nucleic Acids Res 13(13):4699–4717
24. Mannucci PM, Lombardi R, Bader R, Vianello L, Federici AB, Solinas S et al (1985) Heterogeneity of type I von Willebrand disease: evidence for a subgroup with an abnormal von Willebrand factor. Blood 66(4):796–802
25. Haemostasis and Thrombosis Task Force BCfSiH (2001) Investigation and management of heritable thrombophilia. Br J Haematol 114(3):512–528
26. Kutteh WH, Triplett DA (2006) Thrombophilias and recurrent pregnancy loss. Semin Reprod Med 24(1):54–66

5 Inborn Defects of the Coagulative System 83

27. Poort SR, Rosendaal FR, Reitsma PH, Bertina RM (1996) A common genetic variation in the 3′-untranslated region of the prothrombin gene is associated with elevated plasma prothrombin levels and an increase in venous thrombosis. Blood 88(10):3698–3703
28. Gerhardt A, Scharf RE, Beckmann MW, Struve S, Bender HG, Pillny M et al (2000) Prothrombin and factor V mutations in women with a history of thrombosis during pregnancy and the puerperium. N Engl J Med 342(6):374–380
29. Poort SR, Rosendaal FR, Reitsma PH, Bertina RM (1996) A common genetic variation in the 3′-untranslated region of the prothrombin gene is associated with elevated plasma prothrombin levels and an increase in venous thrombosis. Blood 88(10):3698–3703
30. Kierkegaard A (1983) Incidence and diagnosis of deep vein thrombosis associated with pregnancy. Acta Obstet Gynecol Scand 62(3):239–243
31. Tait RC, Walker ID, Perry DJ, Islam SI, Daly ME, McCall F et al (1994) Prevalence of antithrombin deficiency in the healthy population. Br J Haematol 87(1):106–112
32. Adelberg AM, Kuller JA (2002) Thrombophilias and recurrent miscarriage. Obstet Gynecol Surv 57(10):703–709
33. Lockwood CJ (2002) Inherited thrombophilias in pregnant patients: detection and treatment paradigm. Obstet Gynecol 99(2):333–341
34. Frosst P, Blom HJ, Milos R, Goyette P, Sheppard CA, Matthews RG et al (1995) A candidate genetic risk factor for vascular disease: a common mutation in methylenetetrahydrofolate reductase. Nat Genet 10(1):111–113
35. Morelli VM, Lourenco DM, D'Almeida V, Franco RF, Miranda F, Zago MA et al (2002) Hyperhomocysteinemia increases the risk of venous thrombosis independent of the C677T mutation of the methylenetetrahydrofolate reductase gene in selected Brazilian patients. Blood Coagul Fibrinolysis 13(3):271–275
36. Miletich J, Sherman L, Broze G Jr (1987) Absence of thrombosis in subjects with heterozygous protein C deficiency. N Engl J Med 317(16):991–996
37. Foster DC, Yoshitake S, Davie EW (1985) The nucleotide sequence of the gene for human protein C. Proc Natl Acad Sci U S A 82(14):4673–4677
38. Plutzky J, Hoskins JA, Long GL, Crabtree GR (1986) Evolution and organization of the human protein C gene. Proc Natl Acad Sci U S A 83(3):546–550
39. Ploos van Amstel JK, van der Zanden AL, Bakker E, Reitsma PH, Bertina RM (1987) Two genes homologous with human protein S cDNA are located on chromosome 3. Thromb Haemost 58(4):982–987
40. Schmidel DK, Tatro AV, Phelps LG, Tomczak JA, Long GL (1990) Organization of the human protein S genes. Biochemistry 29(34):7845–7852
41. Hiippala ST, Myllyla GJ, Vahtera EM (1995) Hemostatic factors and replacement of major blood loss with plasma-poor red cell concentrates. Anesth Analg 81(2):360–365
42. Stainsby D, MacLennan S, Hamilton PJ (2000) Management of massive blood loss: a template guideline. Br J Anaesth 85(3):487–491
43. Hathcock JJ, Nemerson Y (2004) Platelet deposition inhibits tissue factor activity: in vitro clots are impermeable to factor Xa. Blood 104(1):123–127
44. Mosesson MW (2007) Update on antithrombin I (fibrin). Thromb Haemost 98(1):105–108
45. Brohi K, Cohen MJ, Ganter MT, Matthay MA, Mackersie RC, Pittet JF (2007) Acute traumatic coagulopathy: initiated by hypoperfusion: modulated through the protein C pathway? Ann Surg 245(5):812–818
46. Sniecinski RM, Chen EP, Tanaka KA (2008) Reduced levels of fibrin (antithrombin I) and antithrombin III underlie coagulopathy following complex cardiac surgery. Blood Coagul Fibrinolysis 19(2):178–179
47. Wettstein P, Haeberli A, Stutz M, Rohner M, Corbetta C, Gabi K et al (2004) Decreased factor XIII availability for thrombin and early loss of clot firmness in patients with unexplained intraoperative bleeding. Anesth Analg 99(5):1564–1569
48. Levy JH, Tanaka KA (2008) Prohemostatic agents to prevent perioperative blood loss. Semin Thromb Hemost 34(5):439–444

49. Heindl B, Delorenzo C, Spannagl M (2005) High dose fibrinogen administration for acute therapy of coagulopathy during massive perioperative transfusion. Anaesthesist 54(8):787–790

50. Godje O, Haushofer M, Lamm P, Reichart B (1998) The effect of factor XIII on bleeding in coronary surgery. Thorac Cardiovasc Surg 46(5):263–267

51. Levy JH, Fingerhut A, Brott T, Langbakke IH, Erhardtsen E, Porte RJ (2006) Recombinant factor VIIa in patients with coagulopathy secondary to anticoagulant therapy, cirrhosis, or severe traumatic injury: review of safety profile. Transfusion 46(6):919–933

52. O'Connell KA, Wood JJ, Wise RP, Lozier JN, Braun MM (2006) Thromboembolic adverse events after use of recombinant human coagulation factor VIIa. JAMA 295(3):293–298

53. Sniecinski R, Szlam F, Chen EP, Bader SO, Levy JH, Tanaka KA (2008) Antithrombin deficiency increases thrombin activity after prolonged cardiopulmonary bypass. Anesth Analg 106(3):713–718, table of contents

54. Lo B, Fijnheer R, Castigliego D, Borst C, Kalkman CJ, Nierich AP (2004) Activation of hemostasis after coronary artery bypass grafting with or without cardiopulmonary bypass. Anesth Analg 99(3):634–640

55. Parolari A, Mussoni L, Frigerio M, Naliato M, Alamanni F, Polvani GL et al (2005) The role of tissue factor and P-selectin in the procoagulant response that occurs in the first month after on-pump and off-pump coronary artery bypass grafting. J Thorac Cardiovasc Surg 130(6):1561–1566

56. Douketis JD, Berger PB, Dunn AS, Jaffer AK, Spyropoulos AC, Becker RC et al (2008) The perioperative management of antithrombotic therapy: American College of Chest Physicians Evidence-Based Clinical Practice Guidelines (8th edition). Chest 133(Suppl 6):299S–339S

Inflammation and Coagulation

6

Walter Vessella, Lara Prisco and Giorgio Berlot

6.1 Introduction

In critically ill patients, the activation of blood coagulation occurs in parallel with the release of inflammatory mediators, which characterizes systemic inflammatory response syndrome (SIRS) and sepsis and sepsis-related conditions such as severe sepsis and septic shock. As a consequence, the overall hemostatic balance is shifted toward the activation of the coagulation, due to either the activation of the clotting system or the downregulation of the anticoagulant pathways [1, 2].

The inflammatory reaction interacts with the coagulation at different levels, including the elevation of blood fibrinogen levels and the induction of tissue factor (TF) expression on the cell surface of leukocytes. Thrombin can thus promote coagulation, anticoagulation, cell proliferation, and inflammation by triggering some of the responses summarized in Fig. 6.1 [2, 3].

6.2 Coagulation Disturbances in Sepsis

Systemic inflammation during sepsis leads to the generation of proinflammatory cytokines that, among other things, orchestrate coagulation and fibrinolytic activation. Both coagulation activation and downregulation of fibrinolysis are principally regulated by tumor necrosis factor α (TNF-α), interleukin (IL)-1, and IL-6. Moreover, TNF-α influences coagulation activation via the action of IL-6. The cornerstone of the coagulation disorder in sepsis constitutes the imbalance between intravascular fibrin formation and fibrin removal. Severely reduced

---

W. Vessella (✉)
Anesthesia and Intensive Care Unit, Cattinara Hospital,
University of Trieste, Trieste, Italy
e-mail: walter.vessella@libero.it

G. Berlot (ed.), *Hemocoagulative Problems in the Critically Ill Patient*,
DOI: 10.1007/978-88-470-2448-9_6, © Springer-Verlag Italia 2012

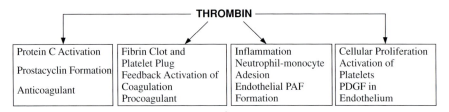

Fig. 6.1 Interaction between coagulation and the inflammatory reaction

anticoagulant capacity and inhibited fibrinolysis are opposed by a massive activation of coagulation, finally leading to overwhelming fibrin formation and consumption of clotting factors and inhibitors as well. Abundant intravascular fibrin formation leads to microvascular thrombosis, which causes widespread ischemic organ damage up to organ necrosis and clinically impresses as widespread skin necrosis and multiple organ dysfunction syndrome [2–4, 5].

Coagulation activation during sepsis is primarily triggered through the Tissue Factor (TF) pathway. In sepsis models, fibrin formation was completely abrogated by blocking this mechanism with anti-TF antibodies and activated factor VII (factor VIIa) inhibiting peptides. Although in a primate model of severe sepsis the contact-phase system was found to be activated, it did not contribute to coagulation activation in sepsis; however, the inhibition of factor XII activation prevented the occurrence of hypotension, indicating that activation of the contact-phase system plays a role for the sepsis-associated hemodynamic changes during sepsis, presumably via the formation of bradykinin [3, 5, 6].

Expression of TF on monocytes and probably on endothelial cells triggers activation of coagulation in sepsis. An additional source of TF might derive from phospholipid fragments originating from activated monocytes, which can be detected in plasma of patients with meningococcal sepsis [5, 7, 8].

After binding to exposed TF, circulating factor VII is activated. The TF/factor VIIa complex then activates factor X to activated factor X (factor Xa), which converts prothrombin to thrombin. These tiny amounts of thrombin formed may activate factor V and factor VIII. Activated factor V (factor Va) enhances the capability of factor Xa to activate prothrombin [7, 9, 10].

However, thrombin generation by the TF/factor VIIa pathway is rapidly abrogated by TF pathway inhibitor, a high-affinity inhibitor of TF/factor VIIa/factor Xa complex present in plasma and on endothelial cells.

However, TF/factor VIIa complex also activates factor IX, which in concert with factor VIIIa takes over the function of TF/factor VIIa to activate factor X, thereby further amplifying the thrombin generation. This amplification of factor X activation by factor IX and factor VIII is important for coagulation in physiologic conditions, as is dramatically demonstrated by the clinical picture of hemophilia A and hemophilia B, which result from deficiency of factor VIII and factor IX, respectively. Thrombin cleaves fibrinogen into fibrin monomers and activates factor XIII, which then covalently cross-links fibrin monomers to form a

6 Inflammation and Coagulation

stable clot. The thrombin generated by the TF/factor VIIa pathway amplified by factor IX and factor VIII in some conditions is still insufficient to overcome fibrinolysis. To surmount this anticoagulant effect of fibrinolysis, activation of a second amplification loop, in addition to that of factor VIII and factor IX, is necessary. This second loop is triggered when the amount of thrombin generated becomes sufficient to activate factor XI, which then generates factor activated factor IX (IXa), which then activates additional factor X, thereby forming additional thrombin. This amplified factor XI dependent thrombin formation will activate thrombin-dependent fibrinolysis inhibitors, which will cleave off binding sites for plasminogen on fibrin, thereby inhibiting fibrinolysis [2, 5, 11, 12].

Although factor IXa/VIIIa and the activated factor XI amplification loop are considered to be important for coagulation activation in sepsis, the evidence for this is scarce. Thrombin is quickly inactivated by antithrombin by forming thrombin–antithrombin complexes, which are rapidly cleared from circulation. Moreover, thrombomodulin (TM) expressed on endothelial cells binds thrombin and abrogates its procoagulant activity.

The thrombin–TM complex activates protein C. Activated protein C rapidly dissociates from the thrombin TM complex and inactivates factor Va and factor VIIIa, thereby decreasing thrombin generation [5, 7, 13].

The function of the activated protein C system is also severely compromised during sepsis. Reduced TM expression on endothelial cells due to inflammatory mediators, such as TNF-α, has been claimed to explain the decreased activated protein C activity. Indeed, expression of TM by the endothelium in purpuric lesions of children with meningococcal sepsis is decreased as compared with expression in control subjects.

Insufficient modulation of thrombin activity by TM and the resulting decreased inactivation of factor VIIIa and factor Va contribute to a severe procoagulant state, which promotes fibrin deposition in the microvasculature.

Thus, together these studies suggest that the reduced activation of protein C in sepsis is due to decreased availability of TM and point to the crucial anticoagulant role of the activated protein C system in the microvasculature. However, this concept is challenged by the observation that infusion of native, plasma-derived protein C in children with severe meningococcal sepsis resulted in the formation of activated protein C in vivo, and in a decrease of D-dimer levels similarly as observed on infusion of recombinant activated protein C in adult patients with sepsis [12, 14, 15].

Sepsis is a clear risk factor for thrombocytopenia in critically ill patients and its severity correlates with the decrease in platelet count. The main factors contributing to thrombocytopenia are (1) the impaired production of platelets, (2) their increased consumption in the tissues, and (3) their sequestration in the spleen. At first glance, the impaired production of platelets from the bone marrow in septic patients, despite high circulating levels of platelet-production-stimulating proinflammatory cytokines and thrombopoietin, might seem contradictory. In a substantial number of patients with sepsis, however, marked hemophagocytosis may occur [16, 17, 18]. This pathological process consists of active phagocytosis of megakaryocytes and other hematopoietic cells by monocytes and macrophages, hypothetically in response to high levels of macrophage colony stimulating factor in sepsis. Platelet consumption probably also plays an important role in patients with sepsis. Thrombin is the most potent activator of platelets in vivo, and intravascular thrombin generation is a ubiquitous event in sepsis with or without evidence of overt disseminated intravascular coagulation (DIC). DIC frequently complicates sepsis. DIC can be found in 25–50% of patients with sepsis and seems to be a strong predictor of mortality. DIC is an acquired syndrome characterized by the activation of intravascular coagulation culminating in intravascular fibrin formation and deposition of fibrin in the microvasculature. Secondary fibrinolysis, or in later stages inhibition of fibrinolysis, accompanies coagulation activation [15, 19].

Although the initial trigger and the dynamics may differ, the clinical picture of severe sepsis or septic shock in latter stages is quite uniform. Fibrin deposition leads to a diffuse obstruction of the microvascular network resulting in progressive organ dysfunction, such as the development of renal insufficiency and acute respiratory distress syndrome, hypotension, and circulatory failure.

Then, it appears that restoration of anticoagulant capacity as well as fibrinolysis might be a promising target for therapy strategies. Since consumption of the biological inhibitors of thrombin may contribute to the formation of thrombin during sepsis, one could speculate that administration of an inhibitor of thrombin formation or a direct inhibitor of the catalytic site of thrombin might be useful in this clinical condition. However, current insights indicate that this view on the efficacy of anticoagulant proteins in sepsis is too simple. The efficacy of clotting inhibitors in sepsis models depends not only on their anticoagulant properties but also on their anti-inflammatory effects [19, 20].

6.3 Clinical Manifestations and Laboratory Investigations

The most common clinical findings in sepsis are related to SIRS (e.g., fever, tachycardia, tachypnea, and leukocytosis) and organ dysfunction (e.g., acute lung injury, acute respiratory distress syndrome, shock). Laboratory markers of the activation of the coagulation cascade are most often manifested by increased D-dimer levels (about 100% patients) and decreased levels of circulating protein C (in more than 90% of patients) [14, 17, 21].

The global coagulation tests which measure the capacity of thrombin generation, such as the prothrombin time and the activated partial thromboplastin time, show prolonged coagulation times because of the decrease of the levels of fibrinogen, prothrombin, and factors II, V, VII, IX, and X as a consequence of consumption and plasmin-induced proteolysis of these factors. Also the reduced platelet count is regarded as an indication for the dysfunction of the hemostatic system. Measurement of antithrombin activity is considered another screening test in patients since its value markedly decline over time owing to consumption [20, 22–24].

6.4 Therapeutic Approach

Based on the pathophysiologic concepts and the striking anticoagulant and anti-inflammatory properties of coagulation inhibitors in models for severe sepsis, administration of these inhibitors has been considered an attractive therapeutic approach for human sepsis. However, despite the sound physiological principles and the indications deriving from preliminary clinical studies, the results of larger trials using these substances have been largely below the expectations, with the exception of recombinant activated human protein C (drotrecogin-α, rh-PAC), which combines anticoagulant and anti-inflammatory properties [25–38]. In the Recombinant Human Activated Protein C Worldwide Evaluation in Severe Sepsis (PROWESS) trial, the administration of this substance was associated with a significant improvement of survival in septic patients (absolute mortality reduction, – 6.1%; relative risk reduction, 19.4%) [29]. Results were so striking that the trial was suspended earlier than expected after the second interim analysis of 1,520 patients, the trial was stopped earlier than expected. Immediately ther after, drotrecogin-alpha was released worldwide, becoming the first drug specifically marketed for the treatment of sepsis.

However, as subsequent trials failed to confirm these initial results and some investigators claimed that the anticipated end of the PROWESS trial constituted an unacceptable bias [30], another large, double-blind, controlled international trial was then launched (PROWESS-SHOCK) in which the administration of the rh-APC was restricted to patients with severe sepsis or septic shock, who were demonstrated to take more advantage from this substance than less sick patients [29, 31]. Since the yet unpublished did not demonstrate any survival difference between treated patients and controls, on October 26, 2011, the manufacturer withdrew the rh-APC from the market, and this substance is no longer available.

6.5 Conclusions

On the basis of many experimental and clinical evidences, one can conclude that inflammation and blood coagulation are intrinsically linked and that sepsis and sepsis-related conditions are associated with the simultaneous activation of both pathways. Despite a number of trials involving several different molecules, the only substance with anticoagulant properties which has been demonstrated to reduce mortality in patients with severe sepsis and septic is drotrecogin-α. However, as confirmatory trials did not confirm the initial beneficial effects on the outcome, recently this substance has been withdrawn.

References

1. Dempfle CE (2004) Coagulopathy of sepsis. Thromb Haemost 91(2):213–224
2. Bone RC, Sibbald WJ, Sprung CL (1992) The ACCP-SCCM consensus conference on sepsis and organ failure. Chest 101(6):1481–1483

3. Esmon CT (2005) The interactions between inflammation and coagulation. Br J Haematol 131(4):417–430
4. McEver RP (2001) Adhesive interactions of leukocytes, platelets, and the vessel wall during hemostasis and inflammation. Thromb Haemost 86(3):746–756
5. Hack CE, Aarden LA, Thijs LG (1997) Role of cytokines in sepsis. Adv Immunol 66:101–195
6. Gando S, Kameue T, Matsuda N, Hayakawa M, Hoshino H, Kato H (2005) Serial changes in neutrophil-endothelial activation markers during the course of sepsis associated with disseminated intravascular coagulation. Thromb Res 116(2):91–100
7. Zeerleder S, Hack CE, Wuillemin WA (2005) Disseminated intravascular coagulation in sepsis. Chest 128(4):2864–2875
8. Levi M, Schultz M (2010) Coagulopathy and platelet disorders in critically ill patients. Minerva Anestesiol 76(10):851–859
9. Aird WC (2003) The hematologic system as a marker of organ dysfunction in sepsis. Mayo Clin Proc 78(7):869–881
10. Aird WC (2003) The role of the endothelium in severe sepsis and multiple organ dysfunction syndrome. Blood 101(10):3765–3777
11. Rocha E, Páramo JA, Montes R, Panizo C (1998) Acute generalized, widespread bleeding, diagnosis and management. Haematologica 83(11):1024–1037
12. Esmon CT, Fukudome K, Mather T, Bode W, Regan LM, Stearns-Kurosawa DJ, Kurosawa S (1999) Inflammation, sepsis, and coagulation. Haematologica 84(3):254–259
13. Gando S, Kameue T, Nanzaki S (1996) Disseminated intravascular coagulation is a frequent complication of systemic inflammatory response syndrome. Thromb Haemost 75:224–228
14. Dellinger RP, Carlet JM, Masur H (2004) Surviving sepsi campaign guidelines for management of severe sepsis and septic shock. Crit Care Med 32:858–873
15. Hack CE (2001) Fibrinolysis in disseminated intravascular coagulation. Semin Thromb Haemost 27:633–638
16. Gando S, Nanzaki S, Kemmotsu O (1999) Disseminated intravascular coagulation and sustained systemic inflammatory response syndrome predict organ dysfunctions after trauma: application of clinical decision analysis. Ann Surg 229:121–127
17. Taylor FB Jr, Toh CH, Hoots WK (2001) Towards definition, clinical and laboratory criteria, and a scoring system for disseminated intravascular coagulation. Thromb Haemost 86:1327–1330
18. Ten Cate H, Timmerman JJ, Levi M (1999) The pathophysiology of disseminated intravascular coagulation. Thromb Haemost 82:713–717
19. Welty-Wolf KE, Carraway MS, Miller DL, Ortel TL, Ezban M, Ghio AJ, Idell S, Piantadosi CA (2001) Coagulation blockade prevents sepsis-induced respiratory and renal failure in baboons. Crit Care Med 164(10 Pt 1):1988–1996
20. Bick RL (1996) Disseminated intravascular coagulation: objective clinical and laboratory diagnosis, treatment, and assessment of therapeutic response. Semin Thromb Haemostas 22:69–88
21. Eisele B, Lamy M, Thijs LG (1998) Antithrombin III in patients with severe sepsis: a randomized, placebo-controlled, double-blind multicenter trial plus meta-analysis on all randomized, placebo-controlled, double-blind trials with antithrombin III in severe sepsis. Intensive Care Med 24:663–672
22. Siegal T, Seligsohn V, Aghal E, Modan M (1978) Clinical and laboratory aspects of disseminated intravascular coagulation (DIC): a study of 118 cases. Thromb Haemostas 39:122–134
23. Hartl WH (1998) Effect of antithrombin III supplementation on inflammatory response in patients with severe sepsis. Shock 10:90–96
24. Baudo F, Caimi TM, de Cataldo F (1998) Antithrombin III (ATIII) replacement therapy in patients with sepsis and/or postsurgical complications: a controlled double-blind, randomized, multicenter study. Intensive Care Med 24:336–342

6 Inflammation and Coagulation 91

25. Bernard GR, Ely EW, Wright TJ, Fraiz J, Stasek JE Jr, Russell JA, Mayers I, Rosenfeld BA, Morris PE, Yan SB, Helterbrand JD (2001) Safety and dose relationship of recombinant human activated protein C for coagulopathy in severe sepsis. Crit Care Med 29(11): 2051–2059

26. Ely EW, Angus DC, Williams MD, Bates B, Qualy R, Bernard GR (2003) Drotrecogin alfa (activated) treatment of older patients with severe sepsis. Crit Care Med 37(2):187–195

27. Laterre PF, Levy H, Clermont G, Ball DE, Garg R, Nelson DR, Dhainaut JF, Angus DC (2004) Hospital mortality and resource use in subgroups of the recombinant human activated protein C worldwide evaluation in severe sepsis (PROWESS) trial. Crit Care Med 32(11): 2207–2218

28. Wheeler A, Steingrub J, Schmidt GA, Sanchez P, Jacobi J, Linde-Zwirble W, Bates B, Qualy RL, Woodward B, Zeckel M (2008) A retrospective observational study of drotrecogin alfa (activated) in adults with severe sepsis: comparison with a controlled clinical trial. Crit Care Med 36(1):14–23

29. Bernard GR, Vincent JL, Laterre PF (2001) Efficacy and safety of recombinant human activated protein C for severe sepsis. N Engl J Med 344:699–709

30. Angus DA (2012) Drotrecogin alpha activated...a sad final fizzle to a roller-coaster party. Crit care 2012 16:107–109

31. Abraham E, Laterre PF, Garg R et al (2005) Drotrecogin alpha (activated) for adults with severe sepsis and low risk of death. New Engl J Med 353:1332–1341

Disseminated Intravascular Coagulation

7

Antonino Gullo, Chiara Maria Celestre and Annalaura Paratore

7.1 Introduction and Definition

Disseminated intravascular coagulation (DIC) is an acquired clinical syndrome characterized by abnormally increased activation of procoagulant pathways. This condition results in intravascular fibrin deposition and decreased levels of hemostatic components, including platelets, fibrinogen, and other clotting factors. DIC may be considered a synonym of consumption coagulopathy; in fact, the syndrome is characterized by pathological dysregulation of the hemostatic and fibrinolytic processes as a consequence of systemic activation of coagulation and fibrinolysis [1].

The coagulation pathway is a physiological response to injury; the development of DIC is a warning signal to the clinician that the primary pathological disease state is decompensating. The extreme form of coagulation activation may complicate a myriad of clinical situations characterized by some form of local or systemic inflammation [2]. Intravascular activation of coagulation, inadequately balanced by physiologic anticoagulant systems and aggravated by impaired endogenous fibrinolysis, may contribute to (micro)vascular fibrin deposition, leading to a disseminated vascular thrombosis.

DIC is a relatively common complication of several underlying conditions, in patients suffering from trauma, sepsis, obstetric calamities, and certain malignancies [3, 4]. The incidence is the same in males and females and occurs at any age; however, no age and race predisposition is known. Morbidity and mortality depend on both the underlying diseases and the severity of coagulopathy.

A. Gullo (✉)
Department of Anesthesia and Intensive Care, Medical School,
"Policlinico" University Hospital, Catania, Italy
e-mail: a.gullo@policlinico.unict.it

G. Berlot (ed.), *Hemocoagulative Problems in the Critically Ill Patient*,
DOI: 10.1007/978-88-470-2448-9_7, © Springer-Verlag Italia 2012

7.2 Pathogenesis of DIC

Several attempts have been made to establish in experimental and clinical settings mechanisms of coagulation useful to understand the evolution of DIC. DIC is a consequence of simultaneous activation of thrombotic and hemorrhagic processes.

Regardless of the type of underlying disease or mechanism, initiation of DIC is caused by enhanced fibrin formation and deposition leading to a spectrum of organ dysfunction failure. The anticoagulant and fibrinolytic systems are simultaneously or consequently depleted or inactivated, by downregulation of thrombomodulin and release of plasminogen activator inhibitor 1 by cytokines. Although chronic DIC can be asymptomatic, acute DIC results in bleeding and intravascular thrombic formation, severe hypoxia, and cellular death. The excess production of thrombin is central to the process of DIC. In addition to the conversion of fibrinogen to fibrin, thrombin has several other effects associated with the coagulation cascade. Thrombin contributes to the activation of factors V, VIII, and XIII (fibrin-stabilizing factor) by a mechanism of an activating effect on platelets. Modulation of anticoagulant molecules is related to a thrombin-dependent mechanism. This element includes generation of activated protein C and protein S and the activation of tissue-type plasminogen activator with subsequent inhibition of activated factors V and VIII, plasminogen activator inhibitor 1, and thrombin-activated fibrinolysis inhibitor [5]. The pathophysiological processes of inflammation and microparticles are not fully understood. Microparticles represent small phospholipid-expressing procoagulant vesicular fragments, released by cellular disruption and apoptosis [6]. They are upregulated and may mediate the hemostatic activation and inflammatory responses. Monocyte and neutrophil activation follow microvascular alteration and deformation of blood components and vessel structure [7].

7.3 Clinical Conditions Associated with DIC

There are various and heterogeneous clinical conditions associated with DIC:
1. Infections
   - Bacterial: meningococcemia, sepsis, Gram-negative sepsis, *Neisseria meningitidis*, *Streptococcus pneumoniae*, malaria
   - Rickettsial: Rocky Mountain spotted fever and others
   - Viral: herpes simplex, hepatitis, cytomegalovirus, varicella, and others
   - Fungal: *Aspergillus* infection, histoplasmosis, cryptococcosis, and others
   - Parasitic: malaria, trypanosomiasis, and others
2. Organ destruction: pancreatitis
3. Obstetric complications
   - Placental abruption
   - Amniotic fluid embolism

- Intrauterine fetal demise
- Preeclampsia
4. Malignancies
  - Acute leukemia: promyelocytic (M3), myelomonocytic (M4), monocytic (M5), lymphoblastic (T cell), and lymphoblastic (Philadelphia-chromosome-positive)
  - Metastatic tumors: neuroblastoma, alveolar rhabdomyosarcoma
  - Cancer of lung, pancreas, prostate, and stomach
5. Collagen vascular disorders
  - Systemic lupus erythematosus
  - Juvenile rheumatoid arthritis
  - Vasculitis
6. Vascular abnormalities
  - Large hemangiomata
  - Vascular aneurysm (aortic aneurysm)
7. Massive tissue injury
  - Severe trauma and shock
  - Burn injuries
  - Major surgery
8. Miscellaneous
  - Liver disease, snake bite, recreational drugs
  - ABO transfusion incompatibility
  - Transplant rejection shock, heat stroke, septic shock, and serotonin syndrome

7.3.1 Critically Ill Patients in an ICU Setting

Coagulations abnormalities occur frequently in critically ill patients and may have a major impact on clinical outcome. There are many causes for deranged coagulation and each of these underlying disorders may require specific therapeutic management. Furthermore, a proper differential diagnosis and the initiation of adequate (supportive or preventive measures) treatment strategies are crucial [8].

Coagulation disorders in critically ill patients may range from isolated thrombocytopenia or prolonged global clotting tests to complex defects, such as DIC (e.g., in the case of patients suffering from severe burn injury causing inflammatory endothelial damage, increased permeability, and disseminated thrombosis as consequence of a high value of intravascular hematocrit). In most critically ill patients, deficiencies of coagulation factors are acquired and may be due to impaired synthesis, massive blood loss, or increased turnover (consumption).

Patients with coagulation defects have a fourfold to fivefold higher risk of bleeding compared with patients with a normal coagulation status. The incidence of thrombocytopenia (platelet count below $150 \times 10^9/L$) in critically ill patients is 35–44%; a platelet count of less than $100 \times 10^9/L$ is seen in 30-50% of patients. A prolonged global coagulation time, such as the prothrombin time (PT) or the

Table 7.1 Differential diagnosis of thrombocytopenia in the ICU

Differential diagnosis	Relative incidence (%)	Additional diagnostic clues
Sepsis	52.4	Positive (blood) cultures, positive sepsis criteria, hematophagocytosis in bone marrow aspirate
DIC	25.3	Prolonged aPTT and PT, increased levels of fibrin degradation products, low level of physiological anticoagulant factors (antithrombin, protein C)
Massive blood loss	7.5	Major bleeding, low hemoglobin level, prolonged aPTT and PT
Thrombotic microangiopathy	0.7	Schistocytes in blood smear, Coombs-negative hemolysis, fever, neurologic symptoms, renal insufficiency
Heparin-induced thrombocytopenia	1.2	Use of heparin, venous or arterial thrombosis, positive heparin-induced thrombocytopenia test (usually ELISA for heparin–platelet factor 4 antibodies), rebound of platelets after cessation of use of heparin
Immune thrombocytopenia	3.4	Antiplatelet antibodies, normal or increased number of megakaryocytes in bone marrow aspirate, decreased thrombopoeitin level
Drug-induced thrombocytopenia	9.5	Decreased number of megakaryocytes in bone marrow aspirate or detection of drug-induced antiplatelet antibodies, rebound of platelet count after cessation of drug use

DIC disseminated intravascular coagulation, *aPTT* activated partial thromboplastin time, *PT* prothrombin time

activated partial thromboplastin time (aPTT) occurs in 14–28% of ICU patients. Regardless of the cause, thrombocytopenia is an independent predictor of ICU mortality.

Other coagulation test abnormalities frequently observed in patients with sepsis include elevated levels of fibrin degradation products and reduced levels of coagulation inhibitors [9]. Seven major causes of thrombocytopenia (platelet count below 150×10^9/L) are listed in Table 7.1.

7.3.2 Severe Infections and Sepsis

The Sepsis Resuscitation and Management Bundles were derived from the 2008 Surviving Sepsis Campaign guidelines.

The Surviving Sepsis Campaign recommends treating hypotension and/or elevated lactate levels [above 4 mmol/L (36 mg/dL)] with fluids:

1. Fluid resuscitation with either natural/artificial colloids (0.2–0.3 g/kg) or crystalloids (20 mL/kg).
2. Fluid resuscitation initially targeting a central venous pressure of at least 8 mmHg (12 mmHg in mechanically ventilated patients).
3. A fluid challenge technique should be applied, wherein fluid administration is continued as long as the hemodynamic improvement (e.g., arterial pressure, heart rate, urine output) continues.

- Fluid challenge in patients with suspected hypovolemia to be started with at least 1,000 mL of crystalloids or 300–500 mL of colloids over 30 min. More rapid administration and greater amounts of fluid may be needed in patients with sepsis-induced tissue hypoperfusion.
- The rate of fluid administration should be reduced substantially when cardiac filling pressures (central venous pressure or pulmonary artery balloon-occluded pressure) increase without concurrent hemodynamic improvement [10].

7.3.3 Obstetrics

There are several obstetric causes of DIC during pregnancy and postpartum.

DIC can occur in several settings, which include emergencies (such as placental abruption and amniotic fluid embolism) as well as complications such as pre-eclampsia [11].

Excessive release of tissue factor (TF) is the primary mechanism involved in DIC resulting from obstetric complications, which include intrauterine fetal demise, amniotic fluid embolism, and placental abruption [12].

The proportionality of the coagulant and fibrinolytic responses may differ between these different conditions. A common theme for pregnancy-associated DIC is the vital role played by the placenta. Removal of the placenta or in severe cases revision of the uterine cavity may be the best option for saving pregnant women, associated with appropriate blood product support [13].

7.3.4 Trauma and Shock

In trauma and shock, tissue damage leads to release of TF and other tissue thromboplastins. High levels of inflammatory cytokines and severe tissue injuries activate the TF-dependent coagulation pathway, followed by massive thrombin generation and its activation. Low levels of protein C and antithrombin induce insufficient coagulation control and the inhibition of the anticoagulation pathway. Primary and secondary fibrin(ogen)olysis is highly activated by the shock-induced tissue hypoxia and disseminated fibrin formation, respectively. Consumption coagulopathy and severe bleeding is frequently combined with diffuse thrombosis in trauma patients [14].

Traumatic coagulopathy is multifactorial. The existence of mixed physiological responses for hemostasis and wound healing and pathological hemostatic responses makes it difficult to understand the mechanisms of the two stages of coagulopathy after trauma.

DIC with the fibrinolytic phenotype is the predominant and initiative pathogenesis of coagulopathy in the early stage of trauma, modified through fibrinogenolysis, contributes to poor prognosis due to massive bleeding. On the other hand, DIC with an antifibrinolytic phenotype characterized by microvascular thrombosis determines a poor outcome in the late stage of trauma [15].

Any alternative to transfusion must minimize the need for transfusion in the first place. This can be done by reducing the volume of blood loss by direct methods where possible, such as hemostasis at the point of bleeding, or by improving the extrinsic coagulation profile. The efficacy and safety of recombinant activated factor VII (factor VIIa) for the treatment of bleeding in trauma has been investigated, and significant reduction of the transfusion requirements in 48 h was found [16, 17].

7.3.5 Stroke

A hypercoagulable state and the activation of the coagulation cascade by cytokines promote coagulation and suppress anticoagulant activities causing stroke. The brain tends to be a target organ of stroke in the conditions of DIC. Nonbacterial thrombotic endocarditis is characterized by the presence of relatively acellular aggregates of fibrin and platelets attached to normal heart valves. Nonbacterial thrombotic endocarditis can be found in DIC [18].

The high risk of thromboembolic events (arterial: myocardial event, cerebral infarction; venous: deep venous thrombosis, pulmonary embolism) by use of recombinant factor VIIa in high-risk patients has been evaluated (intracerebral hemorrhage, advanced age, hypertension, atherosclerosis, diabetes, and immobility) in clinical trials [19]. Higher doses of recombinant factor VIIa in a high-risk population are associated with a small increased risk of what are usually minor cardiac events. Demonstration of the ability of recombinant factor VIIa to improve outcome in future studies should be driven by its effectiveness in slowing bleeding outweighing the risk of a small increase in arterial thromboembolisms [20].

7.4 Diagnosis of DIC

A diagnosis of DIC should be made on the basis of an appropriate clinical suspicion supported by relevant laboratory tests.(grade C, level IV) [21].

The diagnosis of DIC was first based on the detection of microthrombi, but it currently involves analysis of hemostatic abnormalities by laboratory tests.

7 Disseminated Intravascular Coagulation

Diagnosis is usually suggested by the following conditions:

- *Severe cases with hemorrhage.* The PT and the aPTT are usually very prolonged and the fibrinogen level is markedly reduced. High levels of fibrin degradation products, including D-dimer, are found owing to the intense fibrinolytic activity stimulated by the presence of fibrin in the circulation. There is severe thrombocytopenia. The blood film may show fragmented red blood cells (schistocytes).
- *Mild cases without bleeding.* There is increased synthesis of coagulation factors and platelets. PT, aPTT, and platelet counts are normal and the levels of fibrin degradation products are raised.

The International Society on Thrombosis and Haemostasis (ISTH) has developed three diagnostic criteria for DIC. The ISTH diagnostic criteria have high specificity and low sensitivity.

The simple scoring algorithm for DIC as proposed by the ISTH, and using the platelet count, the PT or the internal normalized ratio, and plasma levels of a fibrin related marker, such as D-dimer or other fibrin degradation products, was shown to be a relatively accurate system to establish or reject a diagnosis of DIC. A recent clinical study used the ISTH diagnostic criteria with some modifications for diagnosis of nonovert DIC [22] (Table 7.2).

The scoring systems for DIC are based on a "static" assessment; the "trend" scoring allows longitudinal assessment of the patient's coagulopathy and, when therapy has been instituted, inference on whether the therapy has improved the course of the disease. Adding the scoring system to Acute Physiology and Chronic Evaluation (APACHE II) improved the ability to predict which patients may progress from single to multiple organ dysfunction/failure.

In patients with DIC, a variety of altered coagulation parameters may be detectable, such as thrombocytopenia, prolonged global coagulation times, reduced levels of coagulation inhibitors, and high levels of fibrin degradation products. Several molecular hemostatic markers such as thrombin–antithrombin complex, D-dimer, soluble fibrin, and plasmin–plasmin inhibitor complex have to be adopted for further improvement of diagnostic criteria for DIC [23].

More sophisticated tests for activation of individual factors or pathways of coagulation may point to specific involvement of these components in the pathogenesis of the disorder.

Recently, insights into contributory pathogenetic pathways in DIC have been largely increased, which could result in more precise diagnostic tests for this condition. The diagnosis of DIC should encompass both clinical and laboratory information; however, the clinical and laboratory diagnosis may remain difficult.

Markers used in the diagnosis of DIC involve among others decreased platelet count, which is a sensitive but not specific sign of DIC, PT, which reflects the consumption and depletion of various coagulation factors, and fibrin degradation products (FDPs), which are indicators that plasmin was present, i.e., the fibrinolytic system was activated. In contrast, D-dimers are cross-linked fibrin degradation products, which means that thrombin must have been present to form fibrin and plasmin must have been present to proteolytically digest it. Thrombin–antithrombin complexes form when thrombin binds to antithrombin and forms

Table 7.2 Diagnostic criteria for overt DIC and nonovert DIC of the International Society on Thrombosis and Haemostasis (ISTH)

Overt DIC			Non-overt DIC			
			By original ISTH criteria		By modified ISTH criteria	
	Parameter value	Points	Parameter value	Points	Parameter value	Points
Platelet count (/μL)	50,000–100,000	1	Increased	−1	Only decreased	1
	< 50,000	2	Decreased	1	(<100,000)	
PT (s)	Prolongation of PT:		Not prolonged	−1	Only prolonged	1
	3–6	1	Prolonged	1	(>3 s)	
	≥6	2				
Fibrinogen (mg/dL)	100	1				
D-dimer (μg/mL)	0.5–1	1	Not increased	−1	Always increased	1
	1–3	2	Increased	1	(≥0.5)	
	≥3	3				
Protein C activity (%)			Normal	−1	Decreased	1
			Decreased	1	(<70)	
Antithrombin III (%)			Normal	−1	Decreased	1
			Decreased	1	(<80)	
Calculate score	If ≥ 5 points is compatible with overt DIC; repeat scoring daily		If < 5 is suggestive (not affirmative) of non-overt DIC; repeat scoring next 1–2 days			

In case of underlying disorder associated with DIC add 2 points to the calculate score

7 Disseminated Intravascular Coagulation

irreversible complexes. Elevated thrombin–antithrombin complex levels thus indicate the in vivo presence of thrombin [24].

The PT is a sensitive marker, but fibrinogen levels are not sensitive for DIC due to infectious diseases. The plasmin inhibitor complex in hematologic malignancy, and soluble fibrin monomer complex, antithrombin, and thrombomodulin in patients with infectious disease are sensitive markers for the diagnosis of DIC. Although hemostatic markers are useful for the diagnosis of DIC, the usefulness differs depending on the different underlying diseases.

There is no single clinical or laboratory test that has adequate sensitivity and specificity by itself to confirm or reject a diagnosis of DIC. A combination of widely available tests may be helpful in making the diagnosis of DIC and can also be helpful to guide in the selection of DIC patients who require specific, often expensive, interventions in the coagulation system [25].

Lee and Song [21] developed dynamic algorithms, assessing changes in coagulation parameters over sequential days. This could further increase the diagnostic accuracy for DIC and may be helpful to detect early stages of coagulopathy potentially evolving into DIC. It is important to repeat the tests to monitor the dynamically changing scenario based on laboratory results and clinical observations (grade B, level III).

Thrombocytopenia or a rapidly declining platelet count is an important diagnostic hallmark of DIC. The relevance of thrombocytopenia in patients with DIC is indeed related to an increased risk of bleeding. In particular, patients with a platelet count of less than $50 \times 10^9/L$ have a fourfold to fivefold higher risk of bleeding as compared with patients with a higher platelet count, in particular when anticoagulants are used [26]. The platelet count was shown to be a stronger predictor of ICU mortality than composite scoring systems, such as the APACHE II score or the SOFA score.

It is important to emphasize that global coagulation tests poorly reflect in vivo hemostasis; however, these tests are convenient methods to quickly estimate the concentrations of one or at times multiple coagulation factors for which each test is sensitive. The low value of coagulation factors is reflected by prolonged coagulation screening tests, such as the PT and the aPTT. Several laboratories use the international normalized ratio instead of the PT [27].

Measurement of fibrinogen has been widely advocated as a useful tool for the diagnosis of DIC but it is not very helpful to diagnose DIC in most cases.

Theoretically, measurement of soluble fibrin or fibrin monomers in plasma could be helpful to diagnose intravascular fibrin formation in DIC. The only problem so far is that a reliable test is not available for quantitating soluble fibrin in plasma. Since soluble fibrin in plasma can only be generated intravascularly, this test will not be influenced by extravascular fibrin formation. Other more frequently used tests include tests for elevated levels of fibrin degradation products.

The specificity of high levels of fibrin degradation products is therefore limited and many other conditions, such as trauma, recent surgery, inflammation, and venous thromboembolism, are associated with elevated levels of FDPs, FDP levels are influenced by liver and kidney functions [28].

In severe cases with hemorrhage, the blood film may show fragmented red blood cells (schistocytes in more than 10% of autoptic data).

Plasma levels of physiological coagulation inhibitors, such as antithrombin III and protein C, may be useful indicators of ongoing coagulation activation. Plasma levels of antithrombin have been shown to be potent predictors of survival in patients with sepsis and DIC. Antithrombin levels are markedly decreased not only due to consumption but also due to impaired synthesis, as a result of a negative acute phase response, and degradation by elastase from activated neutrophils.

Protein C levels may also indicate the severity of the DIC. The plasma level of protein C may be regarded as a strong predictor of the outcome in DIC patients. Endothelial dysfunction is even more important in the impairment of the protein C system during DIC [29].

Thromboelastography (TEG) is a method that was developed decades ago and provides an overall picture of ex vivo coagulation. The theoretical advantage of TEG over conventional coagulation assays is that it provides an idea of platelet function as well as fibrinolytic activity. Hyperoagulability and hypocoagulability as demonstrated with TEG were shown to correlate with clinically relevant morbidity and mortality in several studies [30].

There are no systematic studies on the diagnostic accuracy of TEG for the diagnosis of DIC; however, the test may be useful for assessing the global status of the coagulation system in critically ill patients [31].

7.5 Old and New Treatments of Consumption Coagulopathy

Numerous attempts have been made to establish relevant experimental models of DIC to aid in the discovery of new treatment modalities for DIC.

The cornerstone of the treatment of DIC is treatment of the underlying condition. It is evident that the primary focus of attention in the treatment of DIC should be directed toward adequate management of the underlying conditions (e.g., during shock states). In many cases the DIC will spontaneously resolve when the underlying disorder is properly managed (e.g., in obstetric removal of the placenta is the linchpin to treatment in most cases); this emphasizes the critical importance of making a correct diagnosis that underlies the acquired coagulopathy [32].

Despite proper treatment for the underlying disorder, nevertheless, further supportive measures are often required to address the coagulation defect. Assessing morbidity and mortality of DIC is difficult, and treatment strategies are crucial [33]. Hematological interventions such as use of heparins [low molecular weight heparin (LMWH) and unfractionated heparin (UFH)], danaparoid sodium, synthetic protease inhibitor, antithrombin, recombinant human activated protein C, recombinant human soluble thrombomodulin, recombinant TF pathway inhibitor, recombinant factor VIIa, and any other types of hematological interventions for treating DIC during pregnancy and postpartum need to be tested in randomized controlled trials assessing outcomes such as maternal death, perinatal death, and safety [34].

DIC in severely bleeding obstetric patients should be treated aggressively using massive transfusion. Recent studies underline the utility of transfusing these components in defined ratios to prevent dilutional coagulopathy [35, 36].

The literature emphasizes the usefulness of transfusing packed red blood cells, fresh frozen plasma, and platelets earlier and in a defined ratio to prevent dilutional coagulopathy during obstetric hemorrhage. It seems reasonable to use blood products for transfusion earlier and in a 1:1 fresh frozen plasma to red blood cell ratio during acute obstetric hemorrhage. Fibrinogen concentrate should be added if the fibrinogen plasma level remains below 1.0 g/L and perhaps even as soon as it falls below 1.5–2.0 g/L. The addition of tranexamic acid (1 g) is cheap, safe, and likely to be useful. Data on the proactive administration of platelets are insufficient to recommend this practice routinely [37]. The use of recombinant factor VIIa (60–90 µg/kg) is advocated only after failure of other conventional therapies, including embolization and conservative surgery, but prior to obstetric hysterectomy. Prospective randomized controlled trials are highly desirable.

Treatments of DIC involve the surgical repair of the trauma, management of the shock condition, the rapid and sufficient replacement of platelet concentrate, fresh frozen plasma, and depleted coagulation factors. The administration of an antifibrinolytic agent (tranexamic acid) may reduce the risk of death in bleeding trauma patients associated with this type of consumption coagulopathy [38]. Treatment modalities focused on the TF–factor VIIa complex include inactivated factor VII and NAPc2, a member of the nematode family of anticoagulant proteins and an inhibitor of the complex between TF, factor VIIa, and activated factor X, and antibodies against TF/factor VIIa in an experimental setting, and encouraging results have been obtained. Recombinant factor VIIa has been demonstrated to be useful in cases of severe bleeding. However, a careful consideration of the risks and benefits should be undertaken before administration of factor VIIa [39].

Furthermore, antifibrinolytic agents, such as ε-aminocaproic acid and tranexamic acid, can also be considered in patients with DIC if bleeding predominates. These agents should always be administered with heparin (antithrombin effects) to prevent their prothrombotic effects.

However, in spite of this progress, the therapeutic decisions are still controversial and should be individualized on the basis of the nature of DIC and the severity of the clinical .symptoms (Table 7.3).

7.6   Recommendations

The guidelines advocate the followed recommendations:

Recommendation 1: plasma and platelets

Transfusion of platelets or plasma (components) in patients with DIC should not primarily be based on laboratory results and should in general be reserved for patients who present with bleeding (grade C, level IV). In patients with DIC and

Table 7.3 Treatment modalities for DIC

Replacement therapy	Fresh frozen plasma
Anticoagulants	Unfractionated and low molecular weight heparin Danaparoid sodium Recombinant hirudin Recombinant tissue factor pathway inhibitor Recombinant nematode anticoagulant protein c2
Restoration of anticoagulant pathways	Antithrombin Recombinant human activated protein C
Other agents	Recombinant activated factor VII Antifibrinolytic agents Antiselectin antibodies Recombinant interleukin-10 Monoclonal antibodies against TNF and CD14

bleeding or at high risk of bleeding (e.g., postoperative patients or patients due to undergo an invasive procedure) and a platelet count of less than 50×10^9/L, transfusion of platelets should be considered (grade C, level IV).

In nonbleeding patients with DIC, prophylactic platelet transfusion is not given unless it is perceived that there is a high risk of bleeding (grade C, level IV). In bleeding patients with DIC and prolonged PT and aPTT, administration of fresh frozen plasma may be useful. It should not, however, be instituted on the basis of laboratory tests alone but should be considered in those with active bleeding and in those requiring an invasive procedure. There is no evidence that infusion of plasma stimulates the ongoing activation of coagulation (grade C, level IV). If transfusion of fresh frozen plasma is not possible in patients with bleeding because of fluid overload, consider using a factor such as prothrombin complex concentrate, recognizing that this will only partially correct the defect because it contains only a selected factor, whereas in DIC there is a global deficiency of coagulation factors (grade C, level IV). Severe hypofibrinogenemia (below 1 g/L) that persists despite fresh frozen plasma replacement may be treated with fibrinogen concentrate or cryoprecipitate (grade C, level IV).

Recommendation 2: anticoagulants

In cases of DIC where thrombosis predominates, such as arterial or venous thromboembolism, severe purpura fulminans, and vascular skin infarction, therapeutic doses of heparin should be considered. In these patients where there is perceived to be a coexisting high risk of bleeding, there may be benefits in using continuous infusion of UFH because of its short half-life and reversibility. Weight-adjusted doses (e.g., 10 µg/kg/h) may be used without the intention of prolonging the aPTT ratio to 1.5–2.5 times the control value. Monitoring the aPTT in these cases may be complicated and clinical observation for signs of bleeding is important (grade C, level IV). In critically ill, nonbleeding patients with DIC, prophylaxis for venous thromboembolism with prophylactic doses of heparin or LMWH is recommended (grade A, level Ib).

Recommendation 3: anticoagulant factor concentrates

Consider treating patients with severe sepsis and DIC with recombinant human activated protein C (continuous infusion, 24 μg/kg/h for 4 days) (grade A, level Ib). Patients at high risk of bleeding should not be given recombinant human activated protein C. Current manufacturer guidance advises against using this product in patients with platelet counts of less than $30 \times 10^9/L$. In the event of invasive procedures, administration of recombinant human activated protein C should be discontinued shortly before the intervention (elimination half-life approximately 20 min) and may be resumed a few hours later, dependent on the clinical situation (grade C, level IV). In the absence of further prospective evidence from randomized controlled trials confirming a beneficial effect of antithrombin concentrate on clinically relevant end points in patients with DIC and not receiving heparin, administration of antithrombin cannot be recommended (grade A, level Ib).

Recommendation 4: antifibrinolytic treatment

In general, patients with DIC should not be treated with antifibrinolytic agents (grade C, level IV). Patients with DIC that is characterized by a primary hyperfibrinolytic state (e.g., acute pancreatitis) and who present with severe bleeding could be treated with lysine analogues, such as tranexamic acid (e.g., 1 g every 8 h) (grade C, level IV).

Although treatment of DIC is important, adequate treatment differs according to the type of DIC. In asymptomatic DIC, LMWH, synthetic protease inhibitor, and antithrombin are recommended, although these drugs have not yet been proved to have a high degree of effectiveness.

UFH and danaparoid sodium are sometimes administered in this type of consumption coagulopathy, but their usefulness is not clear. In the marked bleeding type, LMWH, synthetic protease inhibitor, and antithrombin are recommended although there is not high-quality evidence for the effectiveness of these drugs. LMWH, UFH, and danaparoid sodium are not recommended in the case of life-threatening bleeding. In the case of severe bleeding, synthetic protease inhibitor is recommended since it does not cause a worsening of bleeding. Blood transfusions, such as fresh frozen plasma and platelet concentrate, are also required in cases of life-threatening bleeding. In the organ dysfunction/failure type, including sepsis, antithrombin has been recommended on the basis of the findings of several clinical trials. DIC is frequently associated with thrombosis and may thus require strong anticoagulant therapy, such as LMWH, UFH, and danaparoid sodium. These data are reported from the Japanese Society of Thrombosis Hemostasis expert consensus for the treatment of DIC [40].

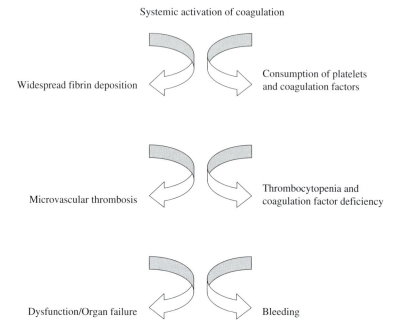

Fig. 7.1 Disseminated intravascular coagulation algorithm

7.7 Conclusion

DIC is a clinicopathological syndrome which complicates a wide range of illnesses. It is characterized by systemic activation of pathways leading to and regulating coagulation, which can result in the generation of fibrin clots that may cause organ failure with concomitant consumption of platelets and coagulation factors that may result frequently in a severe clinical bleeding [41] (Fig. 7.1).

The diagnosis of DIC should encompass both clinical and laboratory information. The ISTH DIC scoring system provides objective measurement of DIC. During a condition of consumption coagulopathy the scoring system correlates with clinical observations and outcome. It is important to monitor the dynamically changing scenario based on laboratory tests and clinical assessment in patients suffering from several syndromes leading to hemorrhagic bleeding and/or thrombosis conditions. However, the cornerstone of the treatment of DIC is treatment of the underlying diseases (e.g., treatment of hypovolemic shock after trauma or severe bleeding in hemorrhagic shock) .

There is no evidence regarding the continuous infusion of UFH. Weight-adjusted doses (e.g., 10 µg/kg/h) may be used without the intention of prolonging the aPTT ratio to 1.5–2.5 times the control value. In critically ill, nonbleeding patients with DIC, prophylaxis for venous thromboembolism with prophylactic doses of heparin or LMWH is recommended [42].

Consumption coagulopathy represents an important challenge for clinical care physicians and intensivists.

References

1. Berthelsen LO, Kristensen AT, Tranholm M (2011) Animal models of DIC and their relevance to human DIC: asystematic review. Thromb Res 128(2):103–116
2. Levi M (2010) Disseminated intravascular coagulation: a disease-specific approach. Semin Thromb Hemost 36(4):363–365
3. Rahman S, Cichon M, Hoppensteadt D et al (2011) Upregulation of microparticles in DIC and its impact on inflammatory processes. Clin Appl Thromb Hemost. [Epub ahead of print]
4. Velez AM, Friedman WA (2011) Disseminated intravascular coagulation during resection of a meningioma. Neurosurgery 68(4):E1165–E1169; discussion E1169
5. Yamakawa K, Fujimi S, Mohri T et al (2011) Treatment effects of recombinant human soluble thrombomodulin in patients with severe sepsis: a historical control study. Crit Care 15(3):R123
6. Chung S, Kim JE, Park S et al (2011) Neutrophil and monocyte activation markers have prognostic impact in disseminated intravascular coagulation: In vitro effect of thrombin on monocyte CD163 shedding. Thromb Res 127(5):450–456
7. Levi M, Schultz M (2010) Coagulopathy and platelet disorders in critically ill patients. Minerva Anestesiol 76(10):851–859
8. Schultz MJ (2009) Early recognition of critically ill patients. Neth J Med 67(9):266–267
9. Levi M, Schouten M, van der Poll T (2008) Sepsis, coagulation, and antithrombin: old lessons and new insights. Semin Thromb Hemost 34(8):742–746
10. Dellinger RP, Levy MM, Carlet JM et al (2008) Surviving sepsis campaign: international guidelines for management of severe sepsis and septic shock: 2008. Crit Care Med 36(1):296–327
11. Uszyński M, Uszyński W (2011) Coagulation and fibrinolysis in amniotic fluid: physiology and observations on amniotic fluid embolism, preterm fetal membrane rupture, and pre-eclampsia. Semin Thromb Hemost 37(2):165–174
12. Thachil J, Toh CH (2009) Disseminated intravascular coagulation in obstetric disorders and its acute haematological management. Blood Rev 23(4):167–176
13. Sugasawa Y, Yamaguchi K, Koh K et al (2011) Successful anesthetic management of a postpartum patient with amniotic fluid embolism. Masui 60(1):91–95
14. Hayakawa M, Sawamura A, Gando S et al (2011) Disseminated intravascular coagulation at an early phase of trauma is associated with consumption coagulopathy and excessive fibrinolysis both by plasmin and neutrophil elastase. Surgery 149(2):221–230
15. Sawamura A, Hayakawa M, Gando S et al (2009) Disseminated intravascular coagulation with a fibrinolytic phenotype at an early phase of trauma predicts mortality. Thromb Res 124(5):608–613
16. Boffard KD, Choong PI, Kluger Y et al (2009) NovoSeven trauma study group.The treatment of bleeding is to stop the bleeding! Treatment of trauma-related hemorrhage. Transfusion 49(Suppl 5):240–247
17. Dutton RP, Parr M, Tortella BJ et al (2011) Recombinant activated factor VII safety in trauma patients: results from the CONTROL Trial. J Trauma 71(1):12–19
18. Terashi H, Uchiyama S, Iwata M (2008) Stroke in cancer patients. Brain Nerve 60(2):143–147

19. Lin Y, Stanworth S, Birchall J et al (2011) Use of recombinant factor VIIa for the prevention and treatment of bleeding in patients without hemophilia: asystematic review and meta-analysis. CMAJ 183(1):E9–19
20. Diringer MN, Skolnick BE, Mayer SA et al (2010) Thromboembolic events with recombinant activated factor VII in spontaneous intracerebral hemorrhage: results from the Factor Seven for Acute Hemorrhagic Stroke (FAST) trial. Stroke 41(1):48–53
21. Lee JH, Song J (2010) Diagnosis of non-overt disseminated intravascular coagulation made according to the International Society on Thrombosis and Hemostasis criteria with some modifications. Korean J Hematol 45(4):260–263
22. Levi M, Schultz M, van der Poll T (2011) Coagulation biomarkers in critically ill patients. Crit Care Clin 27(2):281–297
23. Oh D, Jang MJ, Lee SJ et al (2010) Evaluation of modified non-overt DIC criteria on the prediction of poor outcome in patients with sepsis. Thromb Res 126(1):18–23
24. Levi M, Meijers JC (2011) DIC: which laboratory tests are most useful. Blood Rev 25(1):33–37
25. Kawasugi K, Wada H, Hatada T et al; Japanese Society of Thrombosis Hemostasis/DIC Subcommittee (2011) Prospective evaluation of hemostatic abnormalities in overt DIC due to various underlying diseases. Thromb Res 128(2):186–190
26. Levi MM, Eerenberg E, Löwenberg E, Kamphuisen PW (2010) Bleeding in patients using new anticoagulants or antiplatelet agents: risk factors and management. Neth J Med 68(2):68–76
27. Kim HK, Hong KH, Toh CH (2010) Scientific and standardization committee on DIC of The International Society on Thrombosis and Haemostasis, application of the international normalized ratio in the scoring system for disseminated intravascular coagulation. J Thromb Haemost 8(5):1116–1118
28. Levi M (2008) The coagulant response in sepsis. Clin Chest Med 29(4):627–642
29. Levi M, van der Poll T (2008) The role of natural anticoagulants in the pathogenesis and management of systemic activation of coagulation and inflammation in critically ill patients. Semin Thromb Hemost 34(5):459–468
30. Johansson PI, Stensballe J, Vindeløv N et al (2010) Hypocoagulability, as evaluated by thrombelastography, at admission to the ICU is associated with increased 30-day mortality. Blood Coagul Fibrinolysis 21(2):168–174
31. Park MS, Martini WZ, Dubick MA et al (2009) Thromboelastography as a better indicator of hypercoagulable state after injury than prothrombin time or activated partial thromboplastin time. J Trauma. 67(2):266–275; discussion 275–276
32. Levi M, Toh CH, Thachil J, Watson HG (2009) Guidelines for the diagnosis and management of disseminated intravascular coagulation, British Committee for Standards in Haematology. Br J Haematol 145(1):24–33
33. Sun Y, Wang J, Wu X et al (2011) Validating the incidence of coagulopathy and disseminated intravascular coagulation in patients with traumatic brain injury? Analysis of 242 cases. Br J Neurosurg 25(3):363–368
34. Monteiro RQ (2011) Tissue factor as a target for the treatment of disseminated intravascular coagulation. Thromb Res 127(6):495–496
35. Hossain N, Shah T, Khan N (2011) Transfusion of blood and blood component therapy for postpartum haemorrhage at a tertiary referral center. J Pak Med Assoc 61(4):343–345
36. Padmanabhan A, Schwartz J, Spitalnik SL (2009) Transfusion therapy in postpartum hemorrhage. Semin Perinatol 33(2):124–127
37. Mercier FJ, Bonnet MP (2010) Use of clotting factors and other prohemostatic drugs for obstetric hemorrhage. Curr Opin Anaesthesiol 23(3):310–316
38. Gando S, Sawamura A, Hayakawa M (2011) Trauma, shock, and disseminated intravascular coagulation: lessons from the classical literature. Ann Surg 254(1):10–19

7 Disseminated Intravascular Coagulation

39. Darlington DN, Delgado AV, Kheirabadi BS et al (2011) Effect of hemodilution on coagulation and recombinant factor VIIa efficacy in human blood in vitro. J Trauma 71(5):1152–1163
40. Wada H, Asakura H, Okamoto K et al (2010) Japanese Society of Thrombosis Hemostasis/ DIC subcommittee, expert consensus for the treatment of disseminated intravascular coagulation in Japan. Thromb Res 125(1):6–11
41. Gando S (2011) DIC diagnostic criteria for critical illness. Rinsho Byori Suppl 147:42–48
42. Aikawa N (2011) Revised Surviving Sepsis Campaign guidelines and therapy for severe sepsis. Jpn J Antibiot 64(1):37–44

Coagulative Disturbances in Trauma

8

Giuliana Garufi, Maria Cristina Fiorenza and Giorgio Berlot

8.1 Trauma and Coagulation

Massive bleeding in patients with major trauma is the most common cause of in-hospital mortality during the first 48 h and in the early postoperative period. It interferes with the coagulation process, resulting in a coagulopathy, even in patients with previously normal hemostasis.

Early trauma-induced coagulopathy (TIC) is present in about 20% of patients upon hospital admission and is related to decreased survival [1]. The presence of TIC reflects the severity of injury and is an independent predictor of mortality in trauma [2].

TIC may occur as a nonsurgical, diffuse bleeding from mucosal or damaged tissue, new bleeding from vesical/gastric tubes, or from puncture sites. It is responsible for increased risk of renal insufficiency, multiple organ failure, and longer ventilatory support [3].

Appropriate treatment of the trauma patient with massive bleeding, defined as the loss of one blood volume within 24 h or the loss of 0.5 blood volumes within 3 h, includes the early identification of potential bleeding sources followed by prompt measures to minimize blood loss, restore tissue perfusion, and achieve hemodynamic stability [4]. Accordingly, in patients with traumatic hemorrhage, the time between injury and admission to the hospital should be minimized. In trauma patients without preexisting disease or massive head injury, a number of conditions have been identified as significant risk factors for life-threatening

---

G. Garufi (✉)
Anaesthesia and Intensive Care, Cattinara Hospital,
University of Trieste, Trieste, Italy
e-mail: giugarufi@yahoo.it

G. Berlot (ed.), *Hemocoagulative Problems in the Critically Ill Patient*,
DOI: 10.1007/978-88-470-2448-9_8, © Springer-Verlag Italia 2012

coagulopathy, including an injury severity score of more than 25, a systolic blood pressure of less than 70 mmHg, acidosis with pH below 7.10, and hypothermia with a body temperature below 34°C [5]. The early coagulopathy of trauma primarily occurs in patients with a base deficit greater than 6 mEq/l [4]. After major trauma, protracted reduction in tissue perfusion may impair tissue metabolism, which becomes apparent at cellular, organ, and systemic levels [6]. Uncontrolled posttraumatic bleeding, usually caused by a combination of vascular injury and coagulopathy, is the leading cause of potentially preventable death among trauma patients. The pathogenesis of TIC is complex and multifactorial, involving physiological, biochemical, immunological, and cellular mechanisms. In particular, TIC has a number of causal factors, including dilutional coagulopathy after fluid resuscitation and consumption of clotting factors and platelets due to major blood loss [7]. Increased fibrinolysis, activation of anticoagulant pathways, hypocalcemia, disseminated intravascular coagulation (DIC)-like syndrome may also play a role. Environmental and therapeutic factors may contribute to acidemia, hypothermia, dilution, hypoperfusion, and hemostasis factor consumption [4]. Hypothermia, acidosis, and coagulopathy are commonly referred to as the "lethal triad of trauma" [8]. Acidosis impairs enzyme activity, reduces fibrinogen levels and the platelet count, and prolongs the clotting time [8]; moreover, acidosis interferes with the assembly of the coagulation factor complexes because excess protons destabilize coagulation factor–phospholipid assembly and reduce the activity of the activated factor X–activated factor V prothrombinase complex by 50% at pH 7.2 [9].

Also hypothermia is associated with an increased risk of severe bleeding and death in trauma patients. Actually, different factors cooperate in the occurrence of hypothermia in trauma victims, including the altered central thermoregulation and the decreased heat production due to tissue hypoperfusion, the exposure to low environmental temperatures, and the infusion of cold resuscitation fluids and blood components.

Jurkovich et al. [10] reported that mortality was high when severe bleeding and a core temperature below 32°C occurred in the same individual. Hypothermia prolongs the prothrombin time (PT) and the activated partial thromboplastin time (aPTT) owing to the slowing of the enzymatic reactions and decreased platelet function [11]. In more detail, hypothermia prevents the activation of platelets by traction on the glycoprotein Ib-IX-V complex by von Willebrand factor [12]. It should be remembered that (1) the effect of hypothermia on coagulopathy is difficult to identify by routine coagulation screening tests, such as the PT and the aPTT, because these tests are routinely performed at 37°C, and that (2) a 1°C drop in temperature is associated with roughly a 10% drop in function of clotting factors.

Besides hypothermia and acidosis, other mechanisms contribute to the occurrence of TIC. One theory proposes that tissue factor released during traumatic injuries leads to increased thrombin generation and systemic inflammatory response syndrome. Inflammation and coagulation are strictly related and influence each other. Activation of the coagulation system results in the generation of fibrin with generation of microvascular thrombi and multiple organ dysfunctions [13].

8 Coagulative Disturbances in Trauma

After the massive activation of the coagulation system, the depletion of coagulation factors occurs. The production of new coagulation factors takes 2–4 h and, during this time, there is an anticoagulated state [14]. Another theory postulates that the systemic anticoagulation and fibrinolysis is mediated by activated protein C [15]. Tissue hypoperfusion due to shock causes the release of protein C and reduced thrombin clearance. The activation of the protein C pathway leads to consumption of plasminogen activator inhibitor 1. Moreover, thrombomodulin plays an important role in acute traumatic coagulopathy. Thrombin complexed to thrombomodulin is not free to cleave fibrinogen to form fibrin or activate platelets and also activates thrombin-activated fibrinolysis inhibitor (TAFI); there is also a reduction in TAFI activation by the competitive binding of protein C to the thrombin–thrombomodulin complex, maintaining an anticoagulated state. Fibrinolysis is caused by a combination of low levels of plasminogen activator inhibitor 1, the release of plasminogen activators from the vessel wall, and the decreased activation of TAFI.

Normal activation of the coagulation and fibrinolytic systems results in the consumption of platelets and coagulation factors, and continuing bleeding causes further depletion of these factors. In major blood loss, fibrinogen reaches a critical value earlier than other coagulant factors or platelets. It is present at concentrations of grams per liter, 1000-fold higher than other coagulation factors, which are usually present at levels of milligrams per liter [16]. Nevertheless, hypofibrinogenemia is a usual component of coagulopathies associated with massive bleeding. Martini et al. [17] found that, shortly after a moderate hemorrhagic shock induced in pigs, fibrinogen breakdown was accelerated, whereas fibrinogen synthesis remained unchanged, resulting in a net loss of fibrinogen availability. The acceleration of fibrinogen breakdown was associated with a shortening of the blood clotting time. Hyperfibrinolysis appears to be linked to the severity of the trauma and the organ system affected (e.g., head and urogenital tract injury). In hyperfibrinolysis the coagulopathy can be treated by antifibrinolytic agents before fibrinogen concentrate or cryoprecipitate is given.

Acidosis and hypothermia may also influence fibrinogen metabolism. In a swine model, it was found that acidosis increased fibrinogen breakdown with no effects on fibrinogen synthesis, leading to a depletion of fibrinogen availability [18]. Instead, the potential deficit in fibrinogen availability in hypothermia seems to be due to decreased fibrinogen synthesis with no effect on degradation [19]. Fibrinogen may also reach critical levels at an early stage in trauma patients with massive bleeding because of normovolemic dilution due to fluid replacement therapy that is necessary to prevent shock and acidosis. Polymerization of fibrinogen, and thus total clot strength, can be impaired with colloids, and these effects can be observed with moderate blood loss and infusion of even small quantities of colloids [20].

The critical fibrinogen value is unclear. A threshold of 100 mg/dl fibrinogen has been recommended even though recent clinical data have shown that at fibrinogen levels below 150–200 mg/dl there is an increased tendency for perioperative and postoperative bleeding. The plasma fibrinogen levels often do not agree with functional measurements [20] and can be overestimated in the presence of artificial colloids (see later) [21]. Then, fibrinogen administration using thromboelastometry as guidance may be preferable to measuring plasma fibrinogen levels. A high circulating fibrinogen level exerts a protective effect with regard to blood loss [16], and recent retrospective studies suggest that fibrinogen supplementation may be beneficial [22]. European guidelines for the management of bleeding following major trauma [4] recommend fibrinogen concentrate (dose of 3–4 g) or cryoprecipitate (dose of 50 mg) if bleeding is associated with thromboelastometric signs of functional fibrinogen deficit or a plasma fibrinogen level of less than 150–200 mg/dl.

Because cryoprecipitate is rich in fibrinogen, factor XIII, von Willebrand factor, and factor VIII, it has been used for the treatment of bleeding in acquired fibrinogen or factor XIII deficiency [23]. One unit (15 ml) of cryoprecipitate per 10 kg of body weight is estimated to increase the plasma fibrinogen concentration by 0.5 g/l in the absence of continuing bleeding. In contrast to fresh frozen plasma (1 unit, 250 ml), which contains 0.5–1.0 IU/ml of all plasma factors, the factors contained in prothrombin complex concentrate (about 500 IU, 20 ml) are highly concentrated, at up to 25 times the levels found in fresh frozen plasma. Adverse reactions such as thromboembolic episodes, DIC, and/or hyperfibrinolysis are unlikely.

8.2 Trauma-Induced Coagulopathy and Disseminated Intravascular Coagulopathy

In TIC, unlike what occurs in DIC, there is no generalized intravascular microcoagulation with subsequent consumption. Instead, there is a bleeding-related loss of coagulation factors and platelets. However, DIC may be associated with trauma. DIC is an acquired complex systemic thrombohemorrhagic disorder secondary to the systemic and excessive activation of coagulation, involving the generation of intravascular fibrin and the consumption of procoagulants and platelets. The International Society on Thrombosis and Haemostasis has suggested the following definition for DIC: "An acquired syndrome characterized by the intravascular activation of coagulation with loss of localization arising from different causes. It can originate from and cause damage to the microvasculature, which if sufficiently severe, can produce organ dysfunction" [24].

In trauma patients, the occurrence of a "true" DIC is related to the nature (e.g., brain injury and urogenital tract) and the importance of tissue trauma and to the occurrence and duration of shock and the related tissue hypoxia [25].

8.3 Monitoring Trauma-Induced Coagulopathy

Early monitoring of the coagulative parameters is essential to detect TIC and to define the main causes, including hyperfibrinolysis.

8 Coagulative Disturbances in Trauma

Routine practice to detect posttraumatic coagulopathy includes the measurement of the international normalized ratio, aPTT, fibrinogen, and platelets [4]. PT and aPTT are weak predictors of bleeding tendencies in the critically ill because these tests measure only the first 20–60 s of clot formation and the process is probably not complete for 15–30 min. Moreover, routine laboratory tests cannot assess the effect of hypothermia, acidosis, hypocalcemia, or anemia on hemostasis on coagulation [3].

Thromboelastometry may be helpful to monitor and characterize the coagulopathy and to guide hemostatic therapy [4]. In fact, thromboelastometry provides a real-time graphic representation of clot formation and subsequent lysis.

Thromboelastography is a rapid, simple test that can broadly determine coagulation abnormalities.

8.4 Management of Bleeding and Coagulation in Trauma

Whereas surgical bleeding requires a physical repair, microvascular hemorrhage requires restoration of clotting factors, the administration of clotting cofactors and platelets, and the correction of acidosis and hypothermia. Several approaches have been developed to treat TIC, including:

1. Permissive hypotension. Permissive hypotension may be considered in patients who present with moderate bleeding, but massive volume resuscitation cannot be deferred if patients are in severe hypovolemic shock [23]. A target systolic blood pressure of 80–100 mmHg is recommended until major bleeding has been stopped in the initial phase of trauma [4]. Contraindications to permissive hypotension are head injuries, coronary heart disease, or hypertension [3].

2. Warming. As stated already, in trauma patients hypothermia represents an independent risk factor for bleeding and death. Hypothermia, defined as a core body temperature below 35°C, is associated with acidosis, hypotension and coagulopathy in severely injured patients [4]. In particular, hypothermia is classified as mild (35–32°C), moderate (32–30°C), or severe (below 30°C).

   Hypothermia decreases the enzymatic activity of clotting factors, which are temperature-dependent and function optimally at 37°C. Hypothermia also impairs platelet function, inhibits fibrinogen synthesis, and reduces ATP synthesis [6].

   In trauma patients the early application of measures to reduce heat loss and warm the patient is important to achieve and maintain normothermia. Warmed infusions should also be used for fluid resuscitation via a warming device with a fluid temperature of 40–42°C [3].

3. Correction of acidosis. Acidemia is usually considered as an arterial pH below 7.36. Metabolic acidosis in trauma is believed to be secondary to tissue hypoxia in states of hypovolemia and subsequent inadequate tissue perfusion. The principal indicator of metabolic acidosis in trauma is increased serum concentration of lactate. The use of lactate and base deficit as markers of hypoperfusion

has several limitations: bicarbonate and base deficit levels also assume no pre-existing disturbance in the nonbicarbonate buffers (hemoglobin, magnesium). In a bleeding trauma patient, these buffers are likely to be compromised, and up to 50% of the acid load may be caused by acids other than lactate [26].

4. Correction of ionized calcium. Resuscitation of trauma patients with critical bleeding involves the infusion of large volumes of crystalloid and colloid followed by red blood cell (RBC) transfusion. A reduction in the level of ionized calcium following transfusion is caused by the anticoagulant citrate and is particularly marked when using fresh frozen plasma.

5. Replacement therapy for coagulation. To maintain tissue oxygenation, traditional treatment of trauma patients uses early and aggressive fluid administration to restore blood volume. This approach may, however, increase the hydrostatic pressure on the wound and cause a dislodgement of blood clots, a dilution of coagulation factors, and undesirable cooling of the patient. The aim of the permissive hypotension is to avoid the adverse effects of early aggressive resuscitation while maintaining a level of tissue perfusion that, although lower than normal, is adequate for short periods [4]. Volume resuscitation with crystalloids, colloids, or erythrocytes can lead to dilutional coagulopathy with reduced levels of most hemostatic elements, whereas the administration of fresh frozen plasma dilutes corpuscular elements in blood and restores soluble clotting factors to nearly normal levels [23].

6. Transfusion of erythrocytes. The goal of blood transfusion in trauma settings is to restore RBC mass for adequate tissue oxygen delivery, to mitigate and correct TIC, and to use the minimal number and appropriate choice of blood components; however, an increased hematocrit may also be beneficial for hemostasis. RBCs have been shown to modulate the biochemical and functional responsiveness of activated platelets, suggesting that they contribute to thrombosis and hemostasis and this supports the concept that thrombus formation is a multicellular event [27]. Furthermore, RBCs activate platelet cyclooxygenase, increase the generation of thromboxane A_2 [28], and may directly increase the thrombin burst through exposure of procoagulant phospholipids [29].

The increased acid load from RBC units may also contribute to coagulopathy. The pH of an RBC unit is low, and decreases progressively from around 7.0 initially to around 6.3 at the end of its shelf life during storage, owing to the production of lactic acid by RBCs [30]. Because of the high buffering capacity of plasma in the circulation, transfusion of RBCs with such low pH does not usually cause acid–base disturbance. However, in the case of trauma patients who are already acidotic, massive transfusion of RBCs further increases the acid load, which may in turn exacerbate the ongoing coagulopathy [31].

Whereas the initial insult caused by tissue damage and hypoxia primes the inflammatory system, subsequent transfusion of stored RBCs containing these bioreactive lipids activates a systemic inflammatory response resulting in multiple organ failure [32].

The precise mechanism of RBC-transfusion-related multiple organ failure is yet to be established. Nevertheless, recent evidence supports the hypothesis that,

8 Coagulative Disturbances in Trauma

during storage, bioreactive lipids, which have polymorphonuclear cell priming activity, are generated from aging RBCs [33].

7. Platelets. Platelet dysfunction induced by drugs (acetylsalicylic acid, glycoprotein IIb/IIIa inhibitors, and others) can cause excessive bleeding even with normal platelet counts. When platelet dysfunction is identified or strongly suggested, transfusion of platelet concentrates is strongly advised, even if there is a normal platelet count.

In hemorrhage after trauma or major surgery, the administration of platelet concentrates has to be considered if the platelet count falls below $50 \times 10^3/\mu l$ [23]. A lack of platelets primarily affects clot firmness, which is also influenced by fibrinogen plasma level. To assess an individual's need for replacement therapy, thromboelastographic/thromboelastometric measurements of clot firmness in relation to fibrinogen polymerization can provide valuable information, as strong fibrin polymerization can compensate for the decreased platelet contribution to clot firmness. Thrombocytopenic patients with inflammation-induced elevated fibrinogen levels in thromboelastographic/thromboelastometric monitoring are often not transfused with platelet concentrates because the clot firmness is within the normal range [16].

8. Fresh frozen plasma. Most guidelines recommend the use of fresh frozen plasma either in massive bleeding or in significant bleeding complicated by coagulopathy (PT or aPTT more then 1.5 times the control level) and stipulate one unit of fresh frozen plasma for every four units of RBCs. A fresh frozen plasma to packed RBC ratio of 1:1 conferred a survival advantage in patients requiring massive transfusion [34].The initial recommended dose of fresh frozen plasma is 10–15 ml/kg. Patients treated with oral anticoagulants (vitamin K antagonists) present a particular challenge, and fresh frozen plasma is recommended only when prothrombin complex concentrate is not available [35]. The administration of fresh frozen plasma may be associated with the risk of ABO incompatibility, volume overload, transmission of infectious diseases, transfusion-related acute lung injury, and allergic reactions.

9. Antifibrinolytic agents. Tranexamic acid is a synthetic lysine analogue that is a competitive inhibitor of plasminogen activation, and at much higher concentrations is a noncompetitive inhibitor of plasmin. Aminocaproic acid is also a synthetic lysine analogue that has potency about ten times weaker in vitro than tranexamic acid. In fact, tranexamic acid binds more strongly than aminocaproic acid to both the strong and the weak receptor sites of the plasminogen molecule in a ratio corresponding to the difference in potency between the compounds.

During elective surgery, it is demonstrated that antifibrinolytic drugs, in particular the lysine analogues, provide reductions in blood loss and minimize allogeneic RBC transfusion during and after surgery. Likely, in these situations, where the patient has bleeding vessels, there is a fibrinolytic turnover that exacerbates the bleeding and can be switched off by antifibrinolytic agents. Antifibrinolytic agents reduce blood loss in patients with both normal and exaggerated fibrinolytic responses to surgery apparently free of serious adverse effects [36]. Because major surgery and trauma trigger a hemostatic response similar to that triggered by severe blood loss, tranexamic acid might reduce bleeding and mortality in trauma patients. The effects of early administration of tranexamic acid on death, vascular occlusive events, and blood transfusion were assessed in a randomized controlled trial undertaken in 274 hospitals in 40 countries involving 20,211 trauma patients with, or at risk of, significant hemorrhage [37]. Patients were randomly assigned within 8 h of injury to receive a loading dose of 1 g of tranexamic acid infused over 10 min, followed by an intravenous infusion of 1 g over 8 h, or matching placebo. All-cause mortality was significantly reduced with tranexamic acid; in particular, the risk of death due to bleeding was reduced. Moreover, there was no apparent increase in fatal or nonfatal vascular occlusive events in patients treated with tranexamic acid.

Monitoring of fibrinolysis is recommended in bleeding trauma patients, and the administration of antifibrinolytic agents is suggested in hyperfibrinolysis [4]. Aprotinin, another antifibrinolytic agent, is no longer recommended because it has been associated with patient safety issues: increased rate of renal disease and mortality [38].

10. Recombinant activated coagulation factor VII (rFVIIa) (NovoSeven, Novo Nordisk), structurally nearly identical to the plasma-derived protein, was approved for the treatment of bleeding in patients with hemophilia A or B who have inhibiting antibodies to coagulation factor VIII or IX [39]. Indications have been extended to the treatment and the prevention of episodes of bleeding in patients with congenital and acquired hemophilia, factor VII deficiency, or Glanzmann's thrombasthenia. The use of rFVIIa in severe trauma is controversial. Coagulopathic bleeding may potentially benefit from rFVIIa-enhanced thrombin generation, but many studies indicated that administration of rFVIIa may be associated with an increased risk of thromboembolic events [40]. Levi et al. [41] found an increased risk of arterial thromboembolic events among patients who received off-label high doses (more than 90 $\mu g/kg$) of rFVIIa as compared with patients who received a placebo for bleeding episodes, but not of venous thromboembolic events, especially among the elderly. The off-label use of rFVIIa can be considered if major bleeding in trauma patients persists despite first-line bleeding corrective measures (transfusion therapy, achievement of adequate levels of fibrinogen and platelets, correction of hypothermia, acidosis, and hypocalcemia) [4]. Standard dosing of rFVIIa is 90 mg/kg intravenous bolus every 2–3 h until cessation of bleeding.

11. Prothrombin complex concentrate. Prothrombin complex concentrate is a combination of blood clotting factors prothrombin and factors VII, IX and X, as well as protein C and protein S. It is recommended for the emergency reversal of the effects of oral anticoagulants.

12. Desmopressin. Desmopressin (1-deamino-8-D-arginine), originally approved for treatment of von Willebrand disease, enhances platelet adherence and platelet aggregate growth on subendothelium. The maximal effect occurs after

90 min. It can be considered in refractory microvascular bleeding if the patient has been treated with platelet-inhibiting drugs (e.g., acetylsalicylic acid). Desmopressin partially reverses hypothermia-induced impairment of primary hemostasis in vitro [42].

Studies have investigated the effect of desmopressin in contexts other than trauma and the same concerns arose with possible thromboembolic complications related to the use of this drug.

In diffusely bleeding patients with suspected thrombocytopathy, intravenous desmopressin administration at a dose of 0.3 mg/kg diluted in 50 ml saline, infused over 30 min, may be considered.

13. Factor XIII. Activated factor XIII is a transglutaminase which cross-links fibrin covalently in the presence of calcium ions. Acquired factor XIII deficiency may be caused by increased turnover (e.g., following intravascular clotting, increased blood loss, hyperfibrinolysis) or by increased consumption (e.g., in major surgery). In cases of bleeding, at least 15–20 U/kg body weight may be substituted until hemostasis is achieved [4].

8.5 The Effects of Fluid Resuscitation on Trauma-Induced Coagulopathy

Critically ill patients frequently demonstrate evidence of inadequate tissue perfusion manifested by anaerobic metabolism and lactic acidosis. In these patients, the primary resuscitation goal is to restore tissue perfusion and cellular oxygenation through volume replacement.

Coagulopathy is often a problem after large-volume fluid resuscitation. The origin of this coagulopathy is multifactorial, and resuscitation fluids contribute by cooling the patient and diluting clotting factors. There is also an interaction between resuscitation fluid molecules and the coagulation system. In particular:

1. Crystalloids appear to have no major deleterious effects on coagulation, although it has been shown that hemodilution per se compromises blood coagulation.
2. Gelatins are large molecular weight proteins formed from hydrolysis of bovine bone collagen. They have the property of dissolving in hot water and forming a jelly when cooled. Gelatins are regarded as having minimal effects on coagulation; nevertheless, there are several studies suggesting impaired clot strength and a decreased rate of clot formation when gelatins are used, particularly at dilutions in excess of 40% [43]. This does not demand the imposition of a dose limit since the half-life of gelatins is short and the molecules are rapidly cleared from the circulation. Gelatins can even be considered to be procoagulants [44].
3. Dextrans are synthesized from sucrose by certain lactic acid bacteria and are complex and branched glucans composed of chains of various lengths (from 3 to 2,000 kDa). The straight chain consists of α-1,6 glycosidic linkages between glucose molecules, whereas branches begin from α-1,3 linkages. Dextrans

negatively influence hemostasis either by reducing the level of von Willebrand factor or by impairing platelet function [45]. When dextran is administered, the levels of both von Willebrand factor antigen and ristocetin cofactor decrease, with reduced binding to platelet membrane receptor proteins glycoprotein Ib and glycoprotein IIb/IIIa. This may result in decreased platelet adhesion.

4. Hydroxyethyl starches (HES) are natural polysaccharides structurally similar to glycogen, composed of long chains of branched glucose polymers (amylopectin) substituted by a hydroxyl radical at either the C2 or the C6 position. The C2 substitution rate is higher because C6 is a branch site of the molecule. The glucose subunits are linked within the chain by α-1,4 glycoside bonds and at the branching point by α-1,6 bonds. The branched molecule is called amylopectin, whereas the unbranched molecule is called amylose. HES preparations differ in four characteristics: concentration of HES in solution, mean molecular weight in vitro, and degree and pattern of hydroxyethylation. The most frequently used concentrations are 6 and 10%. The mean molecular weight is an estimate of the average weight of HES molecules in daltons. HES are divided into high, medium, and low molecular weight HES. The number and not the size of the molecules is responsible for the osmotic effect and, at equal concentration, low molecular weight starches contain more osmotically active molecules. In vivo plasma amylase degrades the initial molecule into lower molecular weight molecules that remain oncotically active. Thus, the in vivo molecular weight, resulting from metabolism of the initial molecule, is the main determinant of the pharmacological properties and safety of HES. Other characteristics of HES are the degree and pattern of hydroxyethylation. The number of substituted hydroxyethyl radicals prevents breakdown by amylase and is expressed by the molar substitution rate, which is a number between 0 and 1. Theoretically, intensely substituted high molecular weight HES should ensure a prolonged expansion property, but is responsible for severe adverse effects such as renal failure and coagulopathies. In particular, the high degree of substitution is related to HES-induced coagulopathies. The glucose groups can be hydroxylated at C2, C3, and C6. Substitution occurs more frequently at the C2 and C6 positions and the C2/C6 ratio represents how many hydroxyethyls are substituted at C2 of glucose compared with C6. The C2/C6 ratio correlates with the in vivo stability of the HES. In fact, as amylase acts at position C1, any substitution close to this site, especially at C2, limits breakdown of the HES molecule. Since HES is a polydisperse solution acting as a colloid, its pharmacodynamic action depends on the number of oncotically active molecules, not on the plasma concentration alone. Solutions with a lower in vivo molecular weight contain more molecules at similar plasma concentrations. On the other hand, high plasma concentrations as well as high in vivo molecular weight can affect blood coagulation, especially for factor VIII and von Willebrand factor [46]. The degree of substitution and the C2/C6 ratio are important for the pharmacokinetics of HES. After the beginning of the infusion, the HES molecules are cleaved by α-amylase and this breakdown generates small molecules and the in vivo molecular weight of HES molecules is different from the initial

8   Coagulative Disturbances in Trauma   121

molecular weight. The in vivo molecular weight depends on the initial size of the molecules and especially on the degree of substitution and the C2/C6 ratio. The in vivo molecular weight, and not the in vitro molecular weight, is decisive for the clinical effect and the side effects. Some HES solutions have been associated with clinical coagulopathies and bleeding when administered in large volumes. As mentioned above, HES molecules are typically characterized by the mean molecular weight, the degree of substitution, and the C2/C6 ratio. These characteristics are also important for the coagulation compromising potency. Highly substituted, high molecular weight starches with high C2/C6 ratios are more likely to induce coagulation derangements than lower molecular weight, lesser substituted starches with lower C2/C6 ratios. Furthermore, it has been suggested that colloids suspended in balanced salt solutions are associated with better coagulation profiles than those in saline [47]. The use of HES solutions with lower molecular weight and lower degree of substitution seems to result in fewer side effects. In particular, solutions of HES with a molecular weight of 200,000 and a degree of substitution of 0.5 (HES 200/0.5) and with a molecular weight of 130,000 and a degree of substitution of 0.4 (HES 130/0.4) have been advocated for their superior safety profile. Moreover, HES 130/0.4 may impair blood coagulation less than other HES solutions. It was found that intravascular volume replacement with 6% HES 130/0.4 at a median dose of 49 ml/kg did not increase postoperative blood loss and perioperative blood transfusion requirements in elective coronary artery bypass surgery compared with 6% HES 200/0.5 at the manufacturer's recommended dose of 33 ml/kg [48]. Recent findings show that HES, specifically HES with a molecular weight of 130,000, a degree of substitution of 0.42, and a C2/C6 ratio of 6:1 (Veno-fundin®), a molecular weight of 130,000, a degree of substitution of 0.4, and a C2/C6 ratio of 9:1 (Voluven®), and a molecular weight of 200,000, a degree of substitution of 0.5, and a C2/C6 of 5:1 (Haes-steril®), shorten the clotting time, inducing a mild hypercoagulable state with faster clotting, but with weaker clot strength as assessed by thromboelastometric analysis [49]. The effects on coagulation are related to interference of HES with factor VIII coagulant activity that disturbs platelet aggregability [50]. The available HES are usually obtained from corn and potato starch. An experimental study suggested that potato-starch-derived HES compromises in vitro blood coagulation more than corn-starch-derived HES [51]. Limiting the dose and duration of HES therapy may be helpful in reducing the risk of undesired side effects.

8.6   Conclusions

In trauma patients, multiple factors contribute to the pathogenesis of coagulopathy, which can be further exacerbated by the administrations of large amounts of fluids to restore arterial pressure. Moreover, in this setting the interpretation of blood coagulation tests can be unreliable since they are performed at a normal pH and temperature, whereas these patients are often hypothermic and acidotic. Besides the surgical repair of the bleeding source, if feasible, the prompt recognition and correction of these latter conditions and the administration of both procoagulant and antifibrinolytic substances are the cornerstones of the treatment.

References

1. Cushing M, Shaz BH (2011) Blood transfusion in trauma patients: unresolved questions. Minerva Anestesiol 77(3):349–359
2. MacLeod JB, Lynn M, McKenney MG, Cohn SM, Murtha M (2003) Early coagulopathy predicts mortality in trauma. J Trauma 55(1):39–44
3. Lier H, Böttiger BW, Hinkelbein J, Krep H, Bernhard M (2011) Coagulation management in multiple trauma: a systematic review. Intensive Care Med 37(4):572–582
4. Rossaint R, Bouillon B, Cerny V, Coats TJ, Duranteau J, Fernández-Mondéjar E, Hunt BJ, Komadina R, Nardi G, Neugebauer E, Ozier Y, Riddez L, Schultz A, Stahel PF, Vincent JL, Spahn DR (2010) Task force for advanced bleeding care in Trauma, management of bleeding following major trauma: an updated European guideline. Crit Care 14(2):R52
5. Spahn DR, Rossaint R (2005) Coagulopathy and blood component transfusion in trauma. Br J Anaesth 95(2):130–139
6. Thorsen K, Ringdal KG, Strand K, Søreide E, Hagemo J, Søreide K (2011) Clinical and cellular effects of hypothermia, acidosis and coagulopathy in major injury. Br J Surg. doi: 10.1002/bjs.7497
7. Wafaisade A, Wutzler S, Lefering R, Tjardes T, Banerjee M, Paffrath T, Bouillon B, Maegele M (2010) Trauma registry of DGU, drivers of acute coagulopathy after severe trauma: a multivariate analysis of 1987 patients. Emerg Med J 27(12):934–939
8. Lynn M, Jeroukhimov I, Klein Y, Martinowitz U (2002) Updates in the management of severe coagulopathy in trauma patients. Intensive Care Med 28(Suppl 2):S241–S247
9. Meng ZH, Wolberg AS, Monroe DM 3rd, Hoffman M (2003) The effect of temperature and pH on the activity of factor VIIa: implications for the efficacy of high-dose factor VIIa in hypothermic and acidotic patients. J Trauma 55:886–891
10. Jurkovich GJ, Greiser WB, Luterman A, Curreri PW (1987) Hypothermia in trauma victims: an ominous predictor of survival. J Trauma 27(9):1019–1024
11. Watts DD, Trask A, Soeken K, Perdue P, Dols S, Kaufmann C (1998) Hypothermic coagulopathy in trauma: effect of varying levels of hypothermia on enzyme speed, platelet function, and fibrinolytic activity. J Trauma 44(5):846–854
12. Kermode JC, Zheng Q, Milner EP (1999) Marked temperature dependence of the platelet calcium signal induced by human von Willebrand factor. Blood 94:199–207
13. Hoyt DB, Junger WG, Loomis WH, Liu FC (1994) Effects of trauma on immune cell function: impairment of intracellular calcium signaling. Shock 2(1):23–28
14. Gando S (2001) Disseminated intravascular coagulation in trauma patients. Semin Thromb Hemost 27(6):585–592
15. Brohi K, Cohen MJ, Ganter MT, Schultz MJ, Levi M, Mackersie RC, Pittet JF (2008) Acute coagulopathy of trauma: hypoperfusion induces systemic anticoagulation and hyperfibrinolysis. J Trauma 64(5):1211–1217
16. Fries D, Martini WZ (2010) Role of fibrinogen in trauma-induced coagulopathy. Br J Anaesth 105(2):116–121
17. Martini WZ, Chinkes DL, Pusateri AE, Holcomb JB, Yu YM, Zhang XJ, Wolfe RR (2005) Acute changes in fibrinogen metabolism and coagulation after hemorrhage in pigs. Am J Physiol Endocrinol Metab 289(5):E930–E934

8 Coagulative Disturbances in Trauma

18. Martini WZ, Holcomb JB (2007) Acidosis and coagulopathy: the differential effects on fibrinogen synthesis and breakdown in pigs. Ann Surg 246(5):831–835
19. Martini WZ (2007) The effects of hypothermia on fibrinogen metabolism and coagulation function in swine. Metabolism 56(2):214–221
20. Mittermayr M, Streif W, Haas T, Fries D, Velik-Salchner C, Klingler A, Oswald E, Bach C, Schnapka-Koepf M, Innerhofer P (2007) Hemostatic changes after crystalloid or colloid fluid administration during major orthopedic surgery: the role of fibrinogen administration. Anesth Analg 105(4):905–917
21. Adam S, Karger R, Kretschmer V (2010) Influence of different hydroxyethyl starch (HES) formulations on fibrinogen measurement in HES-diluted plasma. Clin Appl Thromb Hemost 16(4):454–460
22. Stinger HK, Spinella PC, Perkins JG, Grathwohl KW, Salinas J, Martini WZ, Hess JR, Dubick MA, Simon CD, Beekley AC, Wolf SE, Wade CE, Holcomb JB (2008) The ratio of fibrinogen to red cells transfused affects survival in casualties receiving massive transfusions at an army combat support hospital. J Trauma 64(2 Suppl):S79–S85
23. Bolliger D, Görlinger K, Tanaka KA (2010) Pathophysiology and treatment of coagulopathy in massive hemorrhage and hemodilution. Anesthesiology 113(5):1205–1219
24. Taylor FB Jr, Toh CH, Hoots WK, Wada H, Levi M (2001) Scientific subcommittee on disseminated intravascular coagulation (DIC) of the international society on thrombosis and haemostasis (ISTH), towards definition, clinical and laboratory criteria, and a scoring system for disseminated intravascular coagulation. Thromb Haemost 86(5):1327–1330
25. Hardy JF, de Moerloose P, Samama CM, Membres of the Groupe d'Intérêt en Hémostase Péri opératoire (2006) Massive transfusion and coagulopathy: pathophysiology and implications for clinical management. Can J Anaesth 53(6 Suppl):S40–S58
26. Kaplan LJ, Cheung NH, Maerz L, Lui F, Schuster K, Luckianow G, Davis K (2009) A physicochemical approach to acid-base balance in critically ill trauma patients minimizes errors and reduces inappropriate plasma volume expansion. J Trauma 66(4):1045–1051
27. Vallés J, Santos MT, Aznar J, Martínez M, Moscardó A, Piñón M, Broekman MJ, Marcus AJ (2002) Platelet-erythrocyte interactions enhance alpha(IIb)beta(3) integrin receptor activation and P-selectin expression during platelet recruitment: down-regulation by aspirin ex vivo. Blood 99(11):3978-3984
28. Santos MT, Valles J, Marcus AJ, Safier LB, Broekman MJ, Islam N, Ullman HL, Eiroa AM, Aznar J (1991) Enhancement of platelet reactivity and modulation of eicosanoid production by intact erythrocytes, anew approach to platelet activation and recruitment. J Clin Invest 87(2):571–580
29. Peyrou V, Lormeau JC, Hérault JP, Gaich C, Pfliegger AM, Herbert JM (1999) Contribution of erythrocytes to thrombin generation in whole blood. Thromb Haemost 81(3):400–406
30. Knutson F, Lööf H, Högman CF (1999) Pre-separation storage of whole blood: the effect of temperature on red cell 2,3-diphosphoglycerate and myeloperoxidase in plasma. Transfus Sci 21(2):111–115
31. Armand R, Hess JR (2003) Treating coagulopathy in trauma patients. Transfus Med Rev 17(3):223–231
32. Moore FA, Moore EE, Sauaia A (1997) Blood transfusion, an independent risk factor for postinjury multiple organ failure. Arch Surg 132(6):620–624
33. Silliman CC, Clay KL, Thurman GW, Johnson CA, Ambruso DR (1994) Partial characterization of lipids that develop during the routine storage of blood and prime the neutrophil NADPH oxidase. J Lab Clin Med 124(5):684–694
34. Duchesne JC, Hunt JP, Wahl G, Marr AB, Wang YZ, Weintraub SE, Wright MJ, McSwain NE Jr (2008) Review of current blood transfusions strategies in a mature level I trauma center: were we wrong for the last 60 years? J Trauma 65(2):272–276
35. O'Shaughnessy DF, Atterbury C, Bolton Maggs P, Murphy M, Thomas D, Yates S, Williamson LM, British Committee for Standards in Haematology, Blood Transfusion Task

Force (2004) Guidelines for the use of fresh-frozen plasma, cryoprecipitate and cryosupernatant. Br J Haematol 126(1):11–28

36. Henry DA, Carless PA, Moxey AJ, O'Connell D, Stokes BJ, Fergusson DA, Ker K (2011) Anti-fibrinolytic use for minimising perioperative allogeneic blood transfusion. Cochrane Database Syst Rev (1):CD001886

37. CRASH-2 trial collaborators (2010) Effects of tranexamic acid on death, vascular occlusive events, and blood transfusion in trauma patients with significant haemorrhage (CRASH-2): a randomised, placebo-controlled trial. Lancet 376(9734):23–32

38. Fergusson DA, Hébert PC, Mazer CD, Fremes S, MacAdams C, Murkin JM, Teoh K, Duke PC, Arellano R, Blajchman MA, Bussières JS, Côté D, Karski J, Martineau R, Robblee JA, Rodger M, Wells G, Clinch J, Pretorius R (2008) BART investigators a comparison of aprotinin and lysine analogues in high-risk cardiac surgery. N Engl J Med 358(22):2319–2331

39. Ying CL, Tsang SF, Ng KF (2008) The potential use of desmopressin to correct hypothermia-induced impairment of primary haemostasis—an in vitro study using PFA-100. Resuscitation 76(1):129–133

40. Egli GA, Zollinger A, Seifert B et al (1997) Effect of progressive haemodilution with hydroxyethyl starch, gelatin and albumin on blood coagulation. Br J Anaesth 78:684–689

41. Karoutsos S, Nathan N, Lahrimi A, Grouille D, Feiss P, Cox DJ (1999) Thrombelastogram reveals hypercoagulability after administration of gelatin solution. Br J Anaesth 82(2):175–177

42. Wagner BK, D'Amelio LF (1993) Pharmacologic and clinical considerations in selecting crystalloid, colloidal, and oxygen-carrying resuscitation fluids. Part 1. Clin Pharmacol 12:335–346

43. Jungheinrich C, Neff TA (2005) Pharmacokinetics of hydroxyethyl starch. Clin Pharmacokinet 44(7):681–699

44. Roche AM, James MF, Bennett-Guerrero E, Mythen MG (2006) A head-to-head comparison of the in vitro coagulation effects of saline-based and balanced electrolyte crystalloid and colloid intravenous fluids. Anesth Analg 102(4):1274–1279

45. Kasper SM, Meinert P, Kampe S, Görg C, Geisen C, Mehlhorn U, Diefenbach C (2003) Large-dose hydroxyethyl starch 130/0.4 does not increase blood loss and transfusion requirements in coronary artery bypass surgery compared with hydroxyethyl starch 200/0.5 at recommended doses. Anesthesiology 99(1):42–47

46. Zdolsek HJ, Vegfors M, Lindahl TL, Törnquist T, Bortnik P, Hahn RG (2011) Hydroxyethyl starches and dextran during hip replacement surgery: effects on blood volume and coagulation. Acta Anaesthesiol Scand. doi: 10.1111/j.1399-6576.2011.02434

47. Türkan H, Ural AU, Beyan C, Yalçin A (1999) Effects of hydroxyethyl starch on blood coagulation profile. Eur J Anaesthesiol 16(3):156–159

48. Jamnicki M, Zollinger A, Seifert B, Popovic D, Pasch T, Spahn DR (1998) The effect of potato starch derived and corn starch derived hydroxyethyl starch on in vitro blood coagulation. Anaesthesia 53(7):638–644

49. Hedner U (2000) NovoSeven as a universal haemostatic agent. Blood Coagul Fibrinolysis 11:S107–S111

50. Levi M, Levy JH, Andersen HF, Truloff D (2010) Safety of recombinant activated factor VII in randomized clinical trials. N Eng J Med 363:1791–1800

51. Levi M, Peters M, Buller HR (2005) Efficacy and safety of recombinant factor VIIa for treatment of severe bleeding: a systematic review. Crit Care Clin 33:883–890

Hypothermia and Coagulation Disorders

9

Lara Prisco, Vincenzo Campanile and Giorgio Berlot

9.1 Introduction

Hypothermia describes a state in which the body's mechanism for temperature regulation is overwhelmed in the face of a cold stressor. Hypothermia is classified as accidental or intentional, primary or secondary, and according to its severity:

- Accidental hypothermia generally results from unanticipated exposure in an inadequately prepared person.
- Intentional hypothermia is an induced state generally directed at neuroprotection after an at-risk situation (usually after cardiac arrest, see later) [1].
- Primary hypothermia is due to environmental exposure, with no underlying medical condition causing disruption of temperature regulation [2].
- Secondary hypothermia is caused by a medical illness lowering the temperature set-point.
- Mild hypothermia (32–35°C): Between 34 and 35°C, most people shiver vigorously. As the temperature drops below 34°C, patients may develop altered judgment, amnesia, and dysarthria. Respiratory rate may increase. At approximately 33°C, ataxia and apathy may be seen. Patients are generally stable hemodynamically and able to compensate for the symptoms. In this temperature range, hyperventilation, tachypnea, tachycardia, and cold-induced diuresis may also be observed.
- Moderate hypothermia (28–32°C): Oxygen consumption decreases, and the central nervous system (CNS) is further depressed, and hypoventilation,

L. Prisco (✉)
Department of Anaesthesiology, Intensive Care and Emergency Medicine,
Cattinara Hospital, University of Trieste, Trieste, Italy
e-mail: priscolara@gmail.com

G. Berlot (ed.), *Hemocoagulative Problems in the Critically Ill Patient*,
DOI: 10.1007/978-88-470-2448-9_9, © Springer-Verlag Italia 2012

125

hyporeflexia, decreased renal flow, and paradoxical undressing may be observed. As the core temperature reaches 31°C or below, the body loses its ability to generate heat by shivering. At 30°C, patients are at risk of arrhythmias. Atrial fibrillation and other atrial and ventricular rhythms are frequently observed. The heart rate progressively slows, and the cardiac output is reduced. Between 28 and 30°C, pupils may become markedly dilated and minimally responsive to light, a condition that can mimic brain death.

- Severe hypothermia (below 28°C): At 28°C, the body becomes markedly susceptible to ventricular fibrillation and further depression of myocardial contractility. Below 27°C, 83% of patients are comatose. Pulmonary edema, oliguria, coma, hypotension, rigidity, apnea, pulselessness, areflexia, unresponsiveness, fixed pupils, and decreased or absent activity on an electroencephalogram are all seen.

9.2 History

Hypothermia is usually readily apparent in the setting of severe environmental exposure. In elderly patients or "indoor" patients, or in a patient (particularly a wet patient) with exposure to less extreme cold, symptoms may be subtle and less obvious. These patients may have a higher mortality rate secondary to a longer time to diagnosis and increased age and fragility. Mild or moderate hypothermia can present with misleading symptoms, such as confusion, dizziness, chills, and dyspnea.

In an urban environment, the use of alcohol or illicit drugs, drug overdose, psychiatric emergency, and major trauma all are associated with an increased risk of hypothermia.

9.3 Epidemiology

The greatest number of cases of hypothermia occur in an urban setting and are related to environmental exposure attributed to alcoholism, illicit drug use, or mental illness, often exacerbated by concurrent homelessness. Another affected group includes people in an outdoor setting for work or leisure, including hunters, skiers, climbers, boaters/rafters, and swimmers. The estimated overall in-patient mortality in hypothermic patients is 12%. A multicenter survey found a 21% mortality rate for patients with moderate hypothermia (28–32°C body temperature). Mortality is even higher in severe hypothermia (core temperature below 28°C) and despite hospital-based treatment, mortality from moderate or severe hypothermia approaches 40%. Patients experiencing concurrent infection account for most deaths due to hypothermia. Other comorbidities associated with higher mortality rates include homelessness, alcoholism, psychiatric disease, and advanced age.

9 Hypothermia and Coagulation Disorders

9.4 Causes

- Decreased heat production. Several causes related to endocrine derangements may cause decreased heat production, including hypopituitarism, hypoadrenalism, and hypothyroidism. Other causes include severe malnutrition or hypoglycemia and neuromuscular inefficiencies seen in the extremes of age.
- Increased heat loss. This category includes accidental hypothermia due to either immersion or circumstances not associated with immersion, and is the most common cause of hypothermia encountered in the emergency department. Drug- or toxin-induced vasodilatation may facilitate the heat loss. Skin lesion, including erythroderma, burns, or psoriasis, decreases the body's ability to preserve heat.
- Impaired thermoregulation. Many causes may impair the thermoregulation, and, generally, include CNS trauma, strokes, metabolic derangements, intracranial bleeding, Parkinson's disease, CNS tumors, Wernicke disease, and multiple sclerosis.
- Other causes. Miscellaneous causes include sepsis, multiple trauma, pancreatitis, prolonged cardiac arrest, and uremia

  Hypothermia may be related to drug administration; such medications include beta-blockers, clonidine, meperidine, neuroleptics, and general anesthetic agents. Ethanol, phenothiazines, and sedative hypnotics also reduce the body's ability to respond to low ambient temperatures. Another often-overlooked cause of hypothermia is the administration of large amounts intravenous fluids during the resuscitation from hypovolemic shock.

9.5 Pathophysiology

The body's core temperature is tightly regulated in the "thermoneutral zone" between 36.5 and 37.5°C, outside of which thermoregulatory responses are usually activated. The body maintains a stable core temperature through balancing heat production and heat loss. At rest, humans produce 40–60 kcal of heat per square meter of body surface area through generation by cellular metabolism, most prominently in the liver and the heart. Heat production increases with striated muscle contraction; shivering increases the rate of heat production two to five times.

Heat loss occurs via several mechanisms, the most significant of which, under dry conditions, is radiation (55–65% of heat loss). Conduction and convection account for about 15% of additional heat loss, and respiration and evaporation account for the remainder. Conductive and convective heat loss, or direct transfer of heat to another object or circulating air, respectively, are the most common causes of accidental hypothermia. Conduction is a particularly significant mechanism of heat loss in drowning/immersion accidents as the thermal conductivity of water is up to 30 times that of air. The hypothalamus controls

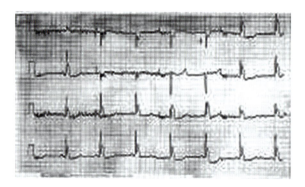

Fig. 9.1 Osborne (J) waves (V_3) in a patient with a rectal core temperature of 26.7°C

thermoregulation via increased heat conservation (peripheral vasoconstriction and behavior responses) and heat production (shivering and increasing levels of thyroxine and epinephrine). Alterations of the CNS may impair these mechanisms. The threshold for shivering is 1°C lower than that for vasoconstriction and is considered a last-resort mechanism by the body to maintain temperature [3]. The mechanisms for heat preservation may be overwhelmed in the face of cold stress and the core temperature can drop secondary to fatigue or glycogen depletion. Hypothermia affects virtually all organ systems. Perhaps the most significant effects are seen in the cardiovascular system and the CNS. Hypothermia results in decreased depolarization of cardiac pacemaker cells, causing bradycardia. Since this bradycardia is not vagally mediated, it can be refractory to standard therapies such as atropine. Mean arterial pressure and cardiac output decrease, and an electrocardiogram may show characteristic J or Osborne waves (see Fig. 9.1). Although it is generally associated with hypothermia, the J wave may be a normal variant and is seen occasionally in sepsis and myocardial ischemia.

Atrial and ventricular arrhythmias can result from hypothermia; asystole and ventricular fibrillation have been noted to begin spontaneously at core temperatures below 25–28°C.

Hypothermia progressively depresses the CNS, decreasing CNS metabolism in a linear fashion as the core temperature drops. At a core temperatures less than 33°C, brain electrical activity becomes abnormal; between 19 and 20°C, an electroencephalogram may appear consistent with brain death. Tissues have decreased oxygen consumption at lower temperatures; it is not clear whether this is due to decreases in metabolic rate at lower temperatures or a greater hemoglobin affinity for oxygen coupled with impaired oxygen extraction of hypothermic tissues.

The term "core temperature afterdrop" refers to a further decrease in core temperature and associated clinical deterioration of a patient after rewarming has been initiated. The current theory of this documented phenomenon is that as peripheral tissues are warmed, vasodilation allows cooler blood in the extremities to circulate back into the body core. Other mechanisms may be in operation as well.

9 Hypothermia and Coagulation Disorders

9.6 Hypothermia-Induced Disturbances of Coagulation

Previous studies reported that hypothermia is accompanied by an impairment of the coagulation system and state that factor activity is severely impaired below 30°C, e.g., at 25°C clotting activity ranges from 0 (factors VIII and IX) to 5% (prothrombin and factor VII). There are also studies showing that standard clotting tests, e.g., activated partial thromboplastin time (aPTT), are impaired at low temperatures [4–6]. Therefore, disturbances of blood coagulation represent a major risk during both accidental and therapeutic hypothermia. Several factors have been proposed to contribute to this coagulopathy in hypothermic patients, including dysregulation of clotting factors and platelets, activation of fibrinolysis, and endothelial injury. Moreover, routine coagulative tests may fail to reveal its presence. Actually, standard clinical clotting assays, including the aPTT, prothrombin time (PT), and thrombin time (TT), are performed on platelet-poor plasma at 37°C. Clotting times of plasma are prolonged when the clotting assays are performed at lower temperatures; hence, it has been suggested that these assays should be performed at the core temperature of the patient to assess the true function of the coagulation system in a given patient. However, this approach does not take into consideration the fact that in vivo coagulation occurs on the surfaces of platelets and endothelial cells, which are also affected by temperature. Thus, traditional clotting times do not reflect any alteration in platelet function that might contribute to a coagulopathy. Several studies, however, have suggested that both quantitative and qualitative platelet abnormalities are involved in hypothermia-related coagulopathy. Studies have suggested that hypothermia-associated thrombocytopenia results from sequestering of platelets in the liver. Likewise, the reduction in coagulation factor enzyme activities and cold-induced platelet abnormalities are reversible on warming; the numbers and half-life of platelets return to normal after rewarming of hypothermic animals and humans. Most of the studies on the effects of hypothermia on platelet functions were done at temperatures below 30°C and therefore may not reflect platelet function at clinically relevant degrees of hypothermia. Therefore, it seems likely that hypothermia-related coagulopathy results from a combined effect of platelet and enzyme dysregulation. Thromboelastographic assays, which evaluate both platelet and enzyme function, show prolonged reaction and coagulation times and decreased clot formation rates at reduced assay temperature. However, few studies have used assay systems that evaluate enzyme and platelet functions simultaneously and attempted to separate the relative contributions of platelet and enzyme function to hypothermic coagulopathy. The impairment is more pronounced for the variables reflecting the humoral part of the coagulation than for maximum clot firmness, which is primarily related to platelet activity. In a rabbit study using thromboelastography (TEG) and Sonoclot analysis, Shimokawa et al. [7] found that coagulation was impaired at 30°C as compared with normal temperature. However, the differences disappeared when coagulation tests were performed at 37°C, even though the blood was drawn at a body temperature of 30°C. They also found that the platelet count decreased after cooling, and speculated whether this could be a contributing cause of the coagulation impairment. However, the effects of hypothermia on single factor activity are known already [4, 5]. The impact of induced hypothermia on coagulation within the range used after cardiac arrest produced minimal effects, but clinical studies have shown a significant increase in blood loss when the temperature was decreased from 36.4 to 35.0°C. However, the effects of relatively mild hypothermia (35.5°C) in trauma patients may have profound effects, and may increase mortality in this patient population [8].

Other studies have also found increased mortality and bleeding in hypothermic patients, and Jeremitsky et al. [9] found hypothermia to independently predict worse outcome after traumatic brain injury. Dirkmann et al. [10] investigated the combined effect on coagulation of hypothermia and acidosis using human whole blood and measurements by thromboelastometry. They showed that initiation and propagation of coagulation, as well as the stability of a formed blood clot, are impaired by hypothermia but not by acidosis under normothermia. However, hypothermia and acidosis occurring together synergistically impair coagulation. Interestingly, when combining hypothermia and acidosis, they found that the impact of acidosis is more important at a lower temperature, and that hypothermia and acidosis interact to impair coagulation variables except clot lysis [10].

9.7 Blood Coagulation Tests in Hypothermic Patients

As stated already, hypothermia both slows the reactions of the coagulation cascade and inhibits platelet function [11]. Since TEG and most other coagulation studies are performed at 37°C regardless of the patient's body temperature, the results of these tests may not be representative of the patient's coagulation status when hypothermia develops. TEG has been recognized as a readily available, qualitative monitor to provide bedside information on the patient's coagulation status. Performing TEG at the patient's actual body temperature rather than 37°C produces significant changes in the reaction time, coagulation time, and clot formation rate.

The maximum amplitude, a reflection of the absolute strength of the clot, was not significantly affected by temperature correction in some investigations [12, 13]. Prolongation of the reaction time and coagulation time and reduction of the clot formation rate in these temperature-corrected thromboelastographic assays on hypothermic patients confirms the observations that hypothermia contributes to coagulopathy. The reaction time (r) represents the time necessary for building up the first fibrin strands, k represents the time to reach a certain clot strength, and α represents the formation rate of the clot. The reaction time is dependent mainly on coagulation factor activity, whereas k and α depend on plasma coagulation and the interaction of platelets with fibrin, increasing clot stability. Impairment of these variables by temperature reduction indicates a reduction in activity of both coagulation factors and platelet function. In patients undergoing cardio-pulmonary bypass (CPB), r, k, and α are affected by a temperature reduction of

9 Hypothermia and Coagulation Disorders

3.7°C, leading to an approximate 50% reduction in coagulation, whereas performing heparinase-modified TEG at 37°C in hypothermic patients may lead to underestimation of coagulopathy during CPB when hypothermia is not considered [14]. Similar results have been reported in hypothermic patients during liver transplantation [12].

However, temperature-adjusted TEG could lead to inappropriate therapeutic interventions if prolongation in TEG is caused by hypothermia and this is treated with administration of coagulation factor. Therefore, it seems appropriate to treat patients with coagulation factors or platelets only when the results of normothermic TEG are abnormal.

In the treatment of hypothermic patients with bleeding disorders, comparison of temperature-adapted and normothermic TEG can help to guide therapeutic interventions, including the administration of coagulation factors, the transfusion of platelets, and active rewarming.

As mentioned already, the maximum amplitude reflects absolute clot strength and not coagulation time, unlike r and k. Temperatures between 33 and 37°C do not affect the maximum amplitude. This finding, together with increased r and k values and a smaller α value, indicates a decrease in the speed of clot formation, but not absolute deterioration in clot quality, which is represented by the maximum amplitude. In the course of surgery, the maximum amplitude decreased for normothermic and temperature-adapted measurements in the same manner. This indicates that TEG is able to detect impairment of platelet function caused by surgery and the extracorporeal circulation.

In a study on active cooling by Kettner et al. [14], the platelet count decreased, however a reduction of the platelet count by the administered fluids seemed unlikely. A decrease in platelet count during active cooling has been described in dogs, where a body temperature reduction to 32°C caused an approximately 70% decrease in platelet count. This decrease was caused by pooling of platelets in the spleen.

Two sets of investigators showed prolongation in plasma coagulation tests caused by in vitro reduction of the assay temperature [4, 6]. The TT was less prolonged than the PT and the aPPT. It was concluded that there may be a cumulative effect in multistep assays, such as the PT and the aPPT, leading to greater prolongation than in one-step assays, such as the TT. Prolongation of approximately 50–60% of the PT and the aPPT was found at 29 and 28°C, respectively. Other studies demonstrated 50–60% prolongation of TEG variables at 33.3°C.

TEG is a global assessment of hemostatic function, documenting the interaction of platelets with the protein of the coagulation cascade from the time of initial fibrin formation through platelet aggregation, clot strengthening, and fibrin cross linkage to eventual clot lysis. It is a multistep assay of many more stages than plasma coagulation tests such as the PT and the aPPT.

The high sensitivity of this technique to temperature may be caused by cumulative slowing of the enzymatic steps of coagulation, as assessed by TEG. Alternatively, either interaction of platelets with coagulation proteins or platelet function per se might be especially sensitive to the efforts of hypothermia.

Hypothermia-induced reversible platelet dysfunction was shown in an animal study by Valeri et al. [11]. In patients undergoing CPB, hypothermia reduced intraoperative platelet function and platelet recovery in the postbypass period [15]. In that study, aprotinin reduced the negative effects of hypothermic CPB on platelet function. Impairment of TEG variables by temperature may be even higher when no aprotinin is given. Furthermore, aprotinin reduces clot lysis, as assessed by TEG. In summary, Kettner et al. [13] demonstrated reductions in coagulation caused by hypothermia, indicating the high sensitivity of TEG to temperature.

All these studies suggest that performing thromboelastographic assays in the standard fashion may overestimate the quality of the coagulation system in vivo when the patient's temperature is less than 37°C. The temperature-corrected TEG may with further study be used to help differentiate a coagulopathy in a hypothermic patient that can be alleviated by warming the patient from one that requires treatment with blood products. Theoretically, the addition of blood products may not improve a hypothermia-induced coagulopathy and may be an unwarranted treatment.

References

1. Polderman KH (2009) Mechanisms of action, physiological effects, and complications of hypothermia. Crit Care Med 37(Suppl 7):S186–S202
2. Long WB 3rd et al (2005) Cold injuries. J Long Term Eff Med Implants 15(1):67–78
3. Sessler DI (2009) Thermoregulatory defense mechanisms. Crit Care Med 37(Suppl 7): S203–S210
4. Reed RL et al (1990) Hypothermia and blood coagulation: dissociation between enzyme activity and clotting factor levels. Circul Shock 32:141–152
5. Wolberg AS et al (2004) A systematic evaluation of the effect of temperature on coagulation enzyme activity and platelet function. J Trauma 56:1221–1228
6. Rohrer MJ, Natale AM (1992) Effect of hypothermia on the coagulation cascade. Crit Care Med 20:1402–1405
7. Shimokawa M et al (2003) The influence of induced hypothermia for hemostatic function on temperature-adjusted measurements in rabbits. Anesth Analg 96:1209–1213
8. Krishna G et al (1998) Physiological predictors of death in exsanguinating trauma patients undergoing conventional trauma surgery. Aust N Z J Surg 68:826–829
9. Jeremitsky E et al (2003) Harbingers of poor outcome the day after severe brain injury: hypothermia, hypoxia, and hypoperfusion. J Trauma 54:312–319
10. Dirkmann D, Hanke AA, Gorlinger K, Peters J (2008) Hypothermia and acidosis synergistically impair coagulation in human whole blood. Anesth Analg 106(6):1627–1632
11. Valeri CR et al (1992) Effect of skin temperature on platelet function in patients undergoing extracorporeal bypass. Cardiovasc Surg 104:108–116
12. Douning LK et al (1995) Temperature corrected thromboelastography in hypothermic patients. Anesth Analg 81:608–611
13. Kettner SC et al (1998) Effects of hypothermia on thromboelastography in patients undergoing cardiopulmonary bypass. Br J Anaesth 80:313–317
14. Kettner SC et al (2003) The effect of graded hypotermia (36°C–32°C) on hemostasis in anesthetized patients without surgical trauma. Anesth Analg 96:1772–1776
15. Boldt J et al (1993) Platelet function in cardiac surgery: influence of temperature and parotinin. Ann Thoracic Surg 55:652–658

Hemostasis in Pregnancy and Obstetric Surgery

10

Marinella Astuto, Valentina Taranto and Simona Grasso

10.1 Hemostatic Changes in Pregnancy

Normal pregnancy is associated with changes in all aspects of hemostasis, including an increase in concentrations of most clotting factors, decreasing concentrations of some of the natural anticoagulants, and diminishing fibrinolytic activity. These changes help in maintaining placental function during pregnancy and meeting delivery's hemostatic challenge, but may predispose to thrombosis and placental vascular complications [1].

10.1.1 Coagulation Factors

Changes in procoagulants

A large number of longitudinal and cross-sectional studies of hemostasis in normal pregnancy have shown that increasing gestation is associated with a progressive increase in the plasma concentrations of fibrinogen (factor I) [2–4], factor VII [2], factor VIII [2–4], von Willebrand factor antigen and ristocetin cofactor activity [3], factor X [2], and factor XII [3, 5]. No consistent change in the concentrations of factor V [2, 3, 6–9] and factor IX [3, 6, 7] occurs, and a reduction in the concentration of factor XI has been reported in several studies [3, 7, 10]. In contrast, a separate study has also shown that during pregnancy the concentrations of coagulation factors V and IX rise significantly (Table 10.1) [1].

M. Astuto (✉)
Department of Anesthesia and Intensive Care,
Pediatric Anesthesia and Intensive Care Section,
"Policlinico" University Hospital, Catania, Italy
e-mail: astmar@tiscali.it

G. Berlot (ed.), *Hemocoagulative Problems in the Critically Ill Patient*,
DOI: 10.1007/978-88-470-2448-9_10, © Springer-Verlag Italia 2012

Table 10.1 Hemostatic change during pregnancy

Systemic changes	Increased concentration	Decreased concentration	No change in concentration
Procoagulant factors	Fibrinogen, factors V, VII, VIII, IX, X	Factor XI	
Anticoagulant factors	Soluble TM	PS	PC
Adhesive proteins	vWF		
Fibrinolytic proteins	PAI-1, PAI-2	t-PA	TAFI
MPs and APAs	MPs		APAs
Local placental changes	TF	TFPI	

MPs microparticles, *APAs* antiphospholipid antibodies, *TM* thrombomodulin, *vWF* von Wille-brand factor, *PAI* plasminogen activator inhibitor, *TF* tissue factor, *PS* protein S, *t-PA* tissue plasminogen activator, *TFPI* tissue factor pathway inhibitor, *PC* protein C, *TAFI* thrombin-activated fibrinolytic inhibitor

Changes in anticoagulations

The physiological anticoagulant system plays a critical role during pregnancy. Neutrophil activation is known to trigger endothelial thrombomodulin proteolysis and to increase soluble thrombomodulin levels in late pregnancy. Thrombomodulin levels at the 12th week of gestation are similar in all pregnancies, but the wide range for each period thereafter makes a thrombomodulin reference curve difficult to use for predicting an adverse event in an individual woman. However, given the thrombomodulin baseline value for a particular woman, a sudden increase could indicate an underlying placental vascular disorder [11].

There are conflicting findings from studies concerning protein C; in fact, some studies show that protein C activity appears to be unaffected by gestation [12–15]. A number of studies have shown no difference in protein C antigen [14, 16–18] or activity [4, 8, 9, 19, 20] in pregnancy. The reason for the disparity reflects the different technologies used [4, 19–21].

Protein S normally exists in plasma in two forms: the functionally active, free protein S and protein S complexes with C4b-binding protein, which is inactive. An increase in the level of C4b-binding protein has been noted during pregnancy. Although the fall in free protein S levels in pregnancy is a physiological event, it is still unresolved whether it contributes to the hypercoagulable state and the increased incidence of gestational thromboembolism. Pregnancy results in a fall in free and total protein S levels [3, 15, 17, 22–25]. In studies conducted before the understanding of the interaction between activated protein C (APC) resistance and protein S functional assays, a reduction in protein S activity was also reported to occur with increasing gestation [20, 23]. Notably, the apparent fall in protein S levels during the first week of pregnancy is a major problem in the diagnosis of inherited protein S deficiency in women. A large body of evidence suggests that APC resistance also plays a key role in pregnancy-related vascular complications [26]. APC resistance is found in association with factor V Leiden mutation or as an acquired state in association with antiphospholipid antibodies (APAs) or cancer [27, 28]. Hormonal changes in pregnancy or during oral contraceptive use or hormone replacement therapy [29, 30] are also associated with APC resistance. The APC sensitivity ratio is reduced during pregnancy [29]; at term, 45% of pregnant women have an APC sensitivity ratio below the 95th percentile of the normal range for nonpregnant women of similar age [31]. Low APC ratios early in pregnancy were observed in subjects who subsequently developed gestational complications, such as pregnancy loss, preeclampsia, and placental abruption [32]. As many as 57% of healthy women developed APC resistance, which reached its lowest value by 28 weeks of gestation. Lower ratios in the classic APC resistance test have been reported during pregnancy, and this phenomenon has been called "acquired" APC resistance [9, 33, 34]. Asymptomatic pregnant carriers of the factor V Leiden mutation did not exhibit a more pronounced coagulation activation than noncarriers, although the higher levels of D-dimer in carriers do indicate an increased fibrin formation and fibrinolytic system activation [35]. A prospective study from Sweden demonstrated an eightfold higher risk of venous thromboembolism (VTE) but a lower rate of profuse intrapartum hemorrhage, which potentially could confer evolutionary advantage [9]. Whereas both factor VIII and protein S could contribute to APC resistance, in a cross-sectional study no correlation was found between the decrease in the classic APC ratio and the free fraction of protein S levels [33]. In pregnancy, a gestation-independent positive relationship of APC resistance with cholesterol, antithrombin, and protein C activity and an inverse relationship with total protein S have also been reported [32].

10.1.2 Thrombin and Fibrin Generation

Thrombin is a serine protease that is responsible for fibrin formation, platelet activation, activation of factor XIII, and the feedback activation of clotting factors V and VIII. As prothrombin is cleaved by activated factor X to form thrombin, a fragment is released. This fragment is called prothrombin fragment $1 + 2$ and can be measured in plasma [36]. Thrombin formation can also be assessed by the circulating level of the complex that it forms with its principal inhibitor, antithrombin (thrombin–antithrombin, TAT, complex) [36]. An increase in TAT complex formation occurs in normal pregnancy. TAT complex levels higher than nonpregnant control values have been reported to be present in 50% of women during the first trimester, with all subjects showing elevated levels in the second and third trimesters [25, 37, 38]. A significant positive correlation between gestational stage and prothrombin fragment $1 + 2$ has also been shown, with levels elevated beyond those of nonpregnant subjects seen early in pregnancy [4, 39, 40]. Delorme et al. [41] have shown that plasma from pregnant women, in in vitro experiments, is capable of more rapid and elevated generation of thrombin than plasma from nonpregnant women. This result, in combination with evidence of an increase in prothrombin activation and TAT complex formation in the absence of any increase in antithrombin levels, suggests that heightened thrombin generation may be a feature of normal pregnancy and, it has been suggested, may indicate a prothrombotic state [42, 43]. Thrombomodulin, a proteoglycan that acts as a thrombin receptor, is found on maternal vascular endothelial cells and on the trophoblastic surface of the placenta [44]. The formation of a thrombin–thrombomodulin complex on the endothelial surface accelerates thrombin activation of the natural anticoagulant protein C approximately 20,000-fold [45]. Formation of this complex directly inhibits the capacity of thrombin to cleave fibrinogen and activate platelets [45–48]. A soluble form of thrombomodulin exists in plasma and urine and has been widely used as a marker of endothelial damage [49, 50]. Normal pregnancy may be associated with an increase in soluble thrombomodulin levels, but the relationship between this cleaved form and the overall anticoagulant effect of thrombin (via APC generation) is unknown [11]. APC is known to be regulated by several inhibitors, including protein C inhibitor 1 [51], α_1-antitrypsin [52], α_2-antiplasmin, C1 esterase inhibitor [53], and α_2-macroglobulin [54]. It is possible to assess the activity of thrombin on protein C activation by measuring APC [55], by measuring the peptide released from protein C on activation [56], or by measuring complexes of APC with its inhibitor α_1-antitrypsin [52]. An increase in the level of APC–α_1-antitrypsin in the third trimester to near double the level observed in the first trimester has been reported to occur in normal pregnancy [18]. In this study, APC–α_1-antitrypsin levels did not correlate with α_1-antitrypsin levels. This suggests that increasing gestation is associated with an increase in the activation of protein C and therefore an increase in thrombin-mediated antithrombotic activity.

10.1.3 Fibrinolytic System

Plasma fibrinolytic activity is reduced during pregnancy, remains low during labor and delivery, but returns to normal shortly after delivery [2]. Tissue plasminogen activator activity decreases during pregnancy [57]. This is due not only to the gradual increase in plasminogen activator inhibitor 1 (PAI-1; normalizes after the postpartum period) [25], but probably mainly to the increasing levels of plasminogen activator inhibitor 2 (PAI-2), originally discovered in human placenta [58–60]. PAI-2 plasma level generally becomes detectable only in pregnant women. Because villus cells are the source of PAI-2 [61, 62], changes in the amount of placental tissue may influence its plasma level [37]; the concentration of PAI-2 differs with birth weight, indicating a dependency not only upon the quantity and quality of the placental tissues but also upon fetal growth and development [37, 63].

10.1.4 Placental Hemostasis

The hemostatic changes that occur in the uteroplacental circulation during pregnancy induce physiological adaptation in uterine spiral arteries, which are required to accommodate the increased maternal blood flow to the intervillus space. Much of the vascular endothelium and the underlying medial smooth muscle is replaced by trophoblasts. Fibrin deposition sites were identified in decidual veins at sites of trophoblast invasion, where villi are implanted into veins [64]. Compared with endothelial vasculature, the trophoblasts lining decidual spiral arteries have a reduced capacity to lyse fibrin, and studies have shown that this is caused by high levels of plasminogen activator inhibitors [65]. In addition, perivascular decidualized human endometrial stromal cells are ideally positioned to prevent postimplantation hemorrhage during endovascular trophoblast invasion by expressing tissue factor (TF), which is a primary cellular mediator of hemostasis. It was demonstrated that paracrine factors, such as endothelial growth factor, are involved in steroid-enhancing TF expression in human endometrial stromal cells through the endothelial growth factor receptor [66].

Notably, several coagulation components, such as TF and thrombomodulin, are involved not only in hemostasis but also in placental blood vessel differentiation. Studies have shown that syncytiotrophoblast cells in primary culture express large amounts of TF that can be modulated by cytokines [67]. Teleologically, the presence of large amounts of TF seems to be essential for the maintenance of hemostasis in the placenta. This, however, may predispose to placental vascular complications, particularly in the setting of maternal thrombophilia [68].

10.1.5 Microparticles

Microparticles (MPs) are membrane nanofragments (0.05–1 µm) with procoagulant and proinflammatory properties [69] that are shed from various cellular surfaces. There are two mechanisms that can result in MP formation: cell activation and apoptosis. They expose membrane antigens that are specific for the cells from which they are derived [70]. Endothelial cells produce MPs when the cells are exposed to cytokines, such as interleukin-1 and tumor necrosis factor. Endothelial MPs are detectable in normal human blood and their levels are increased in patients with a coagulation abnormality associated with the lupus anticoagulant [71], and in acute coronary syndromes [72]. Circulating platelet MP concentration is a marker of platelet activation. Monocyte-derived MPs express TF, P-selectin glycoprotein ligand 1, and CD14. Normal pregnancy is characterized by increased levels of platelets and endothelial MPs compared with the levels in nonpregnant healthy women but the prevalence and the role of MPs in gestational vascular complications remains controversial [73]. Laude et al. [74] found a high prevalence of increased levels of procoagulant MPs in pregnancy loss groups compared with healthy pregnant women. In pathological pregnancies, Bretelle et al. [73] found a significant reduction in the number of platelet MPs in preeclampsia but suggested that the MPs that remain in the circulation are procoagulant. Significantly fewer absolute numbers of platelet MPs were found in women with preeclampsia than in the normal pregnancy control group [75]. Thrombin generation by MPs was similar in normal and preeclamptic pregnancies but the numbers of T-cell and granulocyte MPs were increased in preeclampsia [76, 77]. Syncytiotrophoblast microvilli are shed into the maternal circulation (microvillus deportation) and are present in significantly increased amounts in preeclamptic women [78].

In conclusion, pregnancy is associated with an upregulation of the maternal coagulation cascade that results in an overall increase in thrombin generation. It is likely that placental and maternal thrombin generation have an important function as a cellular growth factor in the developing fetoplacental unit resulting in fibrin formation, which is essential for placental implantation. The maternal alteration in coagulation is clearly a physiological rather than a pathological response. Although there is some evidence that the thrombotic/antithrombotic balance of early pregnancy may be a marker for the development of subsequent vascular disorders such as preeclampsia, a link between the physiological alterations in coagulation and thrombosis remains unproved. Indeed, one study has shown that, despite the progressive changes in coagulation associated with increasing gestation, the risk of venous thrombosis may be equal in the first and second trimesters. It appears likely that the presence of an acquired or inherited thrombophilia will upset this delicate balance of thrombin/fibrin generation and fibrinolysis in pregnancy and increase the risk of thrombosis-linked disorders [79].

10.2 Thrombophilias and Venous Thromboembolism

Pregnancy is considered to be a hypercoagulable state and encompasses all three elements of Virchow's triad. Coagulation anomalies play an important role in adverse pregnancy outcome. Complications which occur during pregnancy are the cause of morbidity and mortality and necessitate medical intervention aimed at improving the fetal and maternal outcome.

Thrombophilias are a hemostatic disorder, classified as inherited or acquired, which affect about 15% of the Caucasian population predisposed to a thrombotic phenomenon [80].

Hereditary disorders include deficiencies of antithrombin III, deficiencies of proteins C and S, genetic mutations such as factor V Leiden, prothrombin gene G20210A, and the thermolabile variant of the methylenetetrahydrofolate reductase (MTHFR) C677T gene [81].

Acquired disorders include thrombophilias and are due to APAs, which include lupus anticoagulant and anticardiolipin antibodies [80]. Data suggest that at least 50% of cases of VTE [82] in pregnant women are associated with an inherited or acquired thrombophilia [83, 84].

Thrombophilias have been investigated in relation to the following obstetric complications: recurrent and nonrecurrent miscarriages in early or late pregnancy, intrauterine death, intrauterine growth retardation (IUGR), placental abruption, hypertensive disorders of pregnancy, and maternal or neonatal thrombosis [81].

10 Hemostasis in Pregnancy and Obstetric Surgery 139

It is important for clinicians to identify which patients are at risk, what the indications for testing are, what laboratory testing should be performed, and which patients should receive treatment. It is best for the clinician to perform a thrombophilia workup pre-conceptually because thrombophilia manifestations can start in early pregnancy [85].

10.2.1 Venous Thromboembolism

VTE is a leading cause of morbidity and mortality during pregnancy and the puerperium. The risk of VTE is five to six times higher among pregnant women than among nonpregnant women of similar age [86–88]. Estimates of the incidence of pregnancy-associated VTE range from one in 1,000 to one in 2,000 deliveries [89]. Pulmonary embolism occurs in approximately 16% of pregnant women with untreated deep vein thrombosis and remains the most frequent cause of maternal death [83, 90]. VTE is also associated with a considerable morbidity in young women, including complications of therapy due to VTE, recurrence of thrombosis, and development of postthrombotic syndrome [91]. It is necessary to estimate the individual probability of thrombosis on the basis of the relative risk associated with single or combined risk factors of hemostasis. During the last 10 years, knowledge of the cause of venous thrombosis has advanced with the discovery of specific genetic defects that contribute to venous thrombogenicity. The coagulation abnormalities include (in addition to deficiencies of antithrombin, protein C, and protein S) the G1691A mutation in the factor V gene (factor V Leiden) and the G20210A mutation in the prothrombin gene. These disorders underlie about 50% of episodes of VTE in pregnant and postpartum women; however, they are also present in at least 10% of Western populations [92, 93]. Thus, the presence of thrombophilic abnormalities alone does not necessarily lead to a clinical event, because many risk factors are common in the general population (e.g., factor V Leiden is present in up to 8% of the population). It is currently considered that VTE is a multifactorial disorder in which acquired and genetic risk factors can interact dynamically [84] (Table 10.2).

10.2.2 Hereditary Disorders

See also Chap. 5.

Antithrombin Deficiency

Antithrombin deficiency has been associated with an increased risk of stillbirth [odds ratio (OR) 5.25%, 95% confidence interval (CI) 1.5–18.1] and fetal loss (OR 1.7; 95% CI 1.0–2.8) [94]. Antithrombin deficiency is diagnosed with an antithrombin–heparin cofactor assay. This assay detects all currently recognized subtypes of familial antithrombin deficiency and is therefore the best single laboratory screening test for this disorder. Antithrombin deficiency should not be screened for in the setting of pregnancy, acute thrombosis, or during anticoagulation [85].

Table 10.2 Expositional (acquired) and dispositional (genetic) risk factors for venous thromboembolism

Acquired	Inherited	Combined/complex
Age	Antithrombin deficiency	Hyperhomocysteinemia
Previous thrombosis	Protein C deficiency	Elevated levels of fibrinogen
Immobilization	Protein S deficiency	Factor VIII
Surgery, trauma	Factor V Leiden	
Pregnancy and puerperium	Prothrombin G20210A mutation	
Oral contraception	Elevated levels of factors IX and XI	
Hormonal replacement therapy	Dysfibrinogenemia	
APA syndrome		
Malignant diseases		
Myeloproliferative disorders		

Protein C Deficiency

Protein C deficiency has been associated with an increased risk of second-trimester miscarriage and stillbirth [94–97]. The inhibitory effect of a protein C is markedly enhanced by protein S, another vitamin K dependent protein. Protein C is affected by pregnancy and therefore should be tested for preconceptually [85].

Protein S Deficiency

Pregnancy reduces the level of protein S by increasing the amount of C4b-binding protein and decreasing the amount of free protein S. Acquired protein S deficiency is also seen in women taking oral contraceptive pills and in those with diabetes mellitus, the lupus anticoagulant, liver disease, sickle cell disease, and inflammatory bowel disease. A meta-analysis by Rey et al. showed an association between idiopathic recurrent pregnancy loss (before 13 weeks) and protein S deficiency at an OR of 14.72, but this did not reach statistical significance (95% CI 0.99–218.01) [124]. Patients with levels of total or free protein S antigen lower than 65 IU/dL are considered to be deficient. Protein S deficiency should be tested for outside pregnancy [99].

Factor V Leiden

Carriers of factor V Leiden mutation are at greater risk of fetal loss and stillbirth than controls with idiopathic recurrent miscarriage [100]. Heterozygotes for the mutation and others with acquired APC resistance have a twofold higher risk of experiencing fetal loss or miscarriage. Factor V Leiden can be accurately diagnosed in pregnancy [95, 96, 101, 102].

Prothrombin G20210A Mutation

An observational study of more than 100 women in the USA with first-trimester pregnancy loss found the prothrombin mutation significantly more frequently than in controls [103]. A study of 87 Middle Eastern women with three or more early pregnancy losses did not show an association with the prothrombin mutation [104]. One meta-analysis of women with early pregnancy loss reported a significant association of the prothrombin mutation, with an OR of 2.0–2.6.14. A recent critical review of 69 published studies suggested a probable association of the prothrombin mutation and recurrent pregnancy loss [96]. The prothrombin gene mutation is associated with elevated plasma levels of prothrombin, but it should not be used for screening. The prothrombin gene mutation can be tested in the setting of pregnancy [87, 105, 106].

Hyperhomocysteinemia

It has been suggested that maternal hyperhomocysteinemia interferes with embryonic development through defective chorionic villus vascularization [107]. A meta-analysis of the association between MTHFR and pregnancy loss before 16 weeks suggests a weak association, with an OR of 1.4 (95% CI 1.0–2.0); however, the association between elevated fasting plasma homocysteine level and early pregnancy loss was significant, with an OR of 2.7 (95% CI 1.4–5.2) [108]. A recent critical review of the literature on thrombophilias and recurrent pregnancy loss suggested a significant association of hyperhomocysteinemia with an increased risk of recurrent pregnancy loss [96].

10.2.3 Acquired Disorders

APAs, primarily lupus anticoagulants and anticardiolipin antibodies (ACAs), are the most common causes of acquired thrombophilia. Approximately 8–14% of venous thromboembolic events are secondary to APAs. The criteria required to establish the diagnosis of lupus anticoagulants have been published [109]. Patients with lupus anticoagulants are at greater risk of thrombosis than patients who are only ACA-positive. Several studies suggest that a level of more than 40 phospholipid units for ACA represents an increased risk factor for venous thrombosis. An international consensus on classification criteria for definite APA syndrome was published in 1999 [110]. According to these criteria, at least one clinical and one laboratory feature must be present for the diagnosis. The presence of APAs during pregnancy is a major risk factor for adverse pregnancy outcome [111]. In large meta-analyses of studies of couples with recurrent abortion, the incidence of APA syndrome was between 15 and 20% compared with approximately 5% in nonpregnant women without a history of obstetric complications [112, 113]. It is not yet understood how APAs arise in patients with the syndrome. Genetic factors and infection may play a role [114].

Recently, another enzyme-linked immunosorbent assay has been introduced to detect antibodies to β_2-glycoprotein I. β_2-Glycoprotein I is a physiologic anticoagulant that is thought to be the true antigenic target for antibodies measured in ACA assays. Although ACA testing is sensitive, it is not a particularly specific indicator for thrombosis. Antibodies against β_2-glycoprotein I have greater specificity in identifying patients at risk of thrombosis but may not be as sensitive in identifying women at risk of obstetric complications. Consequently, patients with moderate- to high-titer ACA (e.g., more than 40 IgG phospholipid units) should be evaluated with anti-β_2-glycoprotein I testing [115]. Several mechanisms have been proposed by which APAs might mediate pregnancy loss. It appears that different coagulation proteins may be involved in binding to phospholipids, which may explain the predisposition to thrombosis. Antibodies against phospholipids could increase thromboxane and decrease prostacyclin synthesis within placental vessels. The resultant prothrombotic environment could promote vascular constriction, platelet adhesion, and placental infarction [113]. APAs appear to interfere with various components of the protein C antithrombotic pathway, including inhibiting the formation of thrombin, decreasing protein C activation by the thrombomodulin–thrombin complex, inhibiting assembly of protein C complex, inhibiting APC activity, and binding to activated factors V and VIII in ways that protect them from proteolysis by activated protein [114]. Another proposed mechanism is the disruption of the placental antithrombotic molecule, annexin V. The levels of annexin V are reduced in placental villi of women with recurrent pregnancy loss who are APA-positive [115]. APAs can also recognize heparin and heparinoid molecules and thereby inhibit antithrombin activity [116]. Heparin has been demonstrated to bind APAs directly in vitro and may facilitate the clearance of APAs in vivo [117, 118]. APAs can interact with cultured human vascular endothelial cells, with resultant injury and/or activation [114]. A more direct action on the trophoblastic cells has been demonstrated and explains how APAs can cause early fetal loss. APAs have been shown to inhibit secretion of human placental chorionic gonadotropin and to inhibit the expression of trophoblast cell adhesion molecules (α_1 and α_5 integrins, E-cadherin, and VE-cadherin) [119]. APAs can activate the complement and an inflammatory reaction; this effect is reversed in vitro by the addition of prophylactic doses of heparin [120].

10.3 Adverse Pregnancy Outcomes

10.3.1 Pregnancy Loss

Pregnancy loss can be separated into two categories: recurrent early pregnancy loss (more than three losses before 10 weeks' gestation) and late fetal loss (one loss after 10 weeks). APA syndrome is associated with both recurrent early pregnancy loss (before 10 weeks) and late fetal loss [121]. A greater proportion of pregnancy losses related to APAs are second- or third-trimester fetal deaths [122]. Alfirevic et al. [123] performed a systematic review and found that unexplained stillbirth, when compared with controls, was more often associated with heterozygous factor V Leiden mutation, protein S deficiency, and APC resistance. A meta-analysis by Rey et al. [124] showed that factor V Leiden, prothrombin gene mutation, and protein S deficiency were

10 Hemostasis in Pregnancy and Obstetric Surgery 143

associated with recurrent early pregnancy loss and late fetal loss. Kovalevsky et al. [101] performed a systematic review on published case–control studies, and the combined ORs for the association between recurrent pregnancy loss, factor V Leiden, and prothrombin gene mutation were 2.0 (95% CI 1.5–2.7, $P < 0.001$) and 2.0 (95% CI 1.0–4.0, P 5.03), respectively [101]. Lissalde-Lavigne et al. [125] performed a case–control study nested in a cohort of 32,683 women, and found that patients with factor V Leiden and prothrombin gene mutation were more likely to have a pregnancy loss after 10 weeks' gestation. In contrast to other studies, Roque et al. [126] examined a cohort of 491 patients with a history of adverse pregnancy outcomes and evaluated the cohort for acquired and inherited thrombophilias. This study showed the presence of one maternal thrombophilia, or more than one thrombophilia was found to be protective of recurrent losses at less than 10 weeks. In contrast, the presence of maternal thrombophilia(s) was modestly associated with an increased risk of losses at greater than 10 weeks. There have been three randomized control trials examining the effect of treatment of APA syndrome patients with recurrent pregnancy loss with low-dose aspirin (acetylsalicylic acid) alone or low-dose aspirin plus heparin [127–129].

Two of these studies showed a significantly better pregnancy outcome and higher rate of live births in women with APA syndrome and recurrent pregnancy loss: 71–80% with the use of heparin and aspirin versus 42–72% with use of aspirin alone [127, 128]. There is some controversy about whether patients with recurrent or late pregnancy loss should be tested for inherited thrombophilias. Only one prospective trial has studied patients with a history of unexplained pregnancy loss and known inherited thrombophilia. Patients were randomized to receive low-dose aspirin or low molecular weight heparin (LMWH). There was a significantly higher number of live births in patients treated with LMWH versus low-dose aspirin (OR 15.5, 95% CI 7–34, $P < 0.0001$). Although this study was not blinded and had no placebo arm, it is the only one looking at history of fetal loss for possible treatment. This positive findings of this study support the argument of testing patients with a history of fetal loss at greater than 10 weeks' gestation for inherited as well as acquired thrombophilias [130].

10.3.2 Severe Preeclampsia and HELLP Syndrome

Preeclampsia (edema–proteinuria–hypertension) is a multisystem disorder of human pregnancy, whose cause remains poorly understood [131]. It is characterized by hypertension (diastolic blood pressure greater than 110 mmHg on one occasion, or greater than 90 mmHg on two or more consecutive occasions at least 4 h apart) and proteinuria (either 30 mg/mmol or greater), occurring after the 20th week of pregnancy in women who have had no previous symptoms [132]. In most instances, preeclampsia occurs during a woman's first pregnancy, although it can recur in a subsequent pregnancy or can occur for the first time in a women with one or more previously unaffected pregnancies. Risk factors for the disorder include, but are not limited to, preeclampsia in a previous pregnancy, a family history of preeclampsia, chronic hypertension, obesity, multifetal gestation, rheumatic disease, and preexisting thrombophilia [133]. A case–control study by Mello et al. [134] suggests that the prevalence of an underlying thrombophilia is significantly higher among women who develop preeclampsia during pregnancy than among those who have an uneventful pregnancy.

The association of severe preeclampsia and thrombophilias is controversial. Branch et al. [135] performed an observational study and showed that 50% of women with APA syndrome developed preeclampsia despite treatment, whereas 25% had severe preeclampsia [113]. A meta-analysis by Robertson et al. [136] showed that the risk of preeclampsia was significantly associated with heterozygous factor V Leiden mutation, heterozygous prothrombin gene mutation, MTHFR homozygosity, ACAs, and hyperhomocysteinemia. However, when the analysis was restricted to severe preeclampsia alone, an OR of 2.04 (95% CI 1.23–3.36) was obtained. A meta-analysis by Alfirevic et al. [123] showed that women with preeclampsia/eclampsia were more likely than controls to have heterozygous factor V Leiden mutation, heterozygous G20210A PT gene mutation, homozygous MTHFR C677T mutation, protein C deficiency, protein S deficiency, or a protein C resistance. Roque et al. [126] showed an increased risk of preeclampsia (OR 3.21, 95% CI 1.20–8.58) among patients with acquired and inherited thrombophilias. HELLP syndrome, defined by hemolysis, elevated liver enzymes levels, and low platelet count, represents a severe variant of preeclampsia. The median age of affected patients is 25 years and the time of presentation during pregnancy ranges from mid-trimester (15%) to term (18%). Thirty percent of patients develop HELLP within 2 days after delivery [137]. Patients typically exhibit vague symptoms such as malaise, fatigue, epigastric or right quadrant pain, nausea, vomiting, and flu-like symptoms. Because of the nonspecific nature of these symptoms, diagnosis is often delayed; one study found an average time to diagnosis of 8 days in women with HELLP syndrome [138]. The clinical findings at the time of diagnosis—weight gain or edema, hypertension, and proteinuria—are similar to those observed in preeclampsia. Martin et al. [137] defined HELLP syndrome on the basis of platelet count. According to this classification, patients with class I HELLP syndrome have a platelet count lower than 50,000/μL, those with class II disease have a platelet count between 50,000 and 100,000/μL, and those with class III have a platelet count higher than 100,000/μL. Although the pathogenesis of preeclampsia is not fully understood, predisposition to endothelial dysfunction is thought to play a crucial role. This may trigger abnormal activation of the hemostatic and/or inflammatory systems. Preeclamptic women are known to have an increased hypercoagulable state compared with those with a normal pregnancy [139–141]. There is a reported increase in levels of factor VIII, von Willebrand factor, TAT complex, D-dimers, soluble fibrin, and thrombomodulin [14, 142–146]. There is also increased resistance to the anticoagulant property of APC [76]. However, antithrombin levels are described as reduced and TF pathway inhibitor levels as unchanged [147, 148]; platelets have a reduced half-life and platelet counts are also decreased [39, 149]. Interestingly, antithrombin and thrombomodulin levels and platelet counts correlate positively with the severity of the disease [146, 147, 149, 150]. The fibrinolytic system is also

10 Hemostasis in Pregnancy and Obstetric Surgery 145

involved in preeclampsia. A significant increase in the level of PAI-1 has been reported [39, 151]. Measurements of the end products of fibrinolysis in both peripheral and uteroplacental circulation in normotensive and preeclamptic pregnancies, including soluble fibrin, TAT complex, plasmin–α_2-antiplasmin complex and D-dimers, showed an abnormal hemostatic pattern occurring in women with preeclampsia compared with normal pregnancy [145]. Expatiated inflammatory reactions occur more often in woman with preeclampsia compared with those with a normal pregnancy [152]. Preeclampsia is associated with circulatory disturbances caused by systematic maternal endothelial cell dysfunction and/or activation. The endothelium is an integral part of the inflammatory network; thus, its activation stimulates leukocytes and vice versa [153]. In preeclampsia both monocytes and granulocytes are activated and proinflammatory cytokines are released into the circulation [154, 155]. Increased cytokine concentration in preeclampsia is a potential stimulus for nicotinamide adenine dinucleotide phosphate oxidase activation, which results in increased superoxide generation [156]. Enhanced superoxide generation by the placenta or neutrophilis leads to an increase in oxidative stress in preeclamptic women [157–159]. Placental ischemia and reperfusion, as a consequence of oxidative stress, have been regarded as a major cause of syncytiotrophoblast apoptosis [160]. Oxidative stress in preeclampsia is not localized to the placenta but disseminates into the maternal circulation [152]. Cellular abnormalities such as those described impair placental implantation and vasculogenesis, leading to fetal hypoxia and the release of vasoactive compounds such as endothelin, nitric oxide, and prostaglandins. High levels of endothelin, a potent vasoconstrictor, are seen in preeclamptic patients. The activity of endothelin, nitric oxide, and prostaglandins leads to hypertension and platelet activation. In turn, injury to the vascular endothelium results in fibrin deposition, further platelet activation, and the release of additional vasoactive agents such as serotonin and thromboxane A_2. The cause of thrombocytopenia in preeclampsia is likely related to increased antiplatelet IgG levels or to activation of the coagulation cascade with subsequent consumption of platelets [161–163].

An additional pathway through which the coagulation and inflammatory system are generally activated is linked to microparticles (MPs). Lok et al. [164] showed that the number of platelet-derived MPs decreased in preeclampsia compared with normal pregnancy, whereas the number of platelet-derived MPs exposing P-selectin increased. These P-selectin-exposing MPs reflect platelet activation, as is found in preeclampsia. Elevated concentrations of erythrocyte-derived MPs have been shown in preeclampsia, and are probably due to hemolysis and hemoconcentration.

These events lead to the multisystem dysfunction seen in patients with HELLP syndrome. Fibrin deposition in the hepatic sinusoids causes hepatocellular injury. Disseminated intravascular coagulation was observed in 21% of patients with HELLP in one series, whereas placental abruption was seen in 16% of patients [165]. Other manifestations of HELLP syndrome include acute renal failure, pulmonary edema, shock, cerebrovascular accident, eclampsia [166], retinal detachment [167], diabetes insipidus [168], and increased incidence of cesarean section [169]. HELLP syndrome is associated with high maternal and neonatal mortality. Maternal mortality ranges from 1.1 to 24.2% [170]. The immediate cause of death is most often rupture of the liver, disseminated intravascular coagulation, acute renal failure, pulmonary edema/acute respiratory distress syndrome, shock, or cerebrovascular accident. Perinatal deaths resulting from placental abruption, asphyxia, or extreme prematurity occur in 10–15% of patients [166]. In the light of the morbidity and mortality associated with preeclampsia and HELLP syndrome, considerable research has focused on prevention of these conditions. The efficacy of various preventive strategies—including magnesium supplementations, low-dose aspirin, zinc supplementation, antihypertensive drugs, and heparin therapy—has been the focus of observational studies, systematic reviews, and randomized trials. Larger, randomized trials failed to confirm the benefit of low-dose aspirin [171, 172]. Antioxidants vitamin C and vitamin E have shown promise in small trials, but further testing needs to be done [173]. A randomized study performed in the USA showed no benefit from calcium supplementation [174]. Some clinicians endorse calcium supplementation in patients with low dietary calcium intake, particularly for those expectant mothers at risk of preeclampsia [175]. Supplemental fish oil may lower the risk of preterm delivery in women with previous preterm delivery, twin pregnancies, IUGR, or preeclampsia, but further studies are needed to confirm this benefit [176].

10.3.3 Intrauterine Growth Retardation

"Intrauterine growth retardation" (IUGR) is a term used to describe a fetus whose estimated weight appears to be less than the tenth percentile for the gestational age. IUGR is associated with an increase in fetal and neonatal mortality and morbidity rates. IUGR has been shown to complicate pregnancies with inherited and acquired thrombophilias [85]. Controversy remains regarding whether there is an association between IUGR and congenital thrombophilias. As preeclampsia is a known risk factor for IUGR, an association between preeclampsia and congenital thrombophilia will indirectly cause an association with IUGR. Fetal thrombophilia has been identified among IUGR infants as an independent risk factor for low birth weight and for preterm birth [177, 178].

IUGR occurs in approximately one third of patients diagnosed with APA syndrome despite treatment seen in retrospective studies [135, 179]. This risk may be higher in untreated pregnancies. Data from Yasuda et al. [180] showed a significant association with IUGR observed with ACAs (OR 6.91, 95% CI 2.70–17.68). IUGR is most often seen in the presence of severe preeclampsia; therefore, it is difficult to establish causality. A prospective cohort study of 95 nulliparous women with elevated antiphospholipid levels on their initial prenatal visit had an increase in fetal loss but no increase in low birth weight or IUGR [181]. A meta-analysis examining the relationship between IUGR and factor V Leiden, prothrombin gene mutation, and MTHFR was recently performed. This analysis showed that the only association seen was with factor V Leiden and MTHFR in case–control studies. Funnel plot analysis suggested the existence of publication bias, given the small number of studies with negative findings [182]. In an Italian study, the association between IUGR (linked to gestational hypertension or idiopathic hypertension) and factor V Leiden, prothrombin mutation A20210, and MTHFR C677T was examined in 61 women with a history of fetal growth retardation and 93 controls of the same race. In all of the patients, antiphospholipid anticoagulants, antithrombins, protein C and total and free protein S antigen were also examined. The results underlined an association between growth retardation and the factor V Leiden mutation (OR 6.9) with the prothrombin mutation (OR 5.9) and with MTHFR C677T homozygosity (OR 1.5). The factor V Leiden and prothrombin mutations were shown to be independent factors for the parameters analyzed [183]. There are limited studies examining antithrombin III, protein C, and protein S and their association with IUGR. Roque et al. [126] found protein C to be associated with an increased risk of IUGR (OR 12.93, 95% CI 2.72–61.45). Alfirevic et al. [123] found that women with IUGR had a higher prevalence of heterozygous G20210A prothrombin gene mutation, homozygous MTHFR C677T gene mutation, protein S deficiency, and antiphospholipid than controls.

10.3.4 Placental Abruption

Some studies have shown a possible association between abruption and thrombophilias. Hyperhomocysteinemia, APC resistance, protein C mutation, MTHRF polymorphism, and the combination of such factors seem to increase the risk as shown in the studies of Wiener-Megnagi et al. [183], van der Molen et al. [184], and Facchinetti et al. [185]. On the other hand, in a study by Prochazka et al. [186], no statistically significant differences related to the analysis of factor V Leiden were found. The association between placenta abruption and thrombophilias was underlined in a recent analysis by Robertson et al. [136] on 922 cases taken from seven studies, particularly with factor V Leiden heterozygosity (OR 4.70, 95% CI 1.13–19.59) and with the prothrombin heterozygosity (OR 7.71, 95% CI 3.01–19.76). Alfirevic et al. found that when compared with controls, placental abruption was more often associated with homozygous and heterozygous factor V Leiden mutation, heterozygous G20210A prothrombin gene mutation, homocysteinemia, APC resistance, or anticardiolipin IgG antibodies. Although there appears to be an association with both inherited and acquired thrombophilia, there are no prospective trials looking at this association and how to prevent recurrence [123].

10.4 Management of Thromboembolism in Pregnancy

Prevention and diagnostic and therapeutic management of VTE in pregnancy are all complicated by the lack of validated approaches in this unique population. Therefore, practice guidelines are developed by extending the evidence from nonpregnant patients, considering the limited data that are available in pregnant patients, and interpreting this evidence with the unique circumstances that surround pregnancy [187].

Table 10.3 Recommendations for thrombophilia testing

Thrombophilia	Indications for testing
Inherited thrombophilia	Personal history of VTE Family history of a diagnosed inherited thrombophilia IUFD (when all other causes have been excluded, severe IUGR, or severe placental lesion)
Acquired thrombophilia	Personal history of VTE Recurrent pregnancy loss (more than 3 losses at before 10 weeks) IUFD (after 10 weeks) Severe preeclampsia (requiring delivery before 34 weeks) Placental insufficiency/IUGR (requiring delivery before 34 weeks)

VTE venous thromboembolism, *IUFD* intrauterine fetal death, *IUGR* intrauterine growth retardation

10.4.1 Screening

Patients with a history of thrombosis, whether it is of idiopathic origin or associated with pregnancy, oral contraceptive use, trauma, obesity, cancer, or underlying medical conditions may benefit from being screened for thrombophilia. Screening patients with a first VTE for thrombophilias is currently the subject of considerable study and debate. Although encouraged by some clinicians, routine testing for thrombophilias may be of limited clinical value. In contrast, patients presenting with recurrent thrombosis or with thrombosis in the setting of a strong family history of VTE may be candidates for thrombophilia testing (Table 10.3).

The basic tests for thrombophilia screening include testing for functional protein C, functional protein S, antithrombin III (functional assay), APC resistance [or factor V Leiden (polymerase chain reaction)], and prothrombin G20210A (polymerase chain reaction). Other screening for acquired thrombophilic conditions can include testing for ACAs IgG and IgM and lupus anticoagulant. Further supplemental screening may consist of testing for homocysteine, other factor V mutations, thrombomodulin gene variants, protein Z levels, PAI-1 activity levels, PAI-1 4G/5G polymorphisms, MTHFR, homocysteine PAI-1 polymorphisms, and factor evaluation (factors VII, VIII, IX, XI) [188]. On the basis of recent literature, hyperhomocysteinemia in connection with MTHFR should not be tested for. The only inherited thrombophilias that should be tested for are factor V Leiden, prothrombin gene mutation, antithrombin, protein C, and protein S. Patients who have had adverse pregnancy outcomes such as early-onset preeclampsia and IUGR requiring delivery before 34 weeks, intrauterine fetal death after 10 weeks, and recurrent pregnancy loss (more than losses before 10 weeks) should undergo APA syndrome testing. The only adverse pregnancy outcome for which an inherited thrombophilia panel should be sent is a fetal loss at greater than 10 weeks [85]. The American College of Obstetrics and Gynecology recommends testing for inherited thrombophilias after an intrauterine fetal death in cases of severe placental lesion, severe IUGR, or a family or personal history of VTE. Factor V Leiden and prothrombin

10 Hemostasis in Pregnancy and Obstetric Surgery

mutations are gene mutations and are not affected by pregnancy. Testing for APA syndrome can also be performed during pregnancy. Thrombophilia screening should be postponed during pregnancy with a new diagnosis of VTE. Thrombophilia testing should be done outside the current thrombotic event and current anticoagulation. Diagnosis of a thrombophilia will not change its management in the setting of a current VTE [189]. Currently, the costs of routine thrombophilia screening for all patients are prohibitive. Clearly, more evidence-based data from prospective randomized trials evaluating the use of anticoagulation for the prevention of adverse patient outcomes are needed before these costs can be justified [85].

10.4.2 Prophylaxis and Treatment

The American College of Chest Physicians (ACCP) recommends clinical antepartum surveillance and prophylactic anticoagulation postpartum in women with a single episode of VTE associated with a temporary risk factor and without a known thrombophilia. If the temporary risk factor is pregnancy, the ACCP recommends prophylactic anticoagulation during pregnancy and postpartum [85].

The ACCP evidence-based clinical practice guidelines (eighth edition) recommend:

- For pregnant women, LMWH rather than unfractionated heparin (UFH) for the prevention and treatment of VTE.
- For pregnant women with acute VTE, initial therapy with either adjusted-dose subcutaneously administered LMWH or adjusted-dose UFH [intravenous bolus, followed by a continuous infusion to maintain the activated partial thromboplastin time (aPTT) within the therapeutic range or subcutaneous therapy adjusted to maintain the aPTT 6 h after injection in the therapeutic range] for at least 5 days. After initial therapy, subcutaneous administration of LMWH or UFH should be continued throughout pregnancy. Use of anticoagulants should be continued for at least 6 weeks postpartum (for a minimum total duration of therapy of 6 months). For pregnant women receiving adjusted-dose LMWH or UFH therapy, discontinuation of heparin therapy at least 24 h prior to elective induction of labor is recommended.
- For pregnant women with a single episode of VTE associated with a transient risk factor that is no longer present and no thrombophilia, clinical surveillance antepartum and anticoagulant prophylaxis postpartum.

If the transient risk factor associated with a previous VTE event is pregnancy- or estrogen-related, the ACCP suggests antepartum clinical surveillance or prophylaxis (prophylactic LMWH/UFH or intermediate-dose LMWH/UFH) plus postpartum prophylaxis rather than routine care:

- For pregnant women with a single idiopathic episode of VTE but without thrombophilia and for pregnant women with thrombophilia (confirmed laboratory abnormality) and a single prior episode of VTE who are not receiving long-term anticoagulant therapy, rather than routine care or adjusted-dose anticoagulation, one of the following is recommended: prophylactic LMWH/

UFH or intermediate-dose LMWH/UFH or clinical surveillance throughout pregnancy plus anticoagulants postpartum.

- For women with "higher-risk" thrombophilias (e.g., antithrombin deficiency, persistent positivity for the presence of APAs, compound heterozygosity for prothrombin G20210A variant and factor V Leiden or homozygosity for these conditions) who have had a single prior episode of VTE and are not receiving long-term anticoagulant therapy, in addition to postpartum prophylaxis, antepartum administration of prophylactic or intermediate-dose LMWH or prophylactic or intermediate-dose UFH is suggested, rather than clinical surveillance.
- For pregnant women with multiple (two or more) episodes of VTE not receiving long-term anticoagulant therapy, antepartum administration of prophylactic, intermediate-dose, or adjusted-dose LMWH or prophylactic, intermediate-dose, or adjusted-dose UFH followed by postpartum administration of anticoagulants is recommended rather than clinical surveillance.
- For pregnant women receiving long-term anticoagulant therapy for prior VTE, LMWH or adjusted dose UFH is recommended throughout pregnancy (either adjusted-dose LMWH or UFH, 75% of adjusted-dose LMWH, or intermediate-dose LMWH) followed by resumption of long-term anticoagulant therapy postpartum.
- For all pregnant women with previous deep vein thrombosis, the use of graduated elastic compression stockings is recommended both antepartum and postpartum.

The underlying values and preferences recommendation places a high value on uncertain incremental benefit with stockings, and a low value on avoiding discomfort and inconvenience:

- For pregnant women with no history of VTE but with antithrombin deficiency, antepartum and postpartum prophylaxis is suggested.
- For all other pregnant women with thrombophilia and no prior VTE, it is recommended that physicians do not use routine pharmacologic antepartum prophylaxis but instead perform an individualized risk assessment.
- For women with recurrent early pregnancy loss (three or more miscarriages) or unexplained late pregnancy loss, screening for APAs is recommended.
- For women with severe or recurrent preeclampsia or IUGR, screening for APAs is suggested.
- For women with APAs and recurrent pregnancy loss (three or more losses) or late pregnancy loss and no history of venous or arterial thrombosis, antepartum administration of prophylactic or intermediate-dose UFH or prophylactic LMWH combined with aspirin is recommended.
- For women considered high risk for preeclampsia, low-dose aspirin therapy throughout pregnancy is recommended.
- For women with a history of preeclampsia, it is suggested that UFH and LMWH should not be used as prophylaxis in subsequent pregnancies.

10 Hemostasis in Pregnancy and Obstetric Surgery 151

There are also recommendations for pregnant women in general:

- For women receiving anticoagulation for the management of VTE who become pregnant, long-term vitamin k antagonist therapy should be substituted with UFH or LMWH.
- For women requiring long-term vitamin K antagonist therapy who are attempting pregnancy and are candidates for UFH or LMWH substitution, it is suggested that frequent pregnancy tests are performed and UFH or LMWH is substituted for long-term vitamin k antagonist therapy when pregnancy is achieved.
- For selected high-risk patients in whom important risk factors persist following delivery, extended prophylaxis (up to 4–6 weeks after delivery) following discharge from hospital is suggested [190].
  - Prophylactic UFH: UFH 5,000 U subcutaneously every 12 h.
  - Intermediate-dose UFH: UFH subcutaneously every 12 h in doses adjusted to target an anti-activated factor X level of 0.1–0.3 U/mL.
  - Adjusted-dose UFH: UFH subcutaneously every 12 h in doses adjusted to target a midinterval aPTT in the therapeutic range.
  - Prophylactic LMWH: e.g., dalteparin 5,000 U subcutaneously every 24 h, tinzaparin 4,500 U subcutaneously every 24h, or enoxaparin 40 mg subcutaneously every 24h (although at extremes of body weight, modification of the dose may be required).
  - Intermediate-dose LMWH: e.g., dalteparin 5,000 U subcutaneously every 12 h or enoxaparin 40 mg subcutaneously every 12 h.
  - Adjusted-dose LMWH: weight-adjusted, full treatment doses of LMWH, given once or twice daily (e.g., dalteparin 200 U/kg or tinzaparin 175 U/kg daily or dalteparin 100 U/kg every 12 h or enoxaparin 1 mg/kg every 12 h).
  - Postpartum administration of anticoagulants: long-term vitamin k antagonist therapy for 4–6 weeks with a target international normalized ratio of 2.0–3.0, with initial UFH or LMWH overlap until the international normalized ratio is 2.0, or prophylactic LMWH for 4–6 weeks.

10.5 Surgery in Pregnancy

During pregnancy it is possible that the future mother is affected by a disease or a clinical problem that can be solved only through surgical measures.

In the past, a surgeon's natural inclination, when faced with a pregnant patient experiencing abdominal pain, was to temporize. This tendency was rooted in the misconception that surgical intervention was likely to injure the fetus, and has been responsible for delays in diagnosis and treatment, which resulted in unfavorable outcomes [191, 192]. Appendicitis, cholecystitis, pancreatitis, bowel obstruction, and trauma are the major nonobstetric abdominal conditions noted in pregnancy that require surgical intervention [193]. Currently, there is evidence that pregnancy should no longer be considered a contraindication to laparoscopic surgery because laparoscopy is not dangerous to either the mother or the fetus [194]. Recovery and return to normal activity is much quicker with laparoscopy than laparatomy [195]. Laparoscopy was first used for evaluation of acute abdominal pain in pregnancy in 1980 by gynecologists [196]. The most commonly reported laparoscopic procedure performed during pregnancy is laparoscopic cholecystectomy [197].

Laparoscopic procedures during pregnancy may provide advantages, particularly in upper abdominal disease, in which visualization and accessibility are not compromised by the expanding uterus [191, 195]. Laparoscopic surgery has the advantage of allowing reduced narcotic use and hence less fetal depression, better intraoperative visualization and exposure, less postoperative pain, early return of bowel function, early ambulation, and shorter postoperative stays. Also, in a perforated appendix, open surgery will require a larger incision, and there is a theoretical increased risk of wound infection and incisional hernia. This may interfere with the delivery of the baby. Several studies have proved that laparoscopic surgery is safe in pregnancy, provided it is done in specialized centers by experienced surgeons [198]. The difficulties are often more concerned with the diagnosis, and some problems occur with symptoms that can be easily confused with those of pregnancy. The possible drawbacks are injury to the uterus during Veress needle insertion, potential reduction of uterine blood flow secondary to increased intra-abdominal pressure, risk of CO_2 absorption by the mother and child, and the technical difficulty of laparoscopic surgery. Physiologic and anatomic changes introduce certain risks unique to the gravid patient, and some associated with laparoscopy in pregnancy. These risks have been postulated to include poor visualization due to gravid uterus, uterine injury during trocar placement, decreased uterine blood flow, or premature labor from the increased intra-abdominal pressure and increased fetal acidosis or other unknown effects due to CO_2 pneumoperitoneum. Decreased uterine blood flow from pneumoperitoneum remains hypothetical [198]. It is reasoned that this is unlikely to be a major concern given the frequent pressure alternations induced during maternal Valsalva maneuver, coughing, and straining. Further, it is maintained that pneumoperitoneum may well be safer than manual uterine retraction during open appendectomy or cholecystectomy. It can be concluded that laparoscopic surgery is now proving to be as safe as open surgery in pregnancy, with no deleterious effects to either mothers or children [199].

References

1. Brenner B (2004) Haemostatic changes in pregnancy. Thromb Res 114(5–6):409–414
2. Stirling Y, Woolf L, North WR, Seghatchian MJ, Meade TW (1984) Haemostasis in normal pregnancy. Thromb Haemost 52(2):176–182
3. Clark P, Brennand J, Conkie JA, McCall F, Greer IA, Walker ID (1998) Activated protein C sensitivity, protein C, protein S and coagulation in normal pregnancy. Thromb Haemost 79(6):1166–1170
4. Kjellberg U, Andersson NE, Rosen S, Tengborn L, Hellgren M (1999) APC resistance and other haemostatic variables during pregnancy and puerperium. Thromb Haemost 81(4):527–531
5. Condie RG (1976) A serial study of coagulation factors XII, XI and X in plasma in normal pregnancy and in pregnancy complicated by pre-eclampsia. Br J Obstet Gynaecol 83(8):636–639

10 Hemostasis in Pregnancy and Obstetric Surgery 153

6. Nilsson IM, Kullander S (1967) Coagulation and fibrinolytic studies during pregnancy. Acta Obstet Gynecol Scand 46(3):273–285
7. Hellgren M, Blomback M (1981) Studies on blood coagulation and fibrinolysis in pregnancy, during delivery and in the puerperium. I. Normal condition. Gynecol Obstet Invest 12(3):141–154
8. Lefkowitz JB, Clarke SH, Barbour LA (1996) Comparison of protein S functional and antigenic assays in normal pregnancy. Am J Obstet Gynecol 175(3 Pt 1):657–660
9. Walker MC, Garner PR, Keely EJ, Rock GA, Reis MD (1997) Changes in activated protein C resistance during normal pregnancy. Am J Obstet Gynecol 177(1):162–169
10. Phillips LL, Rosano L, Skrodelis V (1973) Changes in factor XI (plasma thromboplastin antecedent) levels during pregnancy. Am J Obstet Gynecol 116(8):1114–1116
11. Boffa MC, Valsecchi L, Fausto A, Gozin D, Vigano' D'Angelo S, Safa O et al (1998) Predictive value of plasma thrombomodulin in preeclampsia and gestational hypertension. Thromb Haemost 79(6):1092–1095
12. Gonzalez R, Alberca I, Vicente V (1985) Protein C levels in late pregnancy, postpartum and in women on oral contraceptives. Thromb Res 39(5):637–640
13. Gilabert J, Fernandez JA, Espana F, Aznar J, Estelles A (1988) Physiological coagulation inhibitors (protein S, protein C and antithrombin III) in severe preeclamptic states and in users of oral contraceptives. Thromb Res 49(3):319–329
14. Aznar J, Gilabert J, Estelles A, Espana F (1986) Fibrinolytic activity and protein C in preeclampsia. Thromb Haemost 55(3):314–317
15. Faught W, Garner P, Jones G, Ivey B (1995) Changes in protein C and protein S levels in normal pregnancy. Am J Obstet Gynecol 172(1 Pt 1):147–150
16. Hopmeier P, Halbmayer M, Schwarz HP, Heuss F, Fischer M (1987) Protein C and protein S in mild and moderate preeclampsia. Thromb Haemost 58(2):794–795
17. Lao TT, Yuen PM, Yin JA (1989) Protein S and protein C levels in Chinese women during pregnancy, delivery and the puerperium. Br J Obstet Gynaecol 96(2):167–170
18. Espana F, Gilabert J, Aznar J, Estelles A, Kobayashi T, Griffin JH (1991) Complexes of activated protein C with alpha 1-antitrypsin in normal pregnancy and in severe preeclampsia. Am J Obstet Gynecol 164(5 Pt 1):1310–1316
19. Woodhams BJ, Candotti G, Shaw R, Kernoff PB (1989) Changes in coagulation and fibrinolysis during pregnancy: evidence of activation of coagulation preceding spontaneous abortion. Thromb Res 55(1):99–107
20. Gatti L, Tenconi PM, Guarneri D, Bertulessi C, Ossola MW, Bosco P et al (1994) Hemostatic parameters and platelet activation by flow-cytometry in normal pregnancy: a longitudinal study. Int J Clin Lab Res 24(4):217–219
21. Halligan A, Bonnar J, Sheppard B, Darling M, Walshe J (1994) Haemostatic, fibrinolytic and endothelial variables in normal pregnancies and pre-eclampsia. Br J Obstet Gynaecol 101(6):488–492
22. Malm J, Laurell M, Dahlback B (1988) Changes in the plasma levels of vitamin K-dependent proteins C and S and of C4b-binding protein during pregnancy and oral contraception. Br J Haematol 68(4):437–443
23. Comp PC, Thurnau GR, Welsh J, Esmon CT (1986) Functional and immunologic protein S levels are decreased during pregnancy. Blood 68(4):881–885
24. Fernandez JA, Estelles A, Gilabert J, Espana F, Aznar J (1989) Functional and immunologic protein S in normal pregnant women and in full-term newborns. Thromb Haemost 61(3):474–478
25. Bremme K, Ostlund E, Almqvist I, Heinonen K, Blomback M (1992) Enhanced thrombin generation and fibrinolytic activity in normal pregnancy and the puerperium. Obstet Gynecol 80(1):132–137
26. Bertina RM, Koeleman BP, Koster T, Rosendaal FR, Dirven RJ, de Ronde H et al (1994) Mutation in blood coagulation factor V associated with resistance to activated protein C. Nature 369(6475):64–67

27. Bokarewa MI, Bremme K, Falk G, Sten-Linder M, Egberg N, Blomback M (1995) Studies on phospholipid antibodies, APC-resistance and associated mutation in the coagulation factor V gene. Thromb Res 78(3):193–200
28. Haim N, Lanir N, Hoffman R, Haim A, Tsalik M, Brenner B (2001) Acquired activated protein C resistance is common in cancer patients and is associated with venous thromboembolism. Am J Med 110(2):91–96
29. Cumming AM, Tait RC, Fildes S, Yoong A, Keeney S, Hay CR (1995) Development of resistance to activated protein C during pregnancy. Br J Haematol 90(3):725–727
30. Castoldi E, Brugge JM, Nicolaes GA, Girelli D, Tans G, Rosing J (2004) Impaired APC cofactor activity of factor V plays a major role in the APC resistance associated with the factor V Leiden (R506Q) and R2 (H1299R) mutations. Blood 103(11):4173–4179
31. Mathonnet F, de Mazancourt P, Bastenaire B, Morot M, Benattar N, Beufe S et al (1996) Activated protein C sensitivity ratio in pregnant women at delivery. Br J Haematol 92(1):244–246
32. Clark P, Sattar N, Walker ID, Greer IA (2001) The glasgow outcome, APCR and lipid (GOAL) pregnancy study: significance of pregnancy associated activated protein C resistance. Thromb Haemost 85(1):30–35
33. Vasse M, Leduc O, Borg JY, Chretien MH, Monconduit M (1994) Resistance to activated protein C: evaluation of three functional assays. Thromb Res 76(1):47–59
34. Bokarewa MI, Bremme K, Blomback M (1996) Arg506-Gln mutation in factor V and risk of thrombosis during pregnancy. Br J Haematol 92(2):473–478
35. Eichinger S, Weltermann A, Philipp K, Hafner E, Kaider A, Kittl EM et al (1999) Prospective evaluation of hemostatic system activation and thrombin potential in healthy pregnant women with and without factor V Leiden. Thromb Haemost 82(4):1232–1236
36. Bauer KA, Rosenberg RD (1987) The pathophysiology of the prethrombotic state in humans: insights gained from studies using markers of hemostatic system activation. Blood 70(2):343–350
37. de Boer K, ten Cate JW, Sturk A, Borm JJ, Treffers PE (1989) Enhanced thrombin generation in normal and hypertensive pregnancy. Am J Obstet Gynecol 160(1):95–100
38. Reinthaller A, Mursch-Edlmayr G, Tatra G (1990) Thrombin-antithrombin III complex levels in normal pregnancy with hypertensive disorders and after delivery. Br J Obstet Gynaecol 97(6):506–510
39. Cadroy Y, Grandjean H, Pichon J, Desprats R, Berrebi A, Fournie A et al (1993) Evaluation of six markers of haemostatic system in normal pregnancy and pregnancy complicated by hypertension or pre-eclampsia. Br J Obstet Gynaecol 100(5):416–420
40. Comeglio P, Fedi S, Liotta AA, Cellai AP, Chiarantini E, Prisco D et al (1996) Blood clotting activation during normal pregnancy. Thromb Res 84(3):199–202
41. Delorme MA, Burrows RF, Ofosu FA, Andrew M (1992) Thrombin regulation in mother and fetus during pregnancy. Semin Thromb Hemost 18(1):81–90
42. Weenink GH, Treffers PE, Kahle LH, ten Cate JW (1982) Antithrombin III in normal pregnancy. Thromb Res 26(4):281–287
43. Ramalakshmi BA, Raju LA, Raman L (1995) Antithrombin III levels in pregnancy induced hypertension. Natl Med J India 8(2):61–62
44. Maruyama I, Bell CE, Majerus PW (1985) Thrombomodulin is found on endothelium of arteries, veins, capillaries, and lymphatics, and on syncytiotrophoblast of human placenta. J Cell Biol 101(2):363–371
45. Esmon CT, Owen WG (1981) Identification of an endothelial cell cofactor for thrombin-catalyzed activation of protein C. Proc Natl Acad Sci U S A 78(4):2249–2252
46. Esmon CT, Esmon NL, Harris KW (1982) Complex formation between thrombin and thrombomodulin inhibits both thrombin-catalyzed fibrin formation and factor V activation. J Biol Chem 257(14):7944–7947
47. Esmon NL, Carroll RC, Esmon CT (1983) Thrombomodulin blocks the ability of thrombin to activate platelets. J Biol Chem 258(20):12238–12242

10 Hemostasis in Pregnancy and Obstetric Surgery

48. Hofsteenge J, Taguchi H, Stone SR (1986) Effect of thrombomodulin on the kinetics of the interaction of thrombin with substrates and inhibitors. Biochem J 237(1):243–251
49. Ishii H, Majerus PW (1985) Thrombomodulin is present in human plasma and urine. J Clin Invest 76(6):2178–2181
50. Boffa MC (1996) Considering cellular thrombomodulin distribution and its modulating factors can facilitate the use of plasma thrombomodulin as a reliable endothelial marker? Haemostasis 26(Suppl 4):233–243
51. Suzuki K, Nishioka J, Hashimoto S (1983) Protein C inhibitor. Purification from human plasma and characterization. J Biol Chem 258(1):163–168
52. Heeb MJ, Espana F, Griffin JH (1989) Inhibition and complexation of activated protein C by two major inhibitors in plasma. Blood 73(2):446–454
53. Marlar RA, Kressin DC, Madden RM (1993) Contribution of plasma proteinase inhibitors to the regulation of activated protein C in plasma. Thromb Haemost 69(1):16–20
54. Hoogendoorn H, Toh CH, Nesheim ME, Giles AR (1991) Alpha 2-macroglobulin binds and inhibits activated protein C. Blood 78(9):2283–2290
55. Gruber A, Griffin JH (1992) Direct detection of activated protein C in blood from human subjects. Blood 79(9):2340–2348
56. Bauer KA, Kass BL, Beeler DL, Rosenberg RD (1984) Detection of protein C activation in humans. J Clin Invest 74(6):2033–2041
57. Ishii A, Yamada S, Yamada R, Hamada H (1994) t-PA activity in peripheral blood obtained from pregnant women. J Perinat Med 22(2):113–117
58. Lecander I, Astedt B (1986) Isolation of a new specific plasminogen activator inhibitor from pregnancy plasma. Br J Haematol 62(2):221–228
59. Wright JG, Cooper P, Astedt B, Lecander I, Wilde JT, Preston FE et al (1988) Fibrinolysis during normal human pregnancy: complex inter-relationships between plasma levels of tissue plasminogen activator and inhibitors and the euglobulin clot lysis time. Br J Haematol 69(2):253–258
60. Kruithof EK, Tran-Thang C, Gudinchet A, Hauert J, Nicoloso G, Genton C et al (1987) Fibrinolysis in pregnancy: a study of plasminogen activator inhibitors. Blood 69(2):460–466
61. Booth NA, Bennett B (1994) Fibrinolysis and thrombosis. Baillieres Clin Haematol 7(3):559–572
62. Astedt B, Hagerstrand I, Lecander I (1986) Cellular localisation in placenta of placental type plasminogen activator inhibitor. Thromb Haemost 56(1):63–65
63. Estelles A, Gilabert J, Espana F, Aznar J, Galbis M (1991) Fibrinolytic parameters in normotensive pregnancy with intrauterine fetal growth retardation and in severe preeclampsia. Am J Obstet Gynecol 165(1):138–142
64. Craven CM, Chedwick LR, Ward K (2002) Placental basal plate formation is associated with fibrin deposition in decidual veins at sites of trophoblast cell invasion. Am J Obstet Gynecol 186(2):291–296
65. Sheppard BL, Bonnar J (1999) Uteroplacental hemostasis in intrauterine fetal growth retardation. Semin Thromb Hemost 25(5):443–446
66. Lockwood CJ, Krikun G, Runic R, Schwartz LB, Mesia AF, Schatz F (2000) Progestin-epidermal growth factor regulation of tissue factor expression during decidualization of human endometrial stromal cells. J Clin Endocrinol Metab 85(1):297–301
67. Lanir N, Aharon A, Brenner B (2003) Haemostatic mechanisms in human placenta. Best Pract Res Clin Haematol 16(2):183–195
68. Aharon A, Brenner B, Katz T, Miyagi Y, Lanir N (2004) Tissue factor and tissue factor pathway inhibitor levels in trophoblast cells: implications for placental hemostasis. Thromb Haemost 92(4):776–786
69. Meziani F, Tesse A, Andriantsitohaina R (2008) Microparticles are vectors of paradoxical information in vascular cells including the endothelium: role in health and diseases. Pharmacol Rep 60(1):75–84

70. VanWijk MJ, VanBavel E, Sturk A, Nieuwland R (2003) Microparticles in cardiovascular diseases. Cardiovasc Res 59(2):277–287
71. Combes V, Simon AC, Grau GE, Arnoux D, Camoin L, Sabatier F et al (1999) In vitro generation of endothelial microparticles and possible prothrombotic activity in patients with lupus anticoagulant. J Clin Invest 104(1):93–102
72. Mallat Z, Benamer H, Hugel B, Benessiano J, Steg PG, Freyssinet JM et al (2000) Elevated levels of shed membrane microparticles with procoagulant potential in the peripheral circulating blood of patients with acute coronary syndromes. Circulation 101(8):841–843
73. Bretelle F, Sabatier F, Desprez D, Camoin L, Grunebaum L, Combes V et al (2003) Circulating microparticles: a marker of procoagulant state in normal pregnancy and pregnancy complicated by preeclampsia or intrauterine growth restriction. Thromb Haemost 89(3):486–492
74. Laude I, Rongieres-Bertrand C, Boyer-Neumann C, Wolf M, Mairovitz V, Hugel B et al (2001) Circulating procoagulant microparticles in women with unexplained pregnancy loss: a new insight. Thromb Haemost 85(1):18–21
75. Harlow FH, Brown MA, Brighton TA, Smith SL, Trickett AE, Kwan YL et al (2002) Platelet activation in the hypertensive disorders of pregnancy. Am J Obstet Gynecol 187(3):688–695
76. VanWijk MJ, Boer K, Berckmans RJ, Meijers JC, van der Post JA, Sturk A et al (2002) Enhanced coagulation activation in preeclampsia: the role of APC resistance, microparticles and other plasma constituents. Thromb Haemost 88(3):415–420
77. Knight M, Redman CW, Linton EA, Sargent IL (1998) Shedding of syncytiotrophoblast microvilli into the maternal circulation in pre-eclamptic pregnancies. Br J Obstet Gynaecol 105(6):632–640
78. VanWijk MJ, Nieuwland R, Boer K, van der Post JA, VanBavel E, Sturk A (2002) Microparticle subpopulations are increased in preeclampsia: possible involvement in vascular dysfunction? Am J Obstet Gynecol 187(2):450–456
79. McColl MD, Ramsay JE, Tait RC, Walker ID, McCall F, Conkie JA et al (1997) Risk factors for pregnancy associated venous thromboembolism. Thromb Haemost 78(4):1183–1188
80. Haemostasis and Thrombosis Task Force, British Committee for Standards in Haematology (2001) Investigation and management of heritable thrombophilia. Br J Haematol 114(3):512–528
81. De Santis M, Cavaliere AF, Straface G, Di Gianantonio E, Caruso A (2006) Inherited and acquired thrombophilia: pregnancy outcome and treatment. Reprod Toxicol 22(2):227–233
82. Marik PE, Plante LA (2008) Venous thromboembolic disease and pregnancy. N Engl J Med 359(19):2025–2033
83. Greer IA (1999) Thrombosis in pregnancy: maternal and fetal issues. Lancet 353(9160):1258–1265
84. Rosendaal FR (1999) Venous thrombosis: a multicausal disease. Lancet 353(9159):1167–1173
85. Carbone JF, Rampersad R (2010) Prenatal screening for thrombophilias: indications and controversies. Clin Lab Med 30(3):747–760
86. NIH Consensus Development (1986) Prevention of venous thrombosis and pulmonary embolism. JAMA 256(6):744–749
87. Kierkegaard A (1983) Incidence and diagnosis of deep vein thrombosis associated with pregnancy. Acta Obstet Gynecol Scand 62(3):239–243
88. Treffers PE, Huidekoper BL, Weenink GH, Kloosterman GJ (1983) Epidemiological observations of thrombo-embolic disease during pregnancy and in the puerperium, in 56, 022 women. Int J Gynaecol Obstet 21(4):327–331
89. Rutherford S, Montoro M, Mc Gehee W, Strong T (1991) Thromboembolic disease associated with pregnancy: an 11-year review. Am J Obstet Gynecol 164(Suppl):186
90. Greer IA (1997) Epidemiology, risk factors and prophylaxis of venous thrombo-embolism in obstetrics and gynaecology. Baillieres Clin Obstet Gynaecol 11(3):403–430

10 Hemostasis in Pregnancy and Obstetric Surgery   157

91. McColl MD, Walker ID, Greer IA (1999) The role of inherited thrombophilia in venous thromboembolism associated with pregnancy. Br J Obstet Gynaecol 106(8):756–766
92. Greer IA (2000) The challenge of thrombophilia in maternal-fetal medicine. N Engl J Med 342(6):424–425
93. Seligsohn U, Lubetsky A (2001) Genetic susceptibility to venous thrombosis. N Engl J Med 344(16):1222–1231
94. Preston FE, Rosendaal FR, Walker ID, Briet E, Berntorp E, Conard J et al (1996) Increased fetal loss in women with heritable thrombophilia. Lancet 348(9032):913–916
95. Rai R, Regan L (2000) Thrombophilia and adverse pregnancy outcome. Semin Reprod Med 18(4):369–377
96. Krabbendam I, Franx A, Bots ML, Fijnheer R, Bruinse HW (2005) Thrombophilias and recurrent pregnancy loss: a critical appraisal of the literature. Eur J Obstet Gynecol Reprod Biol 118(2):143–153
97. Coumans AB, Huijgens PC, Jakobs C, Schats R, de Vries JI, van Pampus MG et al (1999) Haemostatic and metabolic abnormalities in women with unexplained recurrent abortion. Hum Reprod 14(1):211–214
98. Kutteh WH, Triplett DA (2006) Thrombophilias and recurrent pregnancy loss. Semin Reprod Med 24(1):54–66
99. MacCallum PK, Cooper JA, Martin J, Howarth DJ, Meade TW, Miller GJ (1998) Associations of protein C and protein S with serum lipid concentrations. Br J Haematol 102(2):609–615
100. Rai R, Backos M, Elgaddal S, Shlebak A, Regan L (2002) Factor V Leiden and recurrent miscarriage-prospective outcome of untreated pregnancies. Hum Reprod 17(2):442–445
101. Kovalevsky G, Gracia CR, Berlin JA, Sammel MD, Barnhart KT (2004) Evaluation of the association between hereditary thrombophilias and recurrent pregnancy loss: a meta-analysis. Arch Intern Med 164(5):558–563
102. Meinardi JR, Middeldorp S, de Kam PJ, Koopman MM, van Pampus EC, Hamulyak K et al (1999) Increased risk for fetal loss in carriers of the factor V Leiden mutation. Ann Intern Med 130(9):736–739
103. Pihusch R, Buchholz T, Lohse P, Rubsamen H, Rogenhofer N, Hasbargen U et al (2001) Thrombophilic gene mutations and recurrent spontaneous abortion: prothrombin mutation increases the risk in the first trimester. Am J Reprod Immunol 46(2):124–131
104. Mahjoub T, Mtiraoui N, Tamim H, Hizem S, Finan RR, Nsiri B et al (2005) Association between adverse pregnancy outcomes and maternal factor V G1691A (Leiden) and prothrombin G20210A genotypes in women with a history of recurrent idiopathic miscarriages. Am J Hematol 80(1):12–19
105. Zotz RB, Gerhardt A, Scharf RE (2003) Inherited thrombophilia and gestational venous thromboembolism. Best Pract Res Clin Haematol 16(2):243–259
106. Poort SR, Rosendaal FR, Reitsma PH, Bertina RM (1996) A common genetic variation in the 3'-untranslated region of the prothrombin gene is associated with elevated plasma prothrombin levels and an increase in venous thrombosis. Blood 88(10):3698–3703
107. Nelen WL, Bulten J, Steegers EA, Blom HJ, Hanselaar AG, Eskes TK (2000) Maternal homocysteine and chorionic vascularization in recurrent early pregnancy loss. Hum Reprod 15(4):954–960
108. Nelen WL, Blom HJ, Steegers EA, den Heijer M, Eskes TK (2000) Hyperhomocysteinemia and recurrent early pregnancy loss: a meta-analysis. Fertil Steril 74(6):1196–1199
109. Brandt JT, Triplett DA, Alving B, Scharrer I (1995) Criteria for the diagnosis of lupus anticoagulants: an update. On behalf of the Subcommittee on Lupus Anticoagulant/Antiphospholipid Antibody of the Scientific and Standardisation Committee of the ISTH. Thromb Haemost 74(4):1185–1190
110. Wilson WA, Gharavi AE, Koike T, Lockshin MD, Branch DW, Piette JC et al (1999) International consensus statement on preliminary classification criteria for definite

antiphospholipid syndrome: report of an international workshop. Arthritis Rheum 42(7):1309–1311

111. Out HJ, Bruinse HW, Christiaens GC, van Vliet M, de Groot PG, Nieuwenhuis HK et al (1992) A prospective, controlled multicenter study on the obstetric risks of pregnant women with antiphospholipid antibodies. Am J Obstet Gynecol 167(1):26–32

112. Kutteh WH (1997) Antiphospholipid antibodies and reproduction. J Reprod Immunol 35(2):151–171

113. ACOG Committee on Practice Bulletins-Obstetrics (2005) ACOG Practice Bulletin #68: Antiphospholipid syndrome. Obstet Gynecol 106(5 Pt 1):1113–1121

114. Rand JH (2003) The antiphospholipid syndrome. Annu Rev Med 54:409–424

115. Rand JH, Wu XX, Guller S, Gil J, Guha A, Scher J et al (1994) Reduction of annexin-V (placental anticoagulant protein-I) on placental villi of women with antiphospholipid antibodies and recurrent spontaneous abortion. Am J Obstet Gynecol 171(6):1566–1572

116. Shibata S, Harpel PC, Gharavi A, Rand J, Fillit H (1994) Autoantibodies to heparin from patients with antiphospholipid antibody syndrome inhibit formation of antithrombin III-thrombin complexes. Blood 83(9):2532–2540

117. Ermel LD, Marshburn PB, Kutteh WH (1995) Interaction of heparin with antiphospholipid antibodies (APA) from the sera of women with recurrent pregnancy loss (RPL). Am J Reprod Immunol 33(1):14–20

118. Franklin RD, Kutteh WH (2003) Effects of unfractionated and low molecular weight heparin on antiphospholipid antibody binding in vitro. Obstet Gynecol 101(3):455–462

119. Di Simone N, Ferrazzani S, Castellani R, De Carolis S, Mancuso S, Caruso A (1997) Heparin and low-dose aspirin restore placental human chorionic gonadotrophin secretion abolished by antiphospholipid antibody-containing sera. Hum Reprod 12(9):2061–2065

120. Girardi G (2005) Heparin treatment in pregnancy loss: potential therapeutic benefits beyond anticoagulation. J Reprod Immunol 66(1):45–51

121. Friederich PW, Sanson BJ, Simioni P, Zanardi S, Huisman MV, Kindt I et al (1996) Frequency of pregnancy-related venous thromboembolism in anticoagulant factor-deficient women: implications for prophylaxis. Ann Intern Med 125(12):955–960

122. Oshiro BT, Silver RM, Scott JR, Yu H, Branch DW (1996) Antiphospholipid antibodies and fetal death. Obstet Gynecol 87(4):489–493

123. Alfirevic Z, Roberts D, Martlew V (2002) How strong is the association between maternal thrombophilia and adverse pregnancy outcome? A systematic review. Eur J Obstet Gynecol Reprod Biol 101(1):6–14

124. Rey E, Kahn SR, David M, Shrier I (2003) Thrombophilic disorders and fetal loss: a meta-analysis. Lancet 361(9361):901–908

125. Lissalde-Lavigne G, Fabbro-Peray P, Cochery-Nouvellon E, Mercier E, Ripart-Neveu S, Balducchi JP et al (2005) Factor V Leiden and prothrombin G20210A polymorphisms as risk factors for miscarriage during a first intended pregnancy: the matched case-control 'NOHA first' study. J Thromb Haemost 3(10):2178–2184

126. Roque H, Paidas MJ, Funai EF, Kuczynski E, Lockwood CJ (2004) Maternal thrombophilias are not associated with early pregnancy loss. Thromb Haemost 91(2):290–295

127. Rai R, Cohen H, Dave M, Regan L (1997) Randomised controlled trial of aspirin and aspirin plus heparin in pregnant women with recurrent miscarriage associated with phospholipid antibodies (or antiphospholipid antibodies). Br Med J 314(7076):253–257

128. Kutteh WH (1996) Antiphospholipid antibody-associated recurrent pregnancy loss: treatment with heparin and low-dose aspirin is superior to low-dose aspirin alone. Am J Obstet Gynecol 174(5):1584–1589

129. Farquharson RG, Quenby S, Greaves M (2002) Antiphospholipid syndrome in pregnancy: a randomized, controlled trial of treatment. Obstet Gynecol 100(3):408–413

130. Gris JC, Mercier E, Quere I, Lavigne-Lissalde G, Cochery-Nouvellon E, Hoffet M et al (2004) Low-molecular-weight heparin versus low-dose aspirin in women with one fetal loss and a constitutional thrombophilic disorder. Blood 103(10):3695–3699
131. Schuiling GA, Koiter TR, Faas MM (1997) Why pre-eclampisa? Hum Reprod 12(10):2087–2091
132. National high blood pressure education program working group report on high blood pressure in pregnancy (1990). Am J Obstet Gynecol 103(5 Pt 1):1691–1712
133. Sibai B, Dekker G, Kupferminc M (2005) Pre-eclampsia. Lancet 365(9461):785–799
134. Mello G, Parretti E, Marozio L, Pizzi C, Lojacono A, Frusca T et al (2005) Thrombophilia is significantly associated with severe preeclampsia: results of a large-scale, case-controlled study. Hypertension 46(6):1270–1274
135. Branch DW, Silver RM, Blackwell JL, Reading JC, Scott JR (1992) Outcome of treated pregnancies in women with antiphospholipid syndrome: an update of the Utah experience. Obstet Gynecol 80(4):614–620
136. Robertson L, Wu O, Langhorne P, Twaddle S, Clark P, Lowe GD et al (2006) Thrombophilia in pregnancy: a systematic review. Br J Haematol 132(2):171–196
137. Martin JN Jr, Blake PG, Lowry SL, Perry KG Jr, Files JC, Morrison JC (1990) Pregnancy complicated by preeclampsia-eclampsia with the syndrome of hemolysis, elevated liver enzymes, and low platelet count: how rapid is postpartum recovery? Obstet Gynecol 76(5 Pt 1):737–741
138. Torry DS, Wang HS, Wang TH, Caudle MR, Torry RJ (1998) Preeclampsia is associated with reduced serum levels of placenta growth factor. Am J Obstet Gynecol 179(6 Pt 1): 1539–1544
139. Brown MA (1995) The physiology of pre-eclampsia. Clin Exp Pharmacol Physiol 22(11):781–791
140. He S, Bremme K, Blomback M (1997) Acquired deficiency of antithrombin in association with a hypercoagulable state and impaired function of liver and/or kidney in preeclampsia. Blood Coagul Fibrinolysis 8(4):232–238
141. McKay DG (1972) Hematologic evidence of disseminated intravascular coagulation in eclampsia. Obstet Gynecol Surv 27(6):399–417
142. Howie PW, Prentice CR, McNicol GP (1971) Coagulation, fibrinolysis and platelet function in pre-eclampsia, essential hypertension and placental insufficiency. J Obstet Gynaecol Br Commonw 78(11):992–1003
143. Redman CW, Denson KW, Beilin LJ, Bolton FG, Stirrat GM (1977) Factor-VIII consumption in pre-eclampsia. Lancet 2(8051):1249–1252
144. Schjetlein R, Abdelnoor M, Haugen G, Husby H, Sandset PM, Wisloff F (1999) Hemostatic variables as independent predictors for fetal growth retardation in preeclampsia. Acta Obstet Gynecol Scand 78(3):191–197
145. Higgins JR, Walshe JJ, Darling MR, Norris L, Bonnar J (1998) Hemostasis in the uteroplacental and peripheral circulations in normotensive and pre-eclamptic pregnancies. Am J Obstet Gynecol 179(2):520–526
146. Dusse LM, Carvalho MG, Getliffe K, Voegeli D, Cooper AJ, Lwaleed BA (2008) Increased circulating thrombomodulin levels in pre-eclampsia. Clin Chim Acta 387(1–2):168–171
147. Weiner CP, Brandt J (1982) Plasma antithrombin III activity: an aid in the diagnosis of preeclampsia-eclampsia. Am J Obstet Gynecol 142(3):275–281
148. Dusse LM, Carvalho MG, Getliffe K, Voegeli D, Cooper AJ, Lwaleed BA (2008) Total plasma tissue factor pathway inhibitor levels in pre-eclampsia. Clin Chim Acta 388(1–2): 230–232
149. Redman CW, Bonnar J, Beilin L (1978) Early platelet consumption in pre-eclampsia. Br Med J 1(6111):467–469
150. Rakoczi I, Tallian F, Bagdany S, Gati I (1979) Platelet life-span in normal pregnancy and pre-eclampsia as determined by a non-radioisotope technique. Thromb Res 15(3–4):553–556

151. Estelles A, Gilabert J, Grancha S, Yamamoto K, Thinnes T, Espana F et al (1998) Abnormal expression of type 1 plasminogen activator inhibitor and tissue factor in severe preeclampsia. Thromb Haemost 79(3):500–508
152. Redman CW, Sacks GP, Sargent IL (1999) Preeclampsia: an excessive maternal inflammatory response to pregnancy. Am J Obstet Gynecol 180(2 Pt 1):499–506
153. Mantovani A, Dejana E (1989) Cytokines as communication signals between leukocytes and endothelial cells. Immunol Today 10(11):370–375
154. Vince GS, Starkey PM, Austgulen R, Kwiatkowski D, Redman CW (1995) Interleukin-6, tumour necrosis factor and soluble tumour necrosis factor receptors in women with preeclampsia. Br J Obstet Gynaecol 102(1):20–25
155. Lim KH, Rice GE, de Groot CJ, Taylor RN (1995) Plasma type II phospholipase A2 levels are elevated in severe preeclampsia. Am J Obstet Gynecol 172(3):998–1002
156. Redman CW, Sargent IL (2003) Pre-eclampsia, the placenta and the maternal systemic inflammatory response–a review. Placenta 24(Suppl A):S21–S27
157. Takagi Y, Nikaido T, Toki T, Kita N, Kanai M, Ashida T et al (2004) Levels of oxidative stress and redox-related molecules in the placenta in preeclampsia and fetal growth restriction. Virchows Arch 444(1):49–55
158. Tsukimori K, Fukushima K, Tsushima A, Nakano H (2005) Generation of reactive oxygen species by neutrophils and endothelial cell injury in normal and preeclamptic pregnancies. Hypertension 46(4):696–700
159. Tsukimori K, Maeda H, Ishida K, Nagata H, Koyanagi T, Nakano H (1993) The superoxide generation of neutrophils in normal and preeclamptic pregnancies. Obstet Gynecol 81(4):536–540
160. Huppertz B, Frank HG, Kingdom JC, Reister F, Kaufmann P (1998) Villous cytotrophoblast regulation of the syncytial apoptotic cascade in the human placenta. Histochem Cell Biol 110(5):495–508
161. Burrows RF, Hunter DJ, Andrew M, Kelton JG (1987) A prospective study investigating the mechanism of thrombocytopenia in preeclampsia. Obstet Gynecol 70(3 Pt 1):334–338
162. Leduc L, Wheeler JM, Kirshon B, Mitchell P, Cotton DB (1992) Coagulation profile in severe preeclampsia. Obstet Gynecol 79(1):14–18
163. McCrae KR, Samuels P, Schreiber AD (1992) Pregnancy-associated thrombocytopenia: pathogenesis and management. Blood 80(11):2697–2714
164. Lok CA, Van Der Post JA, Sargent IL, Hau CM, Sturk A, Boer K et al (2008) Changes in microparticle numbers and cellular origin during pregnancy and preeclampsia. Hypertens Pregnancy 27(4):344–360
165. Sibai BM, Ramadan MK, Usta I, Salama M, Mercer BM, Friedman SA (1993) Maternal morbidity and mortality in 442 pregnancies with hemolysis, elevated liver enzymes, and low platelets (HELLP syndrome). Am J Obstet Gynecol 169(4):1000–1006
166. Miles JF Jr, Martin JN Jr, Blake PG, Perry KG Jr, Martin RW, Meeks GR (1990) Postpartum eclampsia: a recurring perinatal dilemma. Obstet Gynecol 76(3 Pt 1):328–331
167. Nova A, Sibai BM, Barton JR, Mercer BM, Mitchell MD (1991) Maternal plasma level of endothelin is increased in preeclampsia. Am J Obstet Gynecol 165(3):724–727
168. Yamanaka Y, Takeuchi K, Konda E, Samoto T, Satou A, Mizudori M et al (2002) Transient postpartum diabetes insipidus in twin pregnancy associated with HELLP syndrome. J Perinat Med 30(3):273–275
169. Audibert F, Friedman SA, Frangieh AY, Sibai BM (1996) Clinical utility of strict diagnostic criteria for the HELLP (hemolysis, elevated liver enzymes, and low platelets) syndrome. Am J Obstet Gynecol 175(2):460–464
170. Geary M (1997) The HELLP syndrome. Br J Obstet Gynaecol 104(8):887–891
171. CLASP (Collaborative Low-dose Aspirin Study in Pregnancy) Collaborative Group (1994) CLASP: a randomised trial of low-dose aspirin for the prevention and treatment of preeclampsia among 9364 pregnant women. Lancet 343(8898):619–629

172. Rotchell YE, Cruickshank JK, Gay MP, Griffiths J, Stewart A, Farrell B et al (1998) Barbados low dose aspirin study in pregnancy (BLASP): a randomised trial for the prevention of pre-eclampsia and its complications. Br J Obstet Gynaecol 105(3):286–292

173. Chappell LC, Seed PT, Briley AL, Kelly FJ, Lee R, Hunt BJ et al (1999) Effect of antioxidants on the occurrence of pre-eclampsia in women at increased risk: a randomised trial. Lancet 354(9181):810–816

174. Morris CD, Jacobson SL, Anand R, Ewell MG, Hauth JC, Curet LB et al (2001) Nutrient intake and hypertensive disorders of pregnancy: evidence from a large prospective cohort. Am J Obstet Gynecol 184(4):643–651

175. Atallah AN, Hofmeyr GJ, Duley L (2002) Calcium supplementation during pregnancy for preventing hypertensive disorders and related problems. Cochrane Database Syst Rev 10/1002(1):CD001059–1185

176. Olsen SF, Secher NJ, Tabor A, Weber T, Walker JJ, Gluud C (2000) Randomised clinical trials of fish oil supplementation in high risk pregnancies. Fish oil trials in pregnancy (FOTIP) team. Br J Obstet Gynaecol 107(3):382–395

177. von Kries R, Junker R, Oberle D, Kosch A, Nowak-Gottl U (2001) Foetal growth restriction in children with prothrombotic risk factors. Thromb Haemost 86(4):1012–1016

178. Gopel W, Kim D, Gortner L (1999) Prothrombotic mutations as a risk factor for preterm birth. Lancet 353(9162):1411–1412

179. Lima F, Khamashta MA, Buchanan NM, Kerslake S, Hunt BJ, Hughes GR (1996) A study of sixty pregnancies in patients with the antiphospholipid syndrome. Clin Exp Rheumatol 14(2):131–136

180. Yasuda M, Takakuwa K, Tokunaga A, Tanaka K (1995) Prospective studies of the association between anticardiolipin antibody and outcome of pregnancy. Obstet Gynecol 86(4 Pt 1):555–559

181. Lynch A, Marlar R, Murphy J, Davila G, Santos M, Rutledge J et al (1994) Antiphospholipid antibodies in predicting adverse pregnancy outcome. A prospective study. Ann Intern Med 120(6):470–475

182. Facco F, You W, Grobman W (2009) Genetic thrombophilias and intrauterine growth restriction: a meta-analysis. Obstet Gynecol 113(6):1206–1216

183. Wiener-Megnagi Z, Ben-Shlomo I, Goldberg Y, Shalev E (1998) Resistance to activated protein C and the leiden mutation: high prevalence in patients with abruptio placentae. Am J Obstet Gynecol 179(6 Pt 1):1565–1567

184. van der Molen EF, Verbruggen B, Novakova I, Eskes TK, Monnens LA, Blom HJ (2000) Hyperhomocysteinemia and other thrombotic risk factors in women with placental vasculopathy. Br J Obstet Gynaecol 107(6):785–791

185. Facchinetti F, Marozio L, Grandone E, Pizzi C, Volpe A, Benedetto C (2003) Thrombophilic mutations are a main risk factor for placental abruption. Haematologica 88(7):785–788

186. Prochazka M, Happach C, Marsal K, Dahlback B, Lindqvist PG (2003) Factor V Leiden in pregnancies complicated by placental abruption. Br J Obstet Gynaecol 110(5):462–466

187. Rodger M (2010) Evidence base for the management of venous thromboembolism in pregnancy. Hematology Am Soc Hematol Educ Program 2010:173–180

188. Duhl AJ, Paidas MJ, Ural SH, Branch W, Casele H, Cox-Gill J et al (2007) Antithrombotic therapy and pregnancy: consensus report and recommendations for prevention and treatment of venous thromboembolism and adverse pregnancy outcomes. Am J Obstet Gynecol 197(5):457e1–457e21

189. ACOG Practice Bulletin No. 102: management of stillbirth (2009) Obstet Gynecol 113(3):748–761

190. Bates SM, Greer IA, Pabinger I, Sofaer S, Hirsh J (2008) Venous thromboembolism, thrombophilia, antithrombotic therapy, and pregnancy: American college of chest physicians evidence-based clinical practice guidelines (8th edition). Chest 133(6 Suppl):844S–886S

191. Buser KB (2002) Laparoscopic surgery in the pregnant patient–one surgeon's experience in a small rural hospital. J Soc Lap Surg 6(2):121–124
192. Bell RH Jr (2000) Gastrointestinal conditions. J Am Coll Surg 190(2):134–151
193. Angelini DJ (2003) Obstetric triage revisited: update on non-obstetric surgical conditions in pregnancy. J Midwifery Womens Health 48(2):111–118
194. Curet MJ (2000) Special problems in laparoscopic surgery. Previous abdominal surgery, obesity, and pregnancy. Surg Clin North Am 80(4):1093–1110
195. Palanivelu C, Rangarajan M, Senthilkumaran S, Parthasarathi R (2007) Safety and efficacy of laparoscopic surgery in pregnancy: experience of a single institution. J Laparoendosc Adv Surg Tech A 17(2):186–190
196. Amos JD, Schorr SJ, Norman PF, Poole GV, Thomae KR, Mancino AT et al (1996) Laparoscopic surgery during pregnancy. Am J Surg 171(4):435–437
197. Pucci RO, Seed RW (1991) Case report of laparoscopic cholecystectomy in the third trimester of pregnancy. Am J Obstet Gynecol 165(2):401–402
198. Curet MJ, Allen D, Josloff RK, Pitcher DE, Curet LB, Miscall BG et al (1996) Laparoscopy during pregnancy. Arch Surg 131(5):546–550 discussion 50–51
199. Palanivelu C, Rangarajan M, Parthasarathi R (2006) Laparoscopic appendectomy in pregnancy: a case series of seven patients. J Soc Lap Surg 10(3):321–325

Hemostasis During Heart Surgery

11

Luigi Tritapepe, Sara Iannandrea, Michela Generali
and Maria Paola Lauretta

11.1 Introduction

Cardiac surgery is a peculiar setting which requires some expertise in the management of hemostasis alterations. These abnormalities are frequently noticed during the perioperative period, and it is a very challenging task to maintain the delicate balance of the patient's coagulation.

The hemostatic complications generally tend to excessive bleeding or thrombosis. For the former there are usually different options for treatment; in contrast, thrombotic complications are more difficult to treat and result in increased rates of morbidity and hospital mortality (ischemic strokes, thromboembolism) [1]. This is the reason why almost all patients undergoing cardiac surgery arrive in the operating room with a pattern that tends to anticoagulation.

This course of action is sometimes related to an excessive blood loss (during and after the intervention) which requires the transfusion of multiple units of blood components and is independently associated with serious postoperative adverse events, including sepsis, acute respiratory distress syndrome, renal failure, and death.

Factors that contribute to blood loss in cardiac surgery are related to surgical damage of large blood vessels and to acquired defects in hemostasis. The last of these is a consequence of the antiplatelet and anticoagulant therapy administered in the preoperative period, and of the intraoperative management of cardiopulmonary bypass (CPB).

L. Tritapepe (✉)
Department of Anesthesia and Intensive Care, UOD Anesthesia and Intensive
Care in Cardiac Surgery, University of Rome "La Sapienza", Rome, Italy
e-mail: luigi.tritapepe@uniroma1.it

G. Berlot (ed.), *Hemocoagulative Problems in the Critically Ill Patient*,
DOI: 10.1007/978-88-470-2448-9_11, © Springer-Verlag Italia 2012

11.2 Normal Hemostasis

For the correct management of postoperative bleeding some notions of the physiopathological processes of hemostasis are necessary. The clotting process, which includes a primary and a secondary component, is triggered in response to tissue trauma and is initiated by expression of tissue factor. The primary hemostasis consists in the rapid formation of a platelet clot at the site of the lesion. An effective primary hemostasis needs three important events: platelet adhesion, the release of the contents stored in α-granules and dense granules, and platelet aggregation. Within a few seconds of tissue trauma, the platelets adhere to subendothelial matrix proteins, through a specific platelet receptor (glycoprotein Ia/IIa), and von Willebrand factor, an adhesive glycoprotein, stabilizes this interaction (platelet–endothelium). Platelets, after their activation, release into the plasma the contents stored in their granules, among which the most important ones are von Willebrand factor and ADP. ADP activates platelets, through binding platelet surface receptors P2Y1 and P2Y12, and changes the conformation of glycoprotein IIb/IIIa. In this new conformation status, glycoprotein binds fibrinogen and this leads to platelet aggregation and formation of the clot. After the formation of the primary hemostatic clot, the platelets are activated to start the secondary hemostasis, which culminates in the synthesis of a sufficient quantity of thrombin, which converts fibrinogen to fibrin. The secondary coagulation cascade is divided into the extrinsic and intrinsic pathways, which are determined by a chain reaction that converts the inactive precursor to active proteases. These pathways are regulated by cellular and plasmatic factors and by the presence of calcium ions [2]. The extrinsic pathway is triggered in response to tissue trauma and is initiated by expression of tissue factor. The role of the intrinsic pathway is less clear but this pathway plays an important role in the activation of blood by an artificial device such as a CPB circuit or a mechanical circulatory assist device [3]. The point of convergence of the intrinsic and extrinsic pathways is the prothrombinase complex. This complex consists of activated factor X (factor Xa) and activated factor V (factor Va) bound together by calcium ions on a phospholipid membrane and it converts prothrombin (factor II) to thrombin (activated factor II). Finally, thrombin activates factor XIII to activated factor XIII, which stabilizes the fibrin clot by covalently cross-linking fibrin. Regulation of hemostasis also includes various mechanisms essential to limit clot propagation beyond the injury site. One of these is hemodilution. Shear forces within flowing blood quickly destroy the early platelet/fibrin clot, which is highly susceptible to disruption [4]. Other mechanisms initiate their activity to limit clot propagation. Four major counterregulatory pathways have been identified that appear particularly crucial for downregulating hemostasis: fibrinolysis, tissue factor pathway inhibitor (TFPI), the protein C system, and serine protease inhibitors. The fibrinolytic system includes a cascade of chain reactions culminating in plasmin generation and proteolytic degradation of fibrin and fibrinogen. Plasmin is derived from an inactive precursor, plasminogen [5], the conversion being initiated by release of tissue plasminogen activator or urokinase from vascular endothelium, the synthesis of which is stimulated by thrombin. Activated factor XII and kallikrein of the intrinsic pathway activate fibrinolysis after exposure to an artificial device, and the presence of fibrin accelerates plasmin generation [6]. The role of plasmin in the inhibition of hemostasis is not limited to the degradation of fibrin and fibrinogen; indeed, plasmin is also necessary to degrade important cofactors V and VIII as well as to reduce platelet glycoprotein surface receptors essential to adhesion and aggregation. TFPI inhibits the tissue factor/activated factor VII (factor VIIa) complex and thereby the extrinsic coagulation pathway, by forming, together with factor Xa, a phospholipid membrane-bound complex that incorporates and inhibits tissue factor/factor VIIa complexes. TFPI is normally present on the endothelial surface, but heparin administration permits its release into the circulation. This is the way by which heparin catalyzes the inhibitory activity [7]. The third counterregulatory pathway is protein C. It inhibits thrombin and the essential cofactors factor Va and activated factor VIII (factor VIIIa) and is activated by thrombin itself, which, binding a membrane-associated protein, thrombomodulin, activates protein C. Protein C, complexed with the cofactor protein S, degrades cofactors Va and VIIIa. Loss of these critical cofactors limits formation of "tenase" and "prothrombinase" activation complexes, which are essential for formation of factor X and thrombin, respectively. Thrombin, once bound to thrombomodulin, is inactivated and removed from the circulation, providing another mechanism by which protein C downregulates hemostasis. The final regulators of hemostasis are antithrombin and heparin cofactor II. Whereas antithrombin inhibits thrombin as well as activated factor Xa, factor Xa, activated factor XI, and activated factor XII, heparin cofactor II inhibits only thrombin [7]. Antithrombin plays an important role in the downregulation of hemostasis also because by linking with heparin, a catalyst accelerator, it promotes inhibition of targeted enzymes, located on vascular endothelial cells, and provides inhibitory sites for thrombin and factor Xa in vivo.

11.3 The Cardiac Surgery Patient

Patients undergoing cardiac surgery have some acquired alterations of physiologic clotting processes as a consequence of the anticoagulant and antiplatelet therapy administrated during the preoperative period. They can be divided into patients with valves disease and patients with ischemic heart disease. In the first group, patients who have mitral valve disease, associated with atrial fibrillation, usually receive anticoagulant therapy. In contrasts, patients with cardiac ischemic disease take antiplatelet drugs chronically or at the time of their diagnostic cardiac catheterization, frequently within the last week before surgery.

Many studies have demonstrated that most patients receiving aspirin or other nonsteroidal antinflammatory drugs (NSAIDs) therapy do not bleed excessively after surgery. However, the introduction and use of low molecular weight heparin compounds, direct inhibitors of thrombin (e.g., hirudin, argatroban, bivalirudin, dermatan, orgaran), and platelets (e.g., abciximab, eptifibatide, tirofiban, and most importantly long-acting ADP antagonists such as clopidogrel), as well as fibrinolytic agents can potentially increase bleeding and complicate clinical management. The risk of bleeding related to these agents depends on their relative potency, pharmacodynamic half-life, time interval from most recent dose before surgery, and whether or not a reversal agent is available [8].

11.4 Antiplatelet Drugs

The commonly used antiplatelet agents are aspirin, glycoprotein IIb/IIIa inhibitors, and P2Y12 antagonists. Aspirin is commonly used in the setting of acute coronary syndromes and percutaneous coronary intervention and has not been associated with increased bleeding after surgery, so its use should be continued perioperatively. It irreversibly acetylates the catalytic site of cyclooxygenase-1, the enzyme necessary for the processing of thromboxane A_2.

The glycoprotein IIb/IIIa inhibitors abciximab, eptifibatide, and tirofiban are intravenous agents that block aggregation of activated platelets.

In contrast, ticlopidine, clopidogrel, and more recently prasugrel and ticagrelor are oral agents that prevent platelet thrombus formation by inhibiting the ADP receptor P2Y12.

Prasugrel appears to be more potent and is associated with more surgical bleeding than clopidogrel, whereas ticagrelor is associated with less surgical bleeding. Abciximab, clopidogrel, ticlopidine, and prasugrel bind irreversibly to platelets, requiring de novo repopulation of the circulating platelet pool by the bone marrow to recover effective platelet function. The drug dose given, bone marrow turnover, and the size of the circulating platelet pool (itself related to patient size and platelet count) may explain the interpatient variability of the recovery of platelet function. Transfusion of multiple platelet units may be required to achieve hemostasis after CPB.

Reversible receptor binding is seen with the glycoprotein IIb/IIIa inhibitors eptifibatide and tirofiban (both have half-lives of 2 h, with recovery of platelet function occurring 4–8 h after discontinuation) and the P2Y12 receptor antagonist ticagrelor (half-life of 7–8 h and recovery of platelet function after 12 h). It is important to consider the elimination half-life of these drugs because free drugs will bind to and inhibit transfused or native platelets. All approved agents are cleared renally, and renal impairment approximately doubles the time until recovery of platelet function. Even though ticagrelor is cleared mainly through the liver, it has been associated with an increase in the level of creatinine and its use should be avoided in patients with renal dysfunction.

11.5 Antifibrinolytic Drugs

Pharmacological agents used to inhibit conversion of plasminogen to plasmin include aminocaproic acid, tranexamic acid, and aprotinin, which acts by inhibiting plasmin and is used extensively in cardiac surgery [1].

11.6 Acquired Bleeding Disorders

Acquired bleeding disorders are frequently associated with the risk of excessive blood loss in cardiac surgery. Their origin could be a consequence of the use of some drugs, the use of an artificial device (e.g., CPB) and also a direct consequence of the massive tissue destruction and endothelial injury during the surgery.

11.7 Intraoperative Metabolic Abnormalities

Hypothermia has been shown to inhibit coagulation enzymes, decrease platelet count and function, and stimulate fibrinolysis, whereas acidosis impedes fibrin polymerization. Hypocalcemia from citrate toxicity in massively transfused patients must be corrected to permit enzymatic reactions of the coagulation cascade. Anemia further aggravates bleeding diathesis because red cells are thought to assist in platelet margination against an injured vessel wall.

11.8 Disseminated Intravascular Coagulation

Fragmentation of erythrocytes that generates schistocytes and hemolysis, elevated levels of D-dimers, thrombocytopenia, prolonged prothrombin time, partial thromboplastin time, and thrombin time, and decreased fibrinogen levels are typically noted in a disseminated intravascular coagulation. This, initiated by massive tissue destruction and endothelial injury, leads to the release of tissue factors, which triggers widespread thrombus formation in the microcirculation. This further exacerbates endothelial injury by depleting the levels of coagulation factors and platelets while also activating the fibrinolytic system, resulting in a consumptive coagulopathy [1].

11.9 Liver Disease

Advanced liver disease or hypoperfusion ("shock liver") is responsible for a decrease in the levels of circulating procoagulant factors, reflected in a prolonged prothrombin time as the liver is responsible for synthesizing most coagulation factors.

11.10 Vitamin K Deficiency

Malabsorption syndromes can determine deficient states of vitamin K, which is essential for the synthesis of factors II, VII, IX, and X, and therefore increase patients' bleeding tendencies. Coumadin (warfarin) inhibits vitamin K epoxide reductase, which is necessary to "recycle vitamin K" to its reduced state. Only in its reduced state can vitamin K participate in the vital carboxylation of glutamic acid residues of coagulation factors II, VII, IX, and X in the liver [1].

11.11 Renal Disease

A prolonged bleeding time and propensity for bleeding associated with surgery or trauma can lead to chronic renal failure, which commonly occurs in association with platelet dysfunction. The mechanisms appear to be multifactorial and may include accumulation of guanidinosuccinic acid and nitric oxide in uremic plasma [5].

Dialysis and correction of anemia have been reported to shorten bleeding times in patients with chronic renal failure, although the risks associated with these therapies, and the predictive value of the bleeding time for subsequent hemorrhage, remain unclear. Red blood cell concentration has been speculated to play a role as correction of anemia results in shortened bleeding times, presumably related to the role of red blood cells in causing platelet margination along the vessel wall under laminar flow conditions. Traditionally, cryoprecipitate administration occurs in this setting; however, desmopressin (0.3 µg/kg) and conjugated estrogens similarly may shorten bleeding times [9].

11.12 CPB-Mediated Hemostasis Alteration

Among acquired coagulopathy, it is important to discuss the depth the one related to CPB.

This mechanical circulatory assistance device predisposes to an elevated incidence of bleeding, whether in the operating room or immediately after the surgery, which is directly proportional to the duration and the type of intervention and to the anticoagulant/antiplatelet therapy previously administered. Patients who undergo combined procedures (such as heart valve replacement and coronary artery bypass graft) are exposed to the major risks.

The CPB leads to an anticoagulation state due to various factors.

First, the administration of crystalloids for the priming of the circuit and as a component of the cardioplegic solution causes hemodilution and a relative decrease in the levels of coagulation factors and platelets. Moreover, contact of the patient's blood with the extended CPB surfaces leads to the activation of the intrinsic pathway of the coagulation cascade, whereas the endothelium damage, due to surgical trauma, and retransfusion of pericardial blood for the hemore-covery cause the activation of the extrinsic pathway. These conditions cause an alternated activation of hemostasis which requires administration of high doses of heparin to avoid blood clotting. At the end of the procedure the administration of excessive doses of protamine (to antagonize heparin) may also cause inhibition of coagulation factors and platelet consumption and/or dysfunction. In addition, surgical trauma leads to chemotaxis and activation of polymorphonuclear leuko-cytes, which may affect the hemostatic system by releasing elastases.

In the physiopathology of CPB-mediated coagulopathy, an excessive activation of fibrinolysis may also be the considered as a consequence of system activation of factor XII and thrombin, hypothermia, and retransfusion of tissue plasminogen activator from the pericardial cavity blood, which is released from the injured endothelial cells during heart surgery.

A major role is also played by thrombin and plasmin in the hemostatic alter-ations strictly related to the use of CPB. Despite high doses of heparin, thrombin is generated and its activity increases in a way directly proportional to the duration of CPB. It activates factors V, VIII, and XIII and platelets, generates fibrin monomer, and, at the same time, releases tissue plasminogen activator and TFPI. It also activates protein C, which, in conjunction with thrombomodulin, degrades factors Va and VIIIa. On the other hand, excessive plasmin activity may cause hypofri-binogenemia, degradation of factors V, VIII, and XIII, and platelet dysfunction through centralization of granules and proteolytic removal of membrane glyco-protein Ib, with its translocation plasmatic membrane into the canalicular system.

To sum up, CPB-mediated hemostasis alteration can be grouped into four categories: decrease of levels of coagulation factors, primary fibrinolysis, throm-bocytopenia, and transient platelet dysfunction. The last two of these are consid-ered to be the most important causes of bleeding in the postoperative period after cardiac surgery with CPB.

Platelet dysfunction may be due to various factors, such as contact with CPB membranes, use of heparin, and hypothermia, although these abnormalities usually disappear within a few hours after CPB, suggesting that it might result from heparin or inhibition of other plasma factors, rather than an intrinsic defect [10].

11.13 Point of Care

In the preoperative or postoperative period, laboratory-based measures of coagu-lation (such as the prothrombin time and the activated partial thromboplastin time) are still widely adopted; nevertheless, during the intervention a more prompt analysis of coagulation is required. Because of this, in the past few years the use of point-of-care measures has been spreading.

This kind of intraoperative monitoring allows one to administer blood com-ponents and hemostatic drug therapies more specifically and in real time, with proven cost-efficacy.

There are four categories of point-of-care coagulation monitoring:
1 Functional measures of coagulation or tests that measure the intrinsic coagulation pathway
2 Heparin concentration monitors
3 Viscoelastic measures of coagulation
4. Platelet function monitors [11].

11.13.1 Functional Measures of Coagulation

The activated coagulation time (ACT) measures the integrity of the intrinsic and the common coagulation pathways. It is initiated through contact activation using Celite or kaolin, to accelerate clot formation and reduce the time for assay completion. Kaolin is the preferred choice for patients receiving aprotinin (an antifibrinolytic drug) because in such conditions the use of Celite leads to artifactual prolongation of the clotting time [10]. One device commonly used in cardiac surgery setting requires 2 mL of whole blood to be put into a glass test tube containing a small magnet. The tube is consequently placed into the analyzer and rotated slowly at 37°C; by doing so, the magnet can keep contact with a proximity detection switch. The ACT is ended by an alarm triggered when the magnet becomes entrapped and dislodged from the detection switch due to formation of fibrin clot. In another device for measuring the ACT, blood is placed in a cartridge that has an activating agent in it (kaolin) that interacts with the blood. Then the machine drops a plunger that has a small flag attached to it and electronically measures the time it takes for the flag to stop falling, which means it is stopped by the fibrin fibers and sets off an alarm. Because the ACT measures the intrinsic and common pathways of coagulation, heparin and other anticoagulants prolong the ACT itself. In the specific setting of cardiac surgery, it gives precise information about the degree of coagulation of the patient and can also be used to calculate the exact dose of protamine to give at the end of the CPB. The advantages of ACT include ease of use, low cost, and linear operating response at increasing doses of heparin. The disadvantages, on the other hand, are low sensitivity at low heparin concentrations and poor reproducibility. To compensate for this inconvenience, recent ACT devices contain heparinase, which improves the sensitivity for detecting low heparin doses.

The high-dose thrombin time (HiTT) is a modified thrombin time that use a larger dose of thrombin to test for heparin concentration at the doses used during CPB. It supplies an alternative functional measure of heparin anticoagulation by measuring the final common pathway of the coagulation, that is, the conversion of fibrinogen in fibrin, and so it should be less susceptible to the variables that affect the ACT. The method consists in using a test tube containing lyophilized thrombin reagent which is prewarmed and hydrated with 0.5 mL of distilled water and to which 1.5 mL of whole blood is added [12]. The use of high doses of thrombin entails that clot formation is strictly dependent on the presence of fibrinogen, independently of plasma coagulation factors. Therefore, the HiTT is prolonged by heparin (a thrombin inhibitor), severe hypofibrinogenemia or dysfibrinogenemia, and fibrinolysis. During interventions requiring high doses of heparin, such as in the cardiac surgery setting, HiTT prolongation will correlate with the heparin anticoagulant effect.

11.13.2 Heparin Concentration Measurement

Protamine titration is one of the most used point-of-care methods for measurement of heparin concentration during interventions and in perioperative settings. Protamine sulfate is administered to reverse the anticoagulant effects of heparin upon completion of CPB. It is a basic polycationic protein which directly inhibits heparin. The inhibition works approximately in a stoichiometric way, this means that, for example, 1 mg of protamine inhibits 1 mg (approximately 100 U) of heparin, although the optimal protamine-to-heparin ratio is difficult to individualize for each patient because of the great interpatient variability in heparin's metabolism. This device can be used to estimate the heparin dose required to reach proper anticoagulation and, consequently, the exact dose of protamine to administer at the end of CPB [13]. By adding protamine to a sample of heparin-containing blood, the decrease in time to clot formation grows with increasing quantities of protamine, until the concentration of the latter exceeds the concentration of heparin. If blood samples with different concentrations of heparin are analyzed, the first one to clot will be the one with the most closely matched doses of heparin and protamine. Modern devices for point-of-care heparin concentration analysis perform automated measurement. The advantages are sensitivity for low heparin concentrations and relative insensitivity to hemodilution and hypothermia.

11.13.3 Viscoelastic Measures of Coagulation

Thromboelastography (TEG) is a tool for evaluation of bleeding and the effects of blood components and blood products. The ability to evaluate the full spectrum of hemostasis via a single test is very appealing; that is why the use of this assay is spreading. It visualizes the viscoelastic changes that take place during in vitro coagulation, producing a graphical representation of the fibrin polymerization process. The device requires a whole blood sample (usually 0.36 mL), with or without citrate, which is put in a cuvette at 37°C. A pin is suspended in the blood by a torsion wire that is designed to detect any motion within the cup. The cup begins to oscillate every 10 s at a 4°45′ angle, back and forth. The coagulation cascade is activated with the addition of kaolin, leading to thrombin formation, and the fibrinogen is converted to fibrin. Eventually a stable clot is formed when fibrin polymers are stabilized by factor VIII and activated platelets; that is also an effect of thrombin formation. The formed clot disturbs the movement of the pin, letting the sensors produce a curve representing these dynamic changes. Conversely, as the clot breaks down, the amplitude of the curve also diminishes. This curve gives information about the clotting process and fibrinolysis and simplifies qualitative analysis of the individual steps involved. These steps are the following. The period of time starting with the initiation of the test until the beginning of the clot formation is called R (reaction/clotting) time. The following period, starting with the clot formation until the curve reaches an amplitude of 20 mm, is called K time; the K stands for clot kinetics. The angle between the baseline and the tangent to the TEG curve passing through the starting point of coagulation is the α angle (the split after the end point of the R time). The α angle visualizes the acceleration and the kinetics of fibrin formation and cross-linking. The measure of the highest point on the TEG curve is called the maximal amplitude (MA) and represents clot strength. MA increases along with platelet concentration, platelet function, and platelet–fibrin interaction. Another measured parameter is A30, representing the amplitude after 30 min. The difference between MA and A30 reflects the degree of fibrinolysis. This parameter is more often reported as Ly30, an indicator of the fibrinolytic activity during the first 30 min after MA. Ly30 reflects the reduction in the area under the curve. The ratio between the amplitude at a given time point and MA is called the clot lysis index, and it is given as a percentage of MA; therefore, it is a measure of fibrinolysis at a given time. The hemostasis profile is represented by the clot index (CI): it is calculated on the basis of the parameters R, K, α, and MA. The normal range is from -3 to $+3$ [13]. Since the curve represents different phases of coagulation, alterations in its shape allow one to realize a tailored therapy. If the curve shows a prolonged R time, this indicates lack of coagulation factors and, if this is not related to heparin administration, transfusion of plasma may resolve the problem. If it is due to an effect of heparin, protamine sulfate alone or in combination with plasma will be able to reverse the abnormality. A reduced α angle in the curve marks deficiency of fibrinogen, which may be treated with fibrinogen concentrate or plasma, depending on the clinical situation. Low MA suggests reduced platelet function; in this case, always considering the clinical situation, desmopressin and/or platelet concentrates may be indicated. Ly30 and CI, in association with the analysis of the TEG curve shape, give information on the fibrinolytic process. Clearly, there is a difference between the primary and the secondary fibrinolysis, in the same way that the correct treatments differ. If primary fibrinolysis is present, the patient will need antifibrinolytic therapy; on the other hand, if secondary fibrinolysis is present, the patient could benefit from anticoagulation therapy. The information about the fibrinolytic process can be completed by analyzing the TEG curve shape: elevated Ly30 combined with low CI indicates primary fibrinolysis; in contrast, an elevation of both Ly30 and CI suggests secondary fibrinolysis [14].

The Sonoclot is an alternative tool for viscoelastic measurement of coagulation. It responds to mechanical changes that occur within the blood sample (usually 0.4 mL). This device consists of a cylindrical probe that oscillates up and down within a blood sample. The electronic drive and detection circuit senses the resistance to motion that the probe encounters as clot formation occurs and generates an analog electronic signal. The resulting signal is processed by a microcomputer and reported as the clot signal. The record of the clot evolution is saved as a graphic of the clot signal value versus time and is printed on a thermal graphics printer. This graphic is called the Sonoclot signature. In this signature the coagulation cascade begins from the initiation of the signature and continues throughout the liquid phase, which ends when the viscosity of the sample begins to increase as a result of thrombin generation and fibrin formation. The time that the test in the signature remains liquid is called the onset. Once thrombin forms, the fibrinogen converts to fibrin monomers, which spontaneously polymerize into a fibrin gel. The fibrin gel formation is characterized by the slope of the Sonoclot signature during the gel formation (clot rate) and by the height of the signature when gel formation is completed. This information is important to identify hypercoagulable states, for anticoagulant management, and for fibrin hemodilution. Another important function of Sonoclot is its ability to capture the clot retraction that functioning platelets perform on a fibrin clot; in fact they adhere to multiple nodes of the fibrin gel and cause the gel to collapse together or retract. As the clot retracts, it tightens, causing a rise in the curve. When the clot pulls away from the inner surface of the probe the curve falls. Clot retraction is measured by both the time it takes for retraction to occur and the degree of retraction. One useful measurement is the time to peak: the faster the time to peak, the greater the platelet function is intact. Also, a qualitative assessment of the clot retraction is also possible. Sharp, well-defined peaks indicate strong retraction; poorly defined peaks indicate weak retraction. At the end of the coagulation process, fibrin clots dissolve through activation of the fibrinolytic system. This also causes the formation of fibrin split products, which do not polymerize, so, as this fibrinolysis progresses, the fibrin gel dissolves. In a normal blood sample, fibrinolysis usually occurs after many hours. Since most Sonoclot test runs last 45–60 min, lysis will be detected only when hyperfibrinolysis occurs.

Despite their completeness, both TEG and the Sonoclot are not specific for platelet function and are essentially insensitive to cyclooxygenase inhibitors (aspirin, nonsteroidal anti-inflammatory drugs) and P2Y12 antagonists (ticlopidine, clopidogrel) [15].

11.13.4 Platelet Function Monitors

Since platelet dysfunction is one of the most important causes of postoperative bleeding, in the past few years an increasing array of platelet function assays specifically designed as point-of-care instruments have begun to be used [16, 17].

The PFA-100 (platelet function analyzer) measures primary hemostasis by simulating the conditions following vascular wall injury and the coagulation cascade. It requires a whole blood sample (citrate anticoagulated) which is aspirated from a reservoir through a capillary and a biologically active membrane. The membrane, coated with either collagen/epinephrine or collagen/ADP (both platelet activators), contains a central aperture, simulating small vessel wall injury. As blood flows through the aperture, platelets begin to adhere and aggregate. The time until the aperture is completely occluded by the platelet/red blood cell thrombus is reported as the "closure time." It has been proved that the PFA-100 is a highly sensitive screening test for von Willebrand's disease and it can also detect other specific platelet function disorders, such as aspirin-mediated platelet dysfunction. The limitations of the PFA-100 include thrombocytopenia (platelet count below 150,000/uL) and a decreased hematocrit (below 35%), which may prolong the closure time because formation of a platelet/red cell thrombus is directly dependent upon these factors.

The HemoSTATUS platelet function test (or platelet-activated clotting test) works by using platelet activating factor (PAF), which has the ability of accelerating clot formation of the kaolin-activated ACT. The test is performed with a Medtronic HMS coagulation analyzer. A six-channel kaolin ACT cartridge is preloaded with increasing concentrations of PAF. Each individual patient assay gets a clot ratio based on the ratio of the PAF-accelerated ACT to the standard ACT. Normal volunteers are recruited to determine their maximal clot ratio (indicating normal platelet function) so that the patient's ratio can be compared with a standard measure. Higher concentrations of PAF are required to achieve the standard ACT value in patients with platelet dysfunction. A relationship between postoperative bleeding and platelet dysfunction has been reported in cardiac surgery, although recent studies contradicted this relationship [10].

The rapid platelet function analyzer is a turbidimetry-based optical detection system that estimates the ability of activated platelets to bind fibrinogen-coated polystyrene beads. The device works with a whole blood sample with the addition of thrombin receptor activating peptide, which directly activates platelets and stimulates the surface receptor expression of glycoprotein IIb/IIIa. The instrument automatically measures changes in light transmission as activated platelets bind and aggregate fibrinogen-coated beads and generates a signal. Although the rapid platelet function analyzer is a simple to use and provides a rapid bedside measure of platelet function, a baseline reference measurement is required for each patient to calculate the degree of subsequent changes in platelet function [16].

In vivo, in the presence of various agonists, platelets form aggregates that cause a reduction of their number. Plateletworks exploits this characteristic: it is a tool that count platelets at a baseline (whole blood with EDTA) and after the addition of an agonist, such as ADP or collagen. The test is performed in two different tubes. At the end of the test, the difference between platelet counts before and after the addition of the agonist gives a measure of platelet aggregation. The resulting number is reported as "percent aggregation." The advantages of this device include the need for only 1 mL of blood for each tube, the fact that the result is available in less than 5 min, and no need for preparation of the sample [16]. Furthermore, various studies have demonstrated a correlation between platelet count and laboratory-based measures of platelet aggregation. This test can also be used to identify platelet dysfunctions caused by glycoprotein IIb/IIIa antagonists [16].

Another device which can measure different platelet properties is the Hemodyne hemostasis analyzer system. Employing a sample of 0.7 mL of whole blood, it can measure platelet contractile force, i.e., the force generated by platelets during clot formation. The sample is put between two parallel surfaces and various clotting agents are added to begin clot formation. During this process a downward force is imposed from above and the sample begins to change shape. The degree of deformation is measured by a transducer. In this way the device can also calculate another parameter, the elastic modulus, a measure of clot rigidity. During clot formation, the platelets inside retract the clot. The forces generated during the clot retraction move the upper surface and this movement is detected by the displacement transducer. The last parameter measured by the hemostasis analyzer system is the thrombin generation time, a measure of the time between addition of calcium to the sample and initiation of platelet contractile force during clot formation. In preliminary investigations, platelet contractile force was correlated with thrombin production, thrombin inhibitors (such as heparin), and to exposure of glycoprotein IIb/IIIa. The clot elastic modulus is sensitive to changes in clot structure, fibrinogen concentration, the rate of fibrin production, and red cell flexibility. On the other hand, the thrombin generation time is sensitive to clotting factor deficiency [16].

The newer devices developed specifically for the assessment of antiplatelet drugs, such as Platelet Mapping, the cone and plate(let) analyzer, and VerifyNow, are more promising [15].

11.14 Use and Complications of Blood Components

For the postoperative management of hemostasis, it is essential to maintain an adequate state of anticoagulation after heart valve implant and it is also important to avoid the closure of a coronary artery bypass graft, and any thrombotic complications associated with major surgery (deep vein thrombosis, pulmonary embolism, ischemic strokes) [21]. The anticoagulant/antiplatelet therapy used for this purpose obviously increases the risk of bleeding (4–32%), necessitating multiple transfusions of blood components and/or hemostatic agents.

The decision to transfuse red blood cells is primarily based on clinical need to increase the delivering of oxygen, generally the threshold for a transfusion is a hematocrit of 20% and a hemoglobin concentration of 7 g/dL. Several clinical conditions can increase this threshold for transfusion: usually a condition of impaired oxygenation (pulmonary disease, acute anemia with a low offset of 2,3-bisphosphoglycerate, left shift of the hemoglobin dissociation curve due to alkalosis or hypothermia, reduced venous return to the heart, acute myocardial infarction (AMI), myocardial dysfunction, cardiomyopathy, β-adrenergic blockade).

Regarding the administration of concentrated platelets, in cardiac surgery as in any major surgery the platelet count should be between 50,000 and 100,000/mL. Each unit of platelets will increase the count by 5,000–10,000/mL. When patients are receiving a massive blood transfusion, empirical administration of two units of fresh frozen plasma (FFP) for every five units of red blood cells is done. Other indications for use of FFP are the normalization of coagulation factors (15 mL/kg to normalize 30%), the urgent need to antagonize the effect of oral anticoagulant therapy (OAT), and the management of intraoperative bleeding when the ACT is between 480 and 500 s during coronary artery bypass graft or greater than 300 s in the course of deep hypothermic circulatory arrest.

Cryoprecipitate (factor VIII–von Willebrand factor–fibrinogen–fibronectin–factor XIII) is administered in the course of massive microvascular bleeding with a significant reduction of fibrinogen concentration (below 80–100 mg/dL) in patients with congenital or acquired dysfybrinogenemia or a deficit of factor XIII.

There are different complications of massive blood transfusion. Three of these are very severe and can lead to death: transfusion-related acute lung injury (TRALI), ABO incompatibility, and sepsis. Other complications may increase the morbidity of hospital stay: volume overload, hypothermia (which slows down clotting and causes platelet sequestration), dilution coagulopathy, reduction of the level of 2,3-bisphosphoglycerate (which shifts to the left of the hemoglobin dissociation curve), metabolic acidosis, hyperkalemia, and citrate intoxication. In general, the complications of transfusions are classified into infectious and immune-mediated. Among the first are an estimated very low incidence (1:1,600,000) of transmission of hepatitis B virus–hepatitis C virus–human immunodeficiency virus–human T-cell lymphotrophic virus, a highest estimate (4%) of cytomegalovirus transmission and of hepatitis B virus transmission (with and without leukocyte depletion), and bacterial sepsis. Among the immune-mediated complications are hemolytic reaction with acute hemolysis of red blood cells (in patients with hypotension, hemoglobinuria, and massive bleeding) and delayed hemolytic reactions (fever, decreased hematocrit and decreased bilirubin level days after transfusion). Common reactions are related to white blood cells as a result of an antibody response directed against the leukocytes of donor and graft-versus host disease, in which donor lymphocytes trigger an immune response against the host. Very common is the state of generalized immunosuppression of patients after transfusion due to systemic inflammatory response of the body (transfusion-related immunomodulation). Transfusion-related immunomodulation is caused by the progressive release of cytokines from stored blood cells (IL-1, IL-8, TNF) and other bioreactive substances (lipophosphatidylcoline, histamine). Usually allergic reactions such as urticaria, angioedema, and hypotension can occur as a reaction to proteins of the donor. A dreaded complication is TRALI, a noncardiogenic acute pulmonary edema that occurs after transfusion cycles with an incidence of 1:5,000 and a mortality rate of 6–9%. Although the pathogenesis is still much debated, the cause of TRALI seems to be the action of different antibodies directed against HLA antigens and neutrophil count, with the subsequent activation of cytokines and inflammatory response in the lung microvascular bed. A higher incidence of TRALI has been noticed with the administration of plasma derivatives rather than red cell concentrates [18].

During massive postoperative bleeding (more than 150 mL/h) not due to surgical causes, in addition to standard treatment with colloids, crystalloids, blood products, antifibrinolytic drugs (such as tranexamic acid), or protamine, the use of recombinant factor VIIa is gaining approval. It was designed for patients affected by hemophilia A and hemophilia B [19]. Now its use for polytauma, in septic patients, in liver transplantation, and in cardiac surgery is really promising, especially in patients undergoing acute aortic dissection surgery in deep hypothermic circulatory arrest [20], and in patients with aspirin- or clopidogrel-induced platelet dysfunction. Factor VIIa increases the production of thrombin on the platelet surface, a central point for coagulation. It binds tissue factor, forming the factor VII/tissue factor complex which activates factor VIII, and later factors X and V and leads to a prothrombin complex [21]. In this way a rapid and systemic coagulation is achieved and so there is a reduction of blood loss in postoperative period (on average from more than 150 mL/h to less than 100 mL/h 1 h after administration). The transfusion requirements are significantly reduced; in addition, improvements of the international normalized ratio (INR), plated count, fibrinogen level, and antithrombin level are detected after factor VIIa administration [20]. To optimize the effect of factor VIIa, it is necessary to correct hypothermia and acidosis and replace clotting factors by administration of FFP, plated pools, and cryoprecipitates (the fibrinogen level should be greater than 100,000/mL–plated greater than 100,000/mL) [19]. Doses varies from 90 µg/kg in adults in one or two applications to 30–60 µg/kg in pediatric patients. These doses provide a satisfactory margin of safety with no incidence of thromboembolic complication (no higher incidence in deep vein thrombosis, stroke, pulmonary embolism) [20, 21]. Factor VIIa seems to be free from the limitations of other conventional drugs generally used in management of hemorrhage. Protamine has several serious adverse effects, such as hypotension and hypersensitivity reaction; aminocaproic acid and tranexamic acid have an higher antifibrinolytic effectiveness when administrated during the preoperative period; aprotinin is expensive and not useful [21].

Overall, factor VIIa seems to be the most effective and safest drug in acute bleeding also when blood loss is refractory to conventional methods [20, 21].

Another promising drug in the control of massive bleeding is prothrombin complex concentrate (PCC), consisting of prothrombin, factors VII, IX, and X, fibrinogen, proteins C and S, antithrombin, and heparin [22]. This was tested in several surgical settings, and above all to reverse overdose of vitamin K inhibitors before surgery. Therefore, in this context the use of PCC has reduced the need for transfusions, particularly of FFP by normalizing the INR rapidly and significantly, and reducing the massive postoperative bleeding. The optimal doses, still much debated, appear to be 500 IU to correct an INR below 5 and 1,000 IU for an INR above 5 [22]. Currently the main application of PCC seems to be in emergency patients who arrive in the operating room receiving OAT as prophylaxis for chronic atrial fibrillation, arterial and venous thrombosis, and cerebral ischemia, and for the treatment of antiphospholipid syndrome [22]. Numerous studies reported in the literature have compared the effectiveness of PCC and FFP by reporting the INR in range in patients receiving OAT: although the preoperative INR values were similar (2.7 on average) in patients treated with PCC, the normalization of the range was reached in a much shorter time (at 15 min INR 1.6, vs. INR 2.3) [23]. Treatment with PCC has not been associated with adverse events, particularly thrombotic events; in contrast, use of FFP has been associated with refractory bleeding and significant increase in pulmonary arterial pressure, left atrial pressure, increased volume overload, and increased preparation time for therapy because of the group matching tests [23]. On average, in addition, 35% of patients treated with PCC reached the target INR in 15 min, in contrast to 20% of patients reaching the target INR in 60 min for treatment with FFP, demonstrating the effectiveness of PCC in antagonizing in real time the effects of OAT [24]. More and more scientific evidence leads us to conclude that immediate treatment with FFP will be increasingly replaced by treatment with PCC. Even compared with the use of factor VIIa, PCC appears to have important advantages, such as correcting multiple coagulation factors and fibrinogen. The only limitation for its clinical use appears to hypothermia, which slows down the time for the first phase of thrombin formation. PCC is very useful and free from adverse effects: in the literature, there are no reported changes in blood concentrations of creatinine, C-reactive protein, bilirubin, or vital signs at 6 h after administration, nor are there reports of a greater incidence of thrombotic events [24].

References

1. Achneck HE, Sileshi B, Parikh A, Milano CA, Welsby IJ, Lawson JH (2010) Phathophysiology of bleeding and clotting in the cardiac surgery patient. Circulation 122:2068–2077
2. Handin RI (2002) Harrison's principles of internal medicine, vol 1, 14th edn. McGraw-Hill, New York
3. Spanier TB, Chen JM, Oz MC, Edward NM, Kisiel W, Stern DM, Rose EA, Schmidt AM (1998) Selective anticoagulation with active site- blocked factor IX a suggests separate roles for intrinsic and extrinsic coagulation pathways in cardiopulmonary bypass. J Thorac Cardiovasc Surg 116:860–869
4. Furie B, Furie BC (2007) In vivo thrombus formation. J Thromb Haemost 5(Suppl 1):12–17
5. Barshtein G, Ben-Ami R, Yedgar S (2007) Role of red blood cell flow behavior in hemodynamics and hemostasis. Expert Rev Cardiovasc Ther 5:743–752
6. Cesarman-Maus G, Hajjar KA (2005) Molecular mechanisms of fibrinolysis. Br J Haematol 129:307–321
7. Shirk RA, Vlasuk GP (2007) Inhibitors of factor VIIa/tissue factor. Arterioscler Thromb Vasc Biol 27:1895–1900
8. Despobs G, Avidan M, Eby C (2009) Prediction and management of bleeding in cardiac surgery. J Thromb Haemost 7(Suppl 1):111–117
9. Franchini M (2007) The use of desmopressin as a hemostatic agent: a concise review. Am J Hematol 82:731–735
10. Despotis GJ, Joist JH, Goodnough LT (1997) Monitoring of hemostasis in cardiac surgical patients: impact of point-of-care testing on blood loss and transfusion outcomes. Clin Chem 43:1684–1696

11. Miller RD, Eriksson LI, Fleisher LA, Wiener-Kronish JP, Young WL (2010) Miller's anesthesia, 7th edn. Churchill Livingstone, Philadelphia
12. Rochon AG, Shore-Lesserson L (2006) Coagulation monitoring. Anesthesiol Clin 24:839–856
13. Despotis GJ, Gravlee G, Filos K, Levy J (1999) Anticoagulation monitoring during cardiac surgery: a review of current and emerging techniques. Anesthesiology 91:1122–1151
14. Reikvam H, Egil S, Bjørn H, Knut L, Kristin GH, Rolf S, Tor H (2009) Thromboelastography. Transfus Apher Sci 40:119–123
15. Gibbs NM (2009) Point-of-care assessment of antiplatelet agents in the perioperative period: a review. Anaesth Int Care 37(3):354–369
16. Harrison P (2005) Platelet function analysis. Blood Rev 19:111–123
17. Peerschke EI (2002) The laboratory evaluation of platelet dysfunction. Clin Lab Med 22:405–420
18. Barash PG, Cullen BF, Stoelting RK, Cahalan MK, Stock MC (2009) Handbook of clinical anesthesia, 6th edn. Lippincott Williams & Wilkins, Philadelphia
19. Mayo A, Misgav M, Kluger Y, Greenberg R, Pauzner D, Klausner J, Ben-Tal O (2004) Recombinant activated factor VII (NovoSeven): addition to replacement therapy in acute, uncontrolled and life-threatening bleeding. Vox Sang 87:34–40
20. Tritapepe L, De Santis V, Vitale D, Nencini C, Pellegrini F, Landoni G, Toscano F, Miraldi F, Pietropaoli P (2007) Recombinant activated factor VII for refractory bleeding after acute aortic dissection surgery: a propensity score analysis. Crit Care Med 35(7):1685–1690
21. Carrillo-Esper R, Diaz-Medina MI, Carrillo-Cordova JR, Carrillo-Cordova LD (2008) Recombining activated factor VII in cardiac surgery; case report and review of the scientific evidence. Rev Mexi Anestesiol 31(1):45–54
22. Bruce D, Nokes TJC (2008) Prothrombin complex concentrate (Beriplex P/N) in severe bleeding: experience in a large tertiary hospital. Crit Care 12:R105
23. Demeyere R, Gillardin S, Arnout J, Strengers PF (2010) Comparison of fresh frozen plasma and prothrombin complex concentrate for the reversal of oral anticoagulants in patients undergoing cardiopulmonary bypass surgery: a randomized study. Vox Sang 99:251–260
24. Schick KS, Fertmann JM, Jauch KW, Hoffmann JN (2009) Prothrombin complex concentrate in surgical patients: retrospective evaluation of vitamin K antagonist reversal and treatment of severe bleeding. Crit Care 13:R191

Hemocoagulative Aspects of Solid Organ Transplantation

12

Andrea De Gasperi

12.1 Introduction

Transplantation has long been the standard of care for selected patients with end-stage organ disease not responsive to maximal medical treatment. Improvements in basic knowledge, immunosuppression, surgical skills, intraoperative monitoring, and perioperative intensive care have led to extremely high peripostoperative and postoperative survival rates even in the most difficult situations. This is particularly true when results are compared with outcomes of patients on waiting lists [1, 2]. The significant improvement in global results, with an average 5-year survival rate of more than 70% for liver, heart, and kidney transplantation, has created an ever-increasing request for organ transplantation, abdominal grafts (mainly kidney and liver) accounting for more than 70% of all transplant procedures [3, 81].

Absolute contraindications to solid organ transplantation are now few, making transplant procedures also available for older patients (older than 60 years), with increasing complexity both for the comorbidity burden and for the higher risk of perioperative complications [1]. Unfortunately, the need for organ transplantation largely exceeds the number of grafts from cadaveric donors, making organ shortage a worldwide problem. This is why policies to expand the donor pool are among the most addressed items in the field of organ transplantation. In liver transplantation, for example, grafts from living donors or the use of so-called *extended-criteria cadaveric donors* (ECD) or *non-heart beating donors* (NHBD) is increasing [4, 5]. ECD grafts (formerly defined as "*marginal*" grafts, because of the greater risk of failure in the early posttransplant period) [4] were first used in

---

A. De Gasperi (✉)
2 Servizio Anestesia e Rianimazione Ospedale Niguarda Ca' Granda, Milan, Italy
e-mail: andrea.degasperi@ospedaleniguarda.it

G. Berlot (ed.), *Hemocoagulative Problems in the Critically Ill Patient*,
DOI: 10.1007/978-88-470-2448-9_12, © Springer-Verlag Italia 2012

kidney transplantation with encouraging results, and are now considered with increasing confidence in liver transplantation [5]. The use of split livers from living or cadaveric donors and ECD grafts is on the rise, with excellent medium- and long-term results. This policy is consistently contributing to the large worldwide increase of liver transplantation [6, 7]. Double kidney transplant in the case of a marginal (elderly) kidney donor is a new and challenging opportunity for elderly (more than 65 years old) chronic renal failure patients. Of course, in the perspective of achieving the best survival results, the use of ECD makes the donor–recipient matching more complex and crucial. A recognized task and a key challenge for the modern anesthesiologist involved in organ transplantation is the shift from simply getting the patient "out of the operating room alive" to the optimization of the perioperative functional recovery of the grafts, thus contributing to medium- and long-term goals of survival. In this light, preoperative anesthesiological assessment, intraoperative management, and early postoperative intensive care are a dynamic continuum [8–11]. Among the many problems posed to the transplant physician by solid organ transplant procedures, complex hemostatic problems are frequent: they result from defects associated with the preexisting systemic effects of the end-stage organ disease/failure, preoperative antiplatelet/anticoagulant medications, intraoperative bleeding related to surgical technical problems, use of extracorporeal circulation [cardiopulmonary bypass (CPB)], for example, in case of thoracic transplant procedures, metabolic changes during the various phases of the procedures, hypothermic donor grafts, preservation injury, or ischemia reperfusion injury. In this chapter, major perioperative hemostatic derangements and management solutions in subjects undergoing solid organ transplantion will be reviewed and discussed.

12.2 Heart and Lung Transplantation

A combination of factors, and not a single cause, is usually recognized as the base of the frequency and severity of perioperative bleeding during heart transplantation, lung transplantation, or combined heart and lung transplantation [11, 12]. Among them, preoperative medications, underlying disease state, including hepatic and renal (dys)function, type of intrathoracic transplantation, requirement for CPB, and previous cardiac or thoracic surgery are frequently recognized as risk conditions. The use of CPB is known to extensively activate clotting and fibrinolysis during cardiac operations, contributing to an acquired coagulopathy and increased bleeding tendency during and after the operations. In part (but not only), the adverse effects of CPB are related to the blood–material interaction and recirculation of wound blood that may disturb clotting and fibrinolysis [11]. Among them are contact activation through factor XII, complement cascade activation, leukocyte activation, qualitative and quantitative platelet defects, hyperfibrinolysis, hemodilution, hypothermia, systemic heparinization, and the use of protamine to reverse the effects of heparin. These items are specifically addressed in Chap. 11. The effects of CPB on pulmonary function (mainly

12 Hemocoagulative Aspects of Solid Organ Transplantation

interstitial edema due to variable but potentially relevant changes in microvascular permeability) are beyond the scope of this review.

12.2.1 Heart Transplantation

Heart transplantation is currently the therapy of choice for patients with advanced heart failure, with no other therapeutic alternative(s) and no obvious contraindications, the latter mainly related to the patient's ability to withstand surgery and subsequent immunosuppression [12, 13]. Heart failure, whose prevalence in the USA is reported to be close to 7% in people over 65 years old, is defined as a complex clinical syndrome caused by any structural or functional cardiac disorder that impairs the ability of one or both ventricles to maintain adequate cardiac output: heart failure impacts heavily on organ functions and on humoral, neuroendocrine, and inflammatory feedback loops [11]. On the basis of the stages of the syndrome, four classes are recognized: subjects reaching class D heart failure (refractory end-stage heart failure with marked symptoms at rest despite maximal medical therapy) have a 2-year mortality risk of more than 75%. This is why heart transplantation, associated with 1- and 5-year survival rates of more than 85% and more than 70% respectively, is the only effective treatment currently available [12, 13]. Ischemic cardiomyopathy and idiopathic dilated cardiomyopathy are the two most common forms of cardiac disease leading to transplantation. They represent close to 90% of the cases, with the large part of the adult heart transplantations being performed because of nonischemic rather than ischemic cardiomyopathy (51 vs. 38%). Retransplantation (3%), adult congenital heart disease (2%), valve disease (2%), and miscellaneous conditions (viral, infiltrative, and postpartum cardiomyopathy) account for the remaining 4% [12].

Crucial to preventing bleeding in heart transplantation are (1) an adequate and thorough preoperative evaluation, including the use of medication(s) able to affect perioperative hemostasis, (2) the analysis of bleeding or thrombotic tendencies, and (3) a dedicated perioperative strategy, for which expertise in the management of the hemostatic profile during CPB and/or with patients with mechanical circulatory support devices (MCSD).

Preoperative Considerations
The best preoperative screen to identify bleeding disorders in heart transplant candidates is a carefully taken clinical history [14–18]. This is a common feature for all solid organ transplant candidates. Any existing hemostatic defects in patients facing heart transplant surgery will be additive to those associated with antiplatelet agents or induced by CPB, and will increase the likelihood of unexpected hemorrhage. Questions regarding personal/family history, medications, and hemostatic problems with previous surgery and trauma are mandatory. The following items should be considered: preoperative medications, positive personal or family history of bleeding, known bleeding disorder, (i.e., von Willebrand

disease, hemophilia), unexplained anemia, lupus anticoagulant, cyanotic congenital heart disease, recent venous thromboembolisms, severe thrombocytopenia, thrombocytosis, and previous history of heparin-induced thrombocytopenia (HIT). HIT is an idiosyncratic complication of heparin therapy triggered by the development of IgG antibodies to platelet factor 4, leading to a decrease in the platelet count. Bleeding is rare; however, the risk of venous or arterial thrombotic events is high [14]. In heart transplant candidates, HIT could represent a consistent problem. In a cohort of 46 patients, HIT antibodies were detected in 11 patients (39%). Full-blown HIT was diagnosed in ten of 11 patients before transplantation, the mean platelet count at diagnosis being $88,000 \pm 22,000$/ml. HIT with thrombosis syndrome developed in five of 11 patients (45%) (splenic and renal infarctions, renal artery occlusion, coronary artery embolism with myocardial infarction, pulmonary embolism, and femoral and jugular venous occlusions). Early HIT antibody screening and the use of alternative forms of systemic anticoagulation are to be considered as appropriate and safe options in this setting [14].

According to Robinson et al. [15], for patients who are not receiving preoperative anticoagulation therapy, the preoperative activated partial thromboplastin time (aPTT) and prothrombin time (PT) tests constitute a baseline for the interpretation (and possible rational correction) of post-CPB results, even if they are poor predictors by themselves of surgical bleeding. For patients receiving anticoagulants, instead, the tests could provide an indication for preoperative management of anticoagulation [16, 17]. Medications such as unfractionated heparin, low molecular weight heparin, clopidogrel, and ticlopidine are other important preoperative factors able to alter the hemostatic profile. In the case of altered and/or nonconvincing test findings (unexpectedly abnormal prolongation of the PT or aPTT, critical changes in platelet count, the presence of moderate to severe anemia) referral to a hematologist before transplant surgery is mandatory. Heart transplant candidates, often suffering from cardiac dilatation, are prone to mural thrombi formation and potential embolization, particularly in the case of atrial fibrillation. Systemic anticoagulation with warfarin is common; chronic administration of heparin, even if less common, may determine antithrombin deficiency and subsequent problems in maintaining adequate activated clotting time during CPB. HIT and platelet dysfunction are not infrequently associated with the same treatment.

A different but potentially consistent problem very common in patients with severe heart failure could be related to hepatic congestion secondary to right atrial hypertension. Decreased hepatic function and reduced synthesis of coagulation factors and natural anticoagulants are relevant clinical consequences, usually associated with aPTT/PT elevation. Chronic warfarin therapy and passive hepatic congestion are reported to exacerbate the effects introduced by the CPB on the hemostatic profile: together with previous heart surgery, most commonly coronary artery bypass graft procedures, these factors constitute a recognized increased risk of bleeding during and after surgery [12, 15–17].

Heart Transplantation in Patients with Mechanical Circulatory Support Devices

Some of the candidates may have had an MCSD implanted as a bridge to transplantation, the bridging time ranging from a few days to many months [17–19]. Patients supported by an MCSD are at an even greater risk of postoperative bleeding after heart transplantation: chronic activation of the procoagulant and inflammatory pathways induced by the MCSD and the chronic anticoagulation therapy required during the support period play a consistent role. The anticoagulation/antiplatelet regime usually includes warfarin, dipyridamole, and aspirin (or sometimes clopidogrel and ticlopidine) until the time of the operation. Device removal together with the native recipient heart might add considerable complexity and time to the procedure, making bleeding risk greater. In a series of 94 patients, postoperative bleeding and total blood-product use [red blood cell (RBC), fresh frozen plasma (FFP), platelets)] was significantly greater in the MCSD patients than in patients operated on for a primary heart transplant procedure or for a "redo" [17]. A better understanding of the impact of CPB on the compromised hemostatic (and inflammatory) systems of MCSD patients is mandatory to optimize post-CPB hemostasis in this specific setting. A so-called proactive approach aiming at a rational management of perioperative bleeding and at optimization of the hemostatic profile in primary, redo, and MCSD patients undergoing a heart transplant should include the use of thromboelastography (TEG)/thromboelastometry (TEM) before and during CPB to determine the specific hemostatic deficiencies prior to termination of CPB and immediately after: use of blood components, drugs, or both to manipulate the hemostatic profile could be done according to the specific dynamic changes made evident by TEG/TEM—the responses can be verified very rapidly both in vitro and in vivo [19–22]. Since TEG/TEM will be often alluded to in the next sections of this chapter, a short description will be provided now. In contrast to conventional coagulation tests such as the PT/international normalized ratio (INR) and the aPTT, assays of clot formation time in plasma only, TEG assesses in a semiquantitative way overall hemostasis, including the effects of procoagulant proteins, fibrinogen, platelets, and (often forgotten but playing a role) RBCs. Much less clear (if at all) is the role played by the anticoagulant proteins. TEG/TEM measurements reflect specific phases of clot formation [19–22]. The reaction (R) time reflects the latency of activation of the coagulation cascade, and correlates with the PT/INR and aPTT. The kinetic (K) time reflects the rate of initial clot formation, and is proportional to fibrinogen concentrations and platelet count, as is the α angle, which describes the rate of fibrin formation and cross-linking. Finally, the maximum amplitude (MA) reflects maximal clot strength, a sort of representation of the effects caused by all the constituents of the clotting cascade. A schematic representation of a normal TEG trace and a comparison of TEG and TEM traces are shown in Fig. 12.1.

The use of TEG/TEM could lead to important results. According to a recent commentary on the use of TEG to predict and/or decrease bleeding and blood and blood-product use in adult patients undergoing cardiac surgery, TEG might be useful in predicting which patients are likely to bleed postoperatively [21].

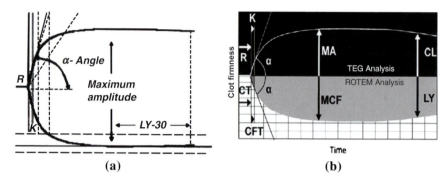

Fig. 12.1 A normal thromboelastography (*TEG*) trace (*left*) and a comparison of TEG and thromboelastometry (*ROTEM*) traces (*right*). *CL* clot lysis, *CFT* clot formation time, *CT* clotting time, *LY* lysis index, *Ly-30* lysis index after 30 min, *MA* maximum amplitude, *MCF*. Reproduced from Ganter and Hofer (2008), Anest Analg 106:1366

Interestingly, it can guide transfusion therapy algorithms in the bleeding cardiac surgical patient, significantly decreasing blood and blood component transfusion requirements [19]. However, some (but now not many) coagulologists are skeptical regarding this approach: further large studies are ongoing to fully validate the use of TEG/TEM and to define the "ideal" treatment algorithms in the various cardiac and noncardiac surgical settings.

As above reported, bleeding tendency in the case of MCSD removal and heart transplantation is not a rare problem and could become a life-threatening complication. A report of a patient who had a biventricular VAD and then had a successful transplant is particularly helpful to understand (1) the problems posed during heart transplantation by the altered hemostasis in this specific setting and (2) the crucial role played by dynamic coagulation monitoring performed with TEM [18]. Immediately before surgery the effects of preoperative oral anticoagulation were reversed with 2,000 IU prothrombin complex concentrates. Platelet transfusion and desmopressin were also administered, aiming, according to the authors' comment, at a safer basal hemostatic profile. TEM and PFA-100 analysis[1] were both used before, during, and after heart transplantation to support every hemostatic manipulation during the entire procedure. Throughout the surgery, the patient received two further platelet concentrates, 15 U of FFP, 0.5 g of tranexamic acid, and 1 g of fibrinogen. Only 6 U of RBC concentrates was needed to maintain adequate hemoglobin concentrations. TEM measurements obtained 1 week after transplantation were within the normal range without any detectable

---

[1] The PFA-100 is a system for analyzing platelet function in which citrated whole blood is aspirated at high shear rates through disposable cartridges containing an aperture within a membrane coated with either collagen and epinephrine or collagen and ADP. These agonists induce platelet adhesion, activation, and aggregation, leading to rapid occlusion of the aperture and cessation of blood flow termed the closure time.

signs of hypercoagulability, and the patient received only 40 mg of low molecular weight heparin [18]. The addition of 0.5–1.0 U/10 kg FFP during CPB and TEG before and during CPB to determine the specific hemostatic deficiencies prior to termination of CPB were also used by Wegner et al. [18] in the same setting to optimize coagulation management. According to these authors, the addition of FFP during CPB appears to optimize the coagulation factor status and eliminates a potential volume overload problem in the post-CPB period.

As already underlined, postoperative bleeding is one of the most frequent complications after cardiac surgery, largely but not only related to the extracorporeal circulation (see Chap. 11). In transplant procedures the use of CPB could lead to an increased use of blood products, early reoperation, long intensive care unit (ICU) and hospital stays, and increased morbidity and mortality [12, 17]. Bleeding related to cardiac surgery can be devastating and life-threatening, with a 5–25% incidence of death. According to Diaz Martin et al. [17], patients who received 6 U or more of blood during heart transplantation had a significantly higher need for continuous renal replacement techniques (50 vs. 12.5%; $P = 0.01$) and higher ICU mortality (33.3 vs. 4%; $P = 0.01$). This significant difference in ICU mortality was also observed when comparing plasma transfusion requirements (35.3 vs. 9.4%; $P = 0.04$). The overall mortality rate was 24.5%, showing significantly higher figures in patients with massive transfusion (83.3 vs. 37.8%; $P = 0.008$). Then, perioperative bleeding and massive transfusion are associated with increased morbidity and mortality also in this specific subsetting of cardiac surgery patients.

12.2.2 Lung Transplantation

Patients admitted for a single or sequential lung transplant for the so-called septic indications (cystic fibrosis or bronchiectasis) could be at increased risk of bleeding. The main causes are vascular pleural adhesion, bulky mediastinal lymph nodes, and recurrent septic complications [22–24]. In the case of a lung transplant for chronic obstructive pulmonary disease, a single lung is often involved: in most of these patients, CPB is not necessary, right-sided heart dysfunction (and the consequent hepatic dysfunction) is much less severe, and the bleeding risk is low. If before the transplant there have been multiple intrathoracic procedures, this is associated with an increased risk of bleeding: once considered as absolute contraindications, previous thoracotomy and/or sternotomy are now considered on an individual basis and are a lesser problem. According to numerous reported series, in spite of the larger number of transfused blood products, morbidity and mortality are not significantly increased when compared with patients who have had no previous thoracic procedures if CPB is not used. According to a recent report from Spain by Paradela et al. [23], postoperative bleeding was the most frequent risk factor and the main cause of reoperation in their series, although it was not associated with increased perioperative mortality. The greater incidence of hemorrhagic complications, as already reported, was associated with the presence of strong adhesions and the use of CPB. In these series, the use of CPB was also significantly associated with mortality (univariate analysis), probably because of its well-known deleterious effects (systemic inflammatory response associated with increased capillary permeability, vasomotor tone disorders, and fluid retention able to jeopardize lung function, together with the risk of bleeding and pulmonary embolism) [23]. Further, in patients who have had lung transplants blood product transfusion may contribute to the overall morbidity and mortality of the population, owing to the adverse pulmonary effects related to transfusion, most notably transfusion-related acute lung injury.

In the late 1990s, when the use of CPB was not infrequent, a bleeding tendency was often recorded: Gu et al. [24] studied this phenomenon. Activation of clotting during lung transplantation, as indicated by the formation of thrombin–antithrombin (TAT) complex, was about twice as high as observed during cardiac operations. According to Gu et al. [24], the pattern and the extent of clotting activation during lung transplantation was different compared with the findings usually reported during cardiac operations. In the latter, increased level of TAT complex was recorded mainly in the late phase of CPB, when suction of the wound blood was more intense. In contrast, in lung transplantation, the level of TAT complex increased significantly after the early phases of the operation: a tempting explanation might reside in the very large wound area created by the surgical separation of pleural adhesion. This was present in patients who underwent a lung transplant without CPB or major thoracic surgery. It was suggested that among the major triggers of clotting activation was the release of tissue factor secondary to the surgical trauma to blood vessels and not the contact activation of blood with the foreign material [24]. According to Gu et al. [24], hyperfibrinolysis might have both an "intrinsic" and an "extrinsic" origin during lung transplantation. Whereas intrinsic activation should have been induced by the contact activation, extrinsic activation of fibrinolysis might also have been triggered during lung transplantation by tissue plasminogen activator (tPA) released from stimulated or injured endothelial cells: tPA is the most potent activator of plasminogen, which initiates fibrinolysis. Together with soluble fibrin, tPA may synergistically cause platelet dysfunction, resulting in impaired hemostasis.

12.2.3 Combined Heart and Lung Transplantation

Combined heart and lung transplantation could be required in cases of complex congenital heart disease and Eisenmenger syndrome or with primary pulmonary hypertension and right-sided heart failure [25–29, 78, 79]. In early series, intraoperative and postoperative bleeding was one of the most frequent and feared complications and impacted both morbidity and mortality [22, 25]. Extensive bleeding, massive perioperative transfusions, early graft dysfunction, and multiple organ failure were common: major bleeding accounted for 36% of intraoperative deaths in one series and blood loss of more than 2 l was associated in another series with a significant risk of early death. As seen for heart transplantation (and the same is true for lung transplantation), bleeding tendency in combined heart and lung transplantation is multifactorial. Preoperative use of medication such as aspirin and dipyridamole is common. Oral anticoagulants are given in selected cases of embolic phenomena and, as in heart transplantation, in the case of ventricular thrombi and atrial fibrillation in patients with heart failure. Owing to the frequent right ventricular dysfunction and/or pulmonary artery hypertension, hepatic congestion is quite common and coagulation disorders associated with decreased coagulation and natural anticoagulation factors are to be considered. The PT and aPTT are frequently prolonged. Owing to the major bleeding during these cases, modification of surgical techniques and local hemostatic agents together with argon beam coagulator were introduced to improve perioperative hemostasis: as result, major surgical improvements made hemorrhage a lesser problem in more recent series [26, 27].

12.2.4 Management

According to a very recent review, RBC transfusion in patients having cardiac surgery is strongly associated with both infection and ischemic postoperative morbidity, hospital stay, increased early and late mortality, and hospital costs [28, 29]. Specifically, in patients undergoing a transplant, transfusion may result in the development of alloantibodies, which may increase the risk of rejection or induce microchimerism or graft-versus-host disease [30, 31]. Measures able to reduce blood loss and transfusion requirements and guidelines to standardize RBC transfusion during heart transplantation are frequently proposed and continuously implemented [13]. As reported earlier, the use of CPB is strongly and uniformly associated with the hemostatic activation and progressive consumption of plasmatic coagulation factors; antiplatelet medication increases perioperative hemorrhage, making frequent the use of transfusion and possible the need for surgical reexploration . Adequate hemostasis has to be achieved before sternotomy closure: FFP, platelets, and cryoprecipitates (or fibrinogen, according to the most recent researches) [82, 83] are to be used according to the coagulation studies, or in their absence in the case of fibrinogen blood concentration below 100 mg/dl. The role of TEG/TEM in this setting has already been discussed [19–21] and its relevance is increasing.

12.2.5 Blood Components

RBC transfusion is mainly indicated to maintain the hemoglobin level between 7 and 10 g/dl in both heart and lung transplantation [13]. According to the most recent available literature [28, 29, 32, 33], more than on a fixed hemoglobin threshold, RBC transfusion should rely upon physiological triggers able to gauge the individual's ability to tolerate and to compensate for the acute decrease in hemoglobin concentration. The decision to transfuse should be guided by multifactorial considerations able to predict which patients could benefit from RBC transfusion: many physiological parameters have been proposed to implement a decision tree, but unfortunately this is not yet available. According to Futier [32] and Orlov et al. [33] (the latter authors in the specific setting of cardiac surgery), "physiologic" transfusion triggers should be based on signs and symptoms of impaired global [lactate, mixed venous O_2 saturation (SvO_2) or central venous O_2 saturation ($ScvO_2$)] or, better, regional tissue oxygenation (ECG ST segment or P300 latency) and not on a hemoglobin threshold [29]. Metabolic markers of global tissue hypoperfusion, such as serum lactate (indicating anaerobic metabolism) or, as a surrogate, base deficit, are easily measured but, as reported, are "each confounded by a range of conditions as well as resuscitative therapies," SvO_2, more easily measured using $ScvO_2$, has proven useful in guiding critical care management and, as reported above, is now championed as a useful physiological marker for the need for RBC transfusion instead of the single hemoglobin value. Orlov et al. [33] reported 74 patients undergoing CPB who received RBC transfusion. The pretransfusion O_2 extraction rate (O_2ER) values were elevated in 27 cases and were normal in 35 cases(56%). Among those who received transfusion for low hemoglobin concentration, 43% (27 of 62) had normal pretransfusion O_2ER values. Whereas the posttransfusion O_2ER values did not change in patients with normal pretransfusion values, O_2ER decreased significantly in patients with elevated pretransfusion values. Inclusion of O_2ER into the decision tree might substantially reduce the post-cardiac-surgery RBC requirement, safely avoiding useless transfusion [28, 34]. CMV seronegative blood to minimize the occurrence of CMV infection is sometimes considered. Leukocyte-depleted blood to reduce HLA alloimmunization and (possible) leukocyte-mediated lung injury, albeit not a routine practice, is sometimes considered in the case of retransplantation [22]. Platelets are considered in the case of persistent bleeding with normal or near-normal activated clotting time. Single-donor apheresis (instead of pooled random-donor platelets) could be a better way to avoid multiple exposure of the recipient. However, the platelet count is not a reliable method to detect qualitative platelet defects, and TEG or TEM or better use of the PFA-100 is to be considered for a more correct and rational correction of the hemostatic defect(s) [20]. Recombinant activated factor VII (rFVIIa; NovoSeven®, Novo Nordisk) is a potent clotting factor currently approved only for the control of bleeding in patients with factor VIII (FVIII) or factor IX inhibitors or patients with factor VII deficiency. However, off-label use of rFVIIa is on the rise for the control of bleeding unresponsive to conventional measures in general, vascular, abdominal, and cardiac surgery patients [35]. In a retrospective case series, Gandhi et al. [36] reported their experience with the use of rFVIIa in the treatment of refractory bleeding in patients with VAD implantation/explantation and an orthotopic heart transplant. Nine patients underwent removal of the bridging VAD followed by a heart transplant, five had VAD implantation, and one patient had only an orthotopic heart transplant. The mean total dose of rFVIIa was 78.3 µg/kg (24–189 µg/kg). Transfusion requirements and blood loss were significantly reduced after rFVIIa administration. Five patients had thromboembolic events, and three died. As stated by the authors, the exact role played by rFVIIa in the development of thromboembolic complications could not be clearly determined. In the most recent retrospective study on the use of rFVIIa in high-risk cardiac surgery, Chapman et al. [80] were able to define this agent as an effective hemostatic drug for intractable bleeding in high-risk cardiac surgery: with respect to the safety profile, rFVIIa does not appear to be associated with increased postoperative complications, including thromboembolic events and death. In the most recent (2011) update of the Society of Thoracic Surgeons and the Society of Cardiovascular Anesthesiologists blood conservation clinical practice guidelines [34] the use of rFVIIa may be considered for the management of intractable nonsurgical bleeding unresponsive to routine hemostatic therapy after cardiac procedures using CPB (level of evidence B). However no large randomized trial data exist to support this use. A recent randomized controlled trial of rFVIIa in 172 patients with bleeding after cardiac surgery reported a significant decrease in reoperation and transfusion need, but a higher incidence of critical serious adverse events, including stroke, in the rFVIIa treatment group [37]. According to the available literature and the most recent reviews, no clear consensus exists on the patients who could be "appropriate candidates" for rFVIIa treatment in this setting; uncertainty exists also in the appropriate dose(s) and in the thrombotic risks associated with its use [34]. In conclusion, as assessed by many authorities in the field, further investigations are needed to define the safety of rFVIIa and its effectiveness in improving postoperative morbidity and mortality in the specific setting of heart and lung transplant procedures.

Antifibrinolytic drugs are frequently used to manipulate the hemostatic profile during cardiothoracic surgery performed with CBP [38]. The use of CPB during lung transplantation has been associated with significantly higher blood loss, transfusion requirements, and mortality. Aprotinin was able to reduce blood loss and RBC transfusion in patients who underwent a lung transplant on CPB, even if different results are present in the literature [39]. Off-pump lung transplantation (OPLT) is becoming the technique of choice at many institutions: among the theoretical benefits of OPLT procedures are less inflammatory activation, reduced coagulopathy and bleeding, and less need for transfusion [40]. The avoidance of air embolization and the elimination of nonpulsatile flow might favorably impact on postoperative neurocognitive, renal, and pulmonary dysfunction. Off-pump double lung transplantation, in spite of being the standard of care on the basis of short- and long-term outcome data, remains a challenging procedure, frequently associated with transfusion of blood products. As for other thoracic surgery performed without the use of CPB, in OPLT bleeding and transfusion have been reported to be reduced by the use of aprotinin. Further, aprotinin was reported to be associated in some series with an improved graft function. However, in a retrospective study recently reported by Balsara et al. [41], the intraoperative administration of aprotinin was associated with a statistically significant reduction in blood product transfusion only in patients with a preoperative diagnosis of chronic obstructive pulmonary disease. Together with the modest reduction of transfusion, the authors were able to demonstrate the absence of any significant improvement in graft function, making questionable the use of aprotinin in routine practice [41]. These results were recently confirmed by Marasco et al. [42] in a retrospective study on single and double lung transplantation. The use of aprotinin, although associated with reduced blood loss, introduced a significantly increased risk of primary graft dysfunction in the early postoperative period. This study further negates support for the use of aprotinin to reduce primary graft dysfunction in lung transplantation and indicates that aprotinin may in fact have a detrimental effect [42]. This is particularly true according to the recent safety concerns regarding aprotinin administration in cardiac surgery. A significant association of adverse effects with the use of aprotinin in cardiac surgery (increased renal failure, increased rate of myocardial infarction and stroke, increased 5-year mortality rate) prompted a worldwide discussion about its safety. Aprotinin was finally suspended from the market in November 2007 after the demonstration of the association with increased mortality in an interim analysis of the BART study. A nonsignificant increase in all-cause mortality but a significant increase in risk of death from a cardiac cause was also evident when patients enrolled in the aprotinin-treated group were compared with patients treated with lysine analogues. With the removal of aprotinin from the market, studies dealing with the safety and efficacy of tranexamic acid and ε-aminocaproic acid in cardiothoracic surgery are increasing in number; however, no study on lung transplantation is currently available [38].

12.3 Liver Transplantation

Liver transplantation is today the treatment of choice for patients with acute or chronic end-stage liver disease (ESLD) not responsive to medical treatment: if they do not receive a transplant, the prognosis of these subjects is poor.

12.3.1 The Liver and the Hemostatic Profile

Acute and chronic liver diseases have been long known to impact the whole hemostatic system, as the liver plays a key role in primary hemostasis and coagulation: it is the organ where (solely or partially) (1) almost all the coagulation factors (fibrinogen, prothrombin, factors V, VII, IX ,X, XI, XII, XIII) apart from FVIII, (2) a large part of the proteins involved in profibrinolysis and antifibrinolysis [apart from tPA, plasminogen activator inhibitor 1 (PAI-1), and urokinase plasminogen activator], (3) the natural anticoagulants (antithrombin, protein C, and protein S) (apart from thrombomodulin), and (4) thrombopoietin, the stimulator factor of platelet production from megakaryocytes, are synthesized [43].

The reticuloendothelial system of the liver plays a major role in the clearance of breakdown products of activated clotting factors such as fibrin-related products, plasmin–α_2-antiplasmin inhibitor complex, and activated platelets [43].

In ESLD patients the hemostatic profile includes [44–46] thrombocytopenia, reduced levels of coagulation factors and inhibitors, reduced levels of fibrinolytic proteins, but increased plasma levels of FVIII and von Willebrand factor. The findings of tests of hemostasis, such as the platelet count, the PT, and the aPTT, are frequently abnormal. Release of cytokines from necrotic liver tissue is one of the causes proposed to explain the increased FVIII blood level of both hepatic and extrahepatic origin [45]. Among patients with chronic liver failure, cholestatic and noncholestatic liver diseases have different hemostatic profiles, the former being characterized by a more favorable hemostatic balance owing to near-normal platelet count and lower reduction in the levels of coagulation factors.

Peripheral vasodilation and impaired vasoconstriction, common in ESLD, are relevant in reducing the role played by the vascular phase of hemostasis in this particular setting. Continuous low-grade activation of endothelial cells results in a quasicontinuous release of several hemostatic proteins: intravascular activation results in consumption of hemostatic factors and, according to Lisman et al. [44], this might contribute to the alterations in the hemostatic system. Elevated plasma levels of the activation markers are due both to decreased clearance secondary to the reduced liver mass (and particularly to the reduced reticuloendothelial system function) and to a low-grade disseminated intravascular coagulation (DIC), with concomitant activation of fibrinolysis (this latter statement is now under discussion). Primary hyperfibrinolysis was reported as sometimes present in ESLD patients [46]. According to the most recent research, true hyperfibrinolysis seems to be present only in the case of a superimposed insult such as sepsis, bleeding, or after surgical stress [45]. Tripodi and Mannucci [46] in the most recent review of the hemostatic profile in chronic liver diseased patients stated that the balance of fibrinolysis is probably restored in patients with liver disease by the parallel changes in profibrinolytic and antifibrinolytic drivers.

Thrombocytopenia is common in cirrhotic patients [43]: the main causes of a reduced platelet count are as follows: (1) *decreased production*, mainly due to bone marrow suppression by hepatitis viruses or alcohol, nutritional deficiencies, and decreased thrombopoietin production; (2) *increased turnover* (accelerated platelet consumption and decreased platelet survival time); (3) *sequestration* secondary to portal hypertension and splenomegaly; and (4) *peripheral consumption*. Hepatorenal syndrome, as all the uremic states, might be involved in the reduced platelet count. Platelet dysfunction (*thrombocytopathy*) is also common and it is not correlated with the platelet count. Further dysfunction might arise from decreased levels of arachidonic acid and adenine nucleotides in the platelets. The net result is the production of undersized and hypofunctional platelets, which impairs their ability to aggregate. The reliability of platelet function studies differs considerably and, according to the most recent reviews, they may not predict a bleeding tendency [47].

As mentioned above, the presence of DIC in ESLD is a matter of discussion. According to Roberts et al. [45], true DIC is characterized by increased thrombin generation and fibrin deposition with resultant consumption of coagulation factors and concomitant fibrinolysis: this is why many early descriptions of DIC in liver disease may be explained by hepatic synthetic failure with altered fibrinolysis (Carr [84], reported by Roberts et al. [45]). Differential diagnosis between DIC and hemostatic profile specific of ESLD could be problematic if prolonged clotting times, low fibrinogen levels, and thrombocytopenia are to be used, being present in both DIC and chronic liver disease [45]. According to Amitrano et al. [48], a diagnosis of DIC in patients with ESLD should be reserved for "those with a known clinical trigger accompanied by progressive decline in coagulation markers and progressive thrombocytopenia."

In summary, in liver disease two opposite hemostatic tendencies are now clearly recognized. On one side there are factors able to impair hemostasis: the reduced synthesis of coagulation factors, hypofibrinogenemia/dysfibrinogenemia, the alteration in the fibrinolytic system (reduced synthesis of FXIII, α_2-antiplasmin, and thrombin-activated fibrinolytic inhibitor; reduced clearance of tPA), thrombocytopenia/thrombocytopathy; on the other side the reduced level of natural anticoagulants, the often elevated level of FVIII, and the reduced synthesis of plasminogen are all conditions able to promote hemostasis [44–47]. The fact that chronic liver diseased patients, in spite of the elevated INR and the sometimes very severe thrombocytopenia, rarely bleed outside the consequences of portal hypertension should be attributed to the so-called rebalanced hemostasis recently introduced by Tripodi and Mannucci, and associated with the parallel reduction of the levels of procoagulant and anticoagulant factors: decreases in the levels of procoagulant proteins are matched by decreases in the levels of anticoagulant proteins, such as proteins C and S, and antithrombin [46].

As is clear from what reported above, in recent years the common belief that patients with liver failure are particularly prone to a bleeding tendency ("autoanticoagulation") has been challenged [44–46]. Widespread clinical observations have supported the statement that bleeding complications are common in patients with advanced liver disease. However, according to most recent clinical and laboratory evidence, the hemostatic system in patients with liver disease has been defined as "more balanced than commonly anticipated" [44–46]. Plasma from patients with cirrhosis generates thrombin as in healthy subjects: thrombin generation in vivo and in vitro is downregulated by thrombomodulin, the main physiologic activator of the natural anticoagulant protein C. This effect is much less evident in ESLD patients as if they are partially resistant to anticoagulation mediated by thrombomodulin. Increased plasma levels of FVIII and the concomitant decrease in the levels of protein C seem to be responsible for this effect. Very high levels of von Willebrand factor, often found in ESLD patients, may contribute to platelet adhesion to the subendothelium at sites of vascular injury, together with the reduced levels of the metalloprotease ADAMTS 13, closely correlated to the severity of chronic liver failure. ADAMTS 13 is a protease synthesized in hepatic stellate cells and able to degrade highly active, large multimers of von Willebrand factor. A platelet count as low as $60 \times 10^9/l$ is usually sufficient in ESLD patients to preserve thrombin generation close to the lower limit of the normal range and might explain the reduced bleeding tendency found in surgical or invasive procedures performed on ESLD patients. Indeed, patients with liver disease develop deep vein thrombosis and pulmonary embolism at nonnegligible rates (0.5–1.9%), making activation of coagulation more frequent than expected. Particularly common in ESLD patients are portal and mesenteric vein thromboses: although hemodynamic changes have been long known to be involved in this specific setting, the observations discussed above, together with the recent demonstration in cirrhotic patients of inherited forms of thrombophilia (prothrombin G20210A mutation), enhance the hypothesis that hypercoagulability too might play a role in thrombotic complications.

In this new light, the most common and critical hemorrhagic problems seen in ESLD patients (e.g., bleeding from ruptured esophageal varices) are today reinterpreted as a consequence of increased splanchnic blood pressure and/or local vascular problems, and not as a direct consequence of the altered hemostasis. As very recently reported by van Veen et al. [47], bleeding tendency is not predicted by the extent of the alterations of both the PT and the INR, neither in a medical nor in a surgical setting. On the contrary, although no evidence supports the use of routine coagulation tests to predict bleeding or thrombotic risk in liver disease, use of global coagulation assays, such as thrombin generation and TEG, is on the rise in this setting [45, 49]. Other important complications associated with ESLD and able to jeopardize the hemostatic profile leading to hypocoagulability and hemorrhage are hemodynamic alterations secondary to portal hypertension, and gastroesophageal tract complications leading to sepsis or septic shock. Among them are spontaneous bacterial peritonitis and renal failure, including hepatorenal syndrome: hemostatic derangements include disorders in platelet–vessel wall interaction (very common in uremic conditions), increased NO production (common with sepsis), and anemia [44–46]. However, even if it is "rebalanced," the coagulation system in ESLD patients is not as stable as in healthy individuals: in the presence of specific risks factors, the balance could be easily shifted toward hemorrhage or thrombosis [46].

Acute liver failure is a clinical syndrome defined by hepatic encephalopathy and coagulopathy (mainly elevated INR). Thrombocytopenia is less frequent and increased levels of PAI-1 shift fibrinolysis toward a hypofibrinolytic state. In spite of an altered INR, clinically significant bleeding and bleeding diathesis are rare, making the "rebalanced theory" applicable also to acute liver failure [49]. According to the most recent data reported by Stravitz et al. [50], patients with acute liver failure were prospectively studied with conventional hemostatic tests and TEG. In spite of a pathological increase in the INR (mean 3.4 ± 1.7, range 1.5–9.6), the mean TEG parameters were normal. Five individual TEG parameters were normal in more than 60% of cases. Smaller MA were present with platelet count below $126 \times 10^9/l$, whereas larger MA were recorded in patients with higher venous ammonia concentrations and with increasing severity of liver injury as assessed by elements of the systemic inflammatory response syndrome. All the patients had a significant decrease of procoagulant factor V and VII levels, proportional to the decreased levels of anticoagulant proteins and inversely proportional to the elevated FVIII levels. The main conclusion was the presence of a normal hemostasis in acute liver failure patients according to both TEG parameters and the almost absent spontaneous bleeding tendency: major evidence was the increased clot strength (MA) associated with (1) increasing severity of liver injury, (2) increased FVIII levels, and (3) concomitant decline in procoagulant and anticoagulant proteins.

12.3.2 Liver Transplantation, the Surgical Phases, and the Changes of the Hemostatic Profile

The "rebalanced theory" has a relevant impact on the management of the hemostatic profile of the ESLD patient, particularly during major liver surgery and liver transplantion [3, 50–51].

In the (recent) past, liver transplantation was known to be at risk of major bleeding complications and massive transfusion requirements, able to heavily impact on patient outcome [22]. Major advances in organ preservation, surgical techniques, intraoperative anesthesiological management (included a better understanding of the pathophysiologic processes of hemostasis in acute or chronic liver diseased patients and a strict hemodynamic monitoring) have contributed to the current relevant results (1-year survival rate today largely exceeds 90% for this highly demanding surgery) [3, 10, 52, 53]. Since the early clinical experiences of human liver transplantation, it was clear that an impaired hemostatic system was further stressed by complex and multiple changes occurring during the various phases of the transplant procedure [22]. For didactic and practical purposes, the surgical procedure is commonly subdivided into three main stages, each characterized by specific physiologic changes, relevant for the proper and finalized anesthesiological management [10, 22, 52, 53].

Stage 1, the *preanhepatic phase*, begins with surgical incision and ends with cross-clamping of the portal vein, the suprahepatic inferior vena cava (IVC), the infrahepatic IVC, and the hepatic artery;

Stage 2, the *anhepatic phase,*, starts after complete occlusion of vascular inflow to the liver, and includes the removal of the native liver and the confection of the vascular anastomoses of the suprahepatic and infrahepatic IVC (if and when needed, according to the surgical technique) and the portal vein and ends with the reperfusion of the newly grafted liver.

Stage 3, the *postanhepatic or neohepatic* phase, extends from the period immediately after the reperfusion of the graft to the end of surgery and includes the arterial anastomosis and the biliary tract reconstruction.

Each stage of the liver transplant procedure is associated with multiple and complex changes of the physiologic profile, including stage-specific changes of hemostasis [10, 22, 53–56].

The choice of blood products, blood components (FFP, cryoprecipitates, fibrinogen, platelets), or drugs aiming at the correction of the various changes during the different stages of liver transplantation has to be driven, if and when needed, by the hemostatic monitoring, now mainly done by TEG/TEM.

Conventional "static" parameters (PT, aPTT, platelet count) are important, but are not completely adequate for an astute intraoperative management: TEG, however, is used in less than 50% of the transplant centers worldwide, in spite of its use being on the rise [10, 52, 53].

Surgical bleeding, when present, could be the main issue during the preanhepatic phase. Bleeding during this phase of surgery is related to the degree of preexisting coagulopathy, the presence and severity of portal hypertension, and the duration and complexity of the surgical procedure [53–56]. Adhesions from previous abdominal surgery and large collateral vessels might add complexity to the surgical dissection, even if surgical skill and technical solutions have dramatically reduced blood loss during this phase. Hypovolemia has to be anticipated and treated with colloid-containing fluid to minimize changes in preload. However, use of restrictive versus more liberal loading policies is now on the rise, even if their use is challenged when they are too restrictive. In the presence of preexisting coagulopathy, FFP is indicated by some soon after incision: its use is, however, challenged by many [50–54]. Fibrinolysis is unusual during this phase. In the case of major blood losses, aggressive fluid resuscitation could result in a dilutional coagulopathy, with a gradual decline in the levels of coagulation factors and platelet count. In contrast, a hypercoagulable state could be seen in primary biliary cirrhosis (PBC) and sclerosing cholangitis (SC). The gradual mild (33–35°C) hypothermia may exacerbate the coagulopathy if it is not counteracted by appropriate measures/devices able to maintain the core temperature close to the normal temperature.

The anhepatic phase is mainly characterized by the hemodynamic changes induced by the cross-clamping of the suprahepatic and infrahepatic IVC and the consequent reduced venous return. During this phase, to ease the hemodynamic impact induced by the reduced venous return (as much as 50%) and the associated critical fall of cardiac output and arterial blood pressure, a venovenous bypass was frequently used: the device evolved from a complicated modified femorofemoral partial CPB (Cambridge liver transplant Unit chaired by Prof Roy Calne experience in the early 1980s) to a dedicated centrifugal force pump (biopump) without systemic heparinization [22, 52]. Diverting IVC and portal venous flows to the axillary vein using the biopump simplified surgery because of the reduced splanchnic congestion, the reduced negative impact on preload, the maintained renal perfusion pressure: a possible positive impact on the development of metabolic acidosis was also demonstrated. Air embolism, thromboembolism, and inadvertent decannulation were among the reported and feared complications, sometimes resulting in an increased relevant morbidity [22]. The use of the "piggyback" technique, with IVC preservation, now used in many centers, has substantially decreased the use of venovenous bypass [52–54]. According to Steadman [53], blood loss is usually limited by vascular clamping of the inflow vessels to the liver. Major changes in the hemostatic profile during stage 2, where the absence of the hepatic clearance might play a crucial role in the accumulation of tissue thromboplastin compounds, are depletion of platelets and the decline in the levels of coagulation factors, possibly due to an activation of coagulation.

Fibrinolysis may start during this stage, owing to an imbalance between reduced PAI-1 level and increased production of tPA, often, but not only, stimulated by endothelial stress secondary to acidosis and cathecolamine release. Even if reported to be frequent, hyperfibrinolysis during the anhepatic phase is evident in less than 40% of the cases in large recent series (including ours) [10, 52–54].

Finally, the neohepatic phase is notable for the reperfusion of the grafted liver and the resultant reperfusion syndrome, which could be extremely challenging [10, 22, 52–54]. A severe coagulopathy is very often seen within minutes after the reperfusion, and is associated with a sensible, diffuse, difficult-to-treat oozing, multifactorial in origin: reperfusion hypothermia, ionized hypocalcemia, quantitative and qualitative platelet defects (platelet activation, trapping of platelets in the graft), dilutional coagulopathy, a heparin-like effect (HLE), hyperfibrinolysis, and the release of a variety of humoral substances from the grafted liver are among the possible causes, alone or in combination. In rare instances, excessive activation of coagulation may also occur at this time. Hyperfibrinolysis is reported as very common (close to 80%), but severe cases associated with extensive bleeding represent less than 40% of cases. In some cases it does not need correction and resolves spontaneously in 60–120 min after reperfusion together with the functional recovery of the graft. In other series the use of antifibrinolytic drugs (mainly aprotinin, but now, after withdrawal of aprotinin from the market, tranexamic acid) has been shown to reduce blood loss during liver transplantation [51–55]. The most recent results for the use of antifibrinolytic drugs will be discussed in the "management" section [56].

The so-called HLE deserves additional discussion. The HLE, owing to heparin (exogenous) or heparin-like substances (endogenous), has been demonstrated after reperfusion of the liver graft for a long time [22, 52–54]. It occurs in close to 70% of cases, even if in the most recent study severe HLE was seen in 30% of cases and treated in 6% of cases [57, 58]. The heparin effect, as demonstrated by heparinase-modified TEG, either resolves spontaneously within 1–2 h of reperfusion or, in the case of continuous, disturbing nonsurgical oozing, is actively treated by administering 50–100 mg protamine sulfate, after the in vitro demonstration of the positive effect of heparinase. In spite of reports of reduced bleeding, a reduced transfusion requirement is not clearly demonstrated [52–54, 58]. This effect could come from exogenous heparin, given to the donor before harvesting (usually 15–20,000 UI), bound to the donor-liver endothelium and subsequently flushed into the systemic circulation of the recipient after reperfusion. However, an endogenous source of heparin-like substances/heparinoids was also postulated, because of the evidence of heparin-like activity reported after reperfusion even in the absence of heparin infusion in the donor liver. According to Senzolo et al. [58], an increased release of heparinoids is correlated with the macrophage activation which follows the ischemia reperfusion injury. A decreased clearance of endogenous and exogenous heparin and heparin-like substances in the severely diseased liver has been proposed: it was demonstrated in an animal model but the effect on coagulation was not reported [57, 58].

12.3.3 Management

As assessed in a recent report from the European Association for Studies on the Liver, management of bleeding complications during liver transplantation (including the "prophylactic" administration of blood, blood components, blood products, or prohemostatic drugs) differs widely between different centers, and general guidelines for patients with liver disease are not yet available [49]. As already mentioned, the use of a lower hemoglobin threshold for packed RBC transfusion in appropriately selected patients is increasing: timing and transfusion triggers of packed RBC still remain an area of great debate in clinical practice in general, and in liver transplantation in particular [52–54, 58–63]. More than a fixed hemoglobin threshold as a transfusion trigger, use of a combination of physiologic parameters able to describe the need for an increase in oxygen-carrying capacity is on the rise also in liver transplantation, changing the strategy which supports the transfusion decision in this context too. According to Ozier and Tsou [63], apart from surgical techniques and different candidate populations, a "center effect" closely correlated with local transfusion practice can be observed, which impacts on the variability of the amount of blood and blood products used in single institutions. What is now evident is the considerably lower transfusion rates with respect to those reported in the late 1990s. The median transfusion requirement in the various institutions (including ours) ranges between 2 and 6 U of packed RBC, whereas successful liver transplant procedures without transfusion have been reported. Dedicated programs for patients refusing blood, such as Jehovah's Witnesses are also active [59]. So far, transfusion triggers in liver transplant surgery have not been studied in randomized controlled trials, but what is evident from the literature in a retrospective analysis is a correlation between the number of RBC transfusions and 1-year survival (hazard ratio of 1.057 per unit of RBC) [63]. In a very recent prospective survey, the transfusion trigger for packed RBC was a hemoglobin level below 6 g/dl [56]. However, as stated by Liu and Niemann [59], the peculiar context of liver transplantation with the possible acute blood loss and the consequent hemodynamic instability make a strict standardization difficult, as proposed for other clinical setting.

According to Lisman et al. [49], recent data show sufficient thrombin production with a platelet count exceeding 50,000/µl. Thus, the efficacy of prophylactic infusions of FFP or platelets has not been demonstrated, and complete normalization of laboratory parameters in cirrhotic patients might not be available even after FFP or platelet administration. Too aggressive efforts to normalize the patient's coagulopathy with large volumes of blood products could also lead to a hypervolemic state. Citrate-associated ionized hypocalcemia might arise, leading to reduced cardiac contractility and vasodilatation, thus making calcium supplementation necessary to overcome hypotension secondary to cardiac output depression [52]. As above mentioned for packed RBC transfusion (worse outcome correlated with blood transfusion), platelets and FFP have also been associated with consistent adverse outcomes. According to Pereboom et al. [61] patient and graft survival rates were significantly reduced in patients who received platelet transfusions when compared with those who did not. Acute lung injury and its major consequences were considered the main reason for the lower survival rate associated with the use of platelets [61]. According to a study by Massicotte et al. [62], abnormal coagulation parameters are not to be corrected perioperatively, unless there is uncontrollable bleeding. No link was found between coagulation defects and bleeding and packed RBC or FFP transfusion. Correction of coagulation defects with plasma transfusion was quoted as "neither useful nor necessary." According to Dalmau et al. [64], no evidence-based threshold values for platelet count and FFP administration are available. For platelets, an option might be to withhold platelet transfusions in a patient with a low platelet count not bleeding and to transfuse platelets only when bleeding occurs. In the case of transfusion, platelet concentrates prepared by apheresis are the best available choice [64]. Instead of FFP in amounts able to determine circulatory overload, in the case of a long reaction time in TEG and a bleeding surgical field, Dalmau et al. [64] in a review on this specific item considered the administration of prothrombin complex concentrate; antithrombin activity, however, must be within the normal range to avoid the risk of thrombosis. Fibrinogen deserves a few words: it plays a key role in achieving a solid coagulation plug, both in a surgical setting and, according to the most recent reports, in trauma coagulopathy [82, 83, 85].

In cirrhotic patients, the fibrinogen level can be low or there can be dysfibrinogenemia or both, so it is advisable to ensure a certain level of fibrinogen during the transplant procedure [85]. Interestingly, in subjects with acquired severe acute hypofibrinogenemia, the 7-day survival was better among those patients with higher fibrinogen levels [64].

Prohemostatic Drugs

A significant decrease in blood loss and blood product requirements has been observed in liver transplant surgery over the last 20 years [3, 10, 58]. Among the contributing factors, apart from a refined surgical approach and better understanding of perioperative hemostatic changes, are the use of prohemostatic drugs, mainly antifibrinolytic drugs [51, 55, 56, 65] and rFVIIa [35, 63, 64, 66–68]. Desmopressin, was able to improve platelet aggregation in patients with platelet dysfunction and blood coagulability of patients undergoing a liver transplant: its use is, however, rare. Antifibrinolytic drugs and rFVIIa can be used either prophylactically or for rescue when there is severe uncontrolled bleeding. In spite of being used per protocol by some centers [55, 56], there is no consensus about the administration of antifibrinolytic drugs, mainly because of the rather different management of perioperative hemostatic problems, which makes it not easy to compare protocols [64].

Antifibrinolytic Drugs

ε-Aminocaproic acid, an antifibrinolytic drug, is used only in the USA. It interferes with plasminogen binding to fibrin, thus inhibiting the conversion of plasminogen to plasmin. In the only prospective randomized trial, it was able to reverse TEG

12 Hemocoagulative Aspects of Solid Organ Transplantation

fibrinolysis, and to reduce blood cell transfusion, without causing thrombotic complications [22].

The antifibrinolytic drugs that have been studied more extensively in liver transplantation are aprotinin and tranexamic acid.

Aprotinin is derived from bovine lung. It is a low molecular weight nonspecific serine protease inhibitor with a primary effect of plasminogen-to-plasmin conversion inhibition. Tranexamic acid is a lysine analogue that inhibits plasminogen-to-plasmin conversion by adhering to lysine binding sites on plasminogen.

Antifibrinolytic drugs were proved to reduce perioperative blood loss in liver transplant recipients by more than 30% compared with controls [44, 52–55]. Hyperfibrinolysis occurring during the anhepatic phase and after reperfusion, due to increased levels of tPA, constituted the basis for the use of antifibrinolytic drugs to improve hemostasis and to reduce blood transfusion needs during liver transplantation [55]. The efficacy of antifibrinolytic drugs in liver transplantation was proven, but many concerns regarding their routine use were raised, mainly because of safety reasons, owing to the risk of thromboembolic complications. In a recent meta-analysis and systematic review of more than 1,400 patients, both aprotinin and tranexamic acid significantly reduced packed RBC transfusion needs during liver transplantation [55]. Aprotinin, but not tranexamic acid, also significantly reduced intraoperative use of FFP. The systematic review did not demonstrate an increased risk of hepatic artery thrombosis, venous thromboembolic events, or mortality in patients who received an antifibrinolytic drug while undergoing a liver transplant [55].

The most recent prospective survey on the use of antifibrinolytic drugs was by Massicotte et al. [56]. Well-known protocols of prophylactic administration of antifibrinolytic agents were used to reduce blood loss during liver transplantation. Aprotinin and tranexamic acid were compared in 400 consecutive liver transplants (different use according to the local protocols and the drug availability): 300 patients received aprotinin (2002–2007) and 100 patients received tranexamic acid (2007–2009, after withdrawal of aprotinin) . Among the goals of the study were research into the independent predictors of intraoperative transfusion requirement and of 1-year patient mortality. Intraoperative blood loss (aprotinin group 1,082 ± 1,056 ml vs. tranexamic acid group 1,007 ± 790 ml) and packed RBC transfusion per patient (0.561.4 vs. 0.561.0 U, respectively) were similar in the two groups. The final hemoglobin concentrations (aprotinin group 9.29 + 1.98 g/dl vs. tranexamic acid group 9.5 + 2.17 g/dl) were similar. Outstandingly high and similar was the percentage of liver transplant patients who did not have transfusion during surgery (80 vs. 82%). The 1-year survival rate (85.1 vs. 87.4%) was not different. No major changes in serum creatinine concentration were also evident [56]. Two variables, baseline hemoglobin level and intraoperative phlebotomy findings, correlated with the two primary outcome measures (transfusion needs and 1-year survival). According to these results, the hemoglobin level before liver transplantation is proposed by Massicotte et al. [56] as a predictor of blood product/transfusion requirements: the higher the baseline hemoglobin level, the lower the risk of transfusion. Low starting hemoglobin and high starting INR values were linked to decreased survival rate.

Recombinant Factor VIIa

Recombinant factor VIIa (rFVIIa) is a potent procoagulant agent, initially developed for bleeding episodes in hemophilia A and hemophilia B patients who developed inhibitors against standard-factor replacements. As reported in the previous sections, rFVIIa binds to tissue factor, stimulating the formation of fibrin, and therefore plays a central role in the activation of coagulation [46]. It has been studied and used, mainly off label, in different surgical procedures associated with a high risk of bleeding and large blood transfusion. The efficacy and safety of prophylactic administration of rFVIIa during liver transplantation has been investigated in two large, placebo-controlled, multicenter trials, with different doses [66–69].

In the repeated perioperative dose trial chaired by Lodge et al. [66] 183 cirrhotic patients, Child-Pugh class B or C, received a repeated intravenous bolus regimen of rFVIIa, 60 or 120 µg/kg or a placebo. No significant effect of rFVIIa was observed on the number of packed RBC units transfused or intraoperative blood loss compared with the placebo group: however, more patients in the rFVIIa study groups avoided packed RBC transfusion. The hospitalization rate and the total surgery time were similar in the two groups. There was not a significant difference in the rate of thromboembolic events.

Planinsic et al. [67] randomized 165 patients with ESLD scheduled for a liver transplant to one of four parallel study groups (single intravenous bolus of rFVIIa, 20, 40, or 80 µg/kg or a placebo prior to surgery), the primary assessment end point being the total number of RBC units transfused perioperatively. Safety was evaluated by the number of adverse events reported. There were no significant differences in the number of packed RBC units required between the placebo and rFVIIa study groups. The number of adverse events was comparable between the study groups. Thus, in spite of the good safety profile in patients undergoing a liver transplant, the authors concluded there was an absence of an effect of rFVIIa on the number of RBC transfusions required. The same results were also obtained by us in a small preliminary single center experience [68] According to the most recent reviews in the field [35, 69], there is a trend across studies toward reduced RBC transfusion requirements with rFVIIa prophylaxis, but neither the operating room time nor the length of stay in the ICU was reduced. On the other side, no effect of rFVIIa on mortality or thromboembolism was evident.

According to the most recent meta-analysis [69], prophylactic administration of rFVIIa failed to significantly modify any of the outcomes studied. This has implications for clinical practice, because there appears to be no clear evidence to promote its use in liver transplantation (or liver resection), apart from in specific cases, after having ruled out other possible alternative causes of bleeding. Even if more trials are to be considered to adequately evaluate the use of prophylactic rFVIIa in liver transplantation, room for a specific role does not seem to be likely: as mentioned by Yank et al. [69] however, the available evidence of low strength is too limited to compare the harms and benefits of rFVIIa in liver transplantation.

12.4 Kidney Transplantation

Improvements in immunosuppressive medication, organ procurement, patient preparation, and surgical techniques have resulted in a significant increase in survival rates after kidney transplantation. Furthermore, kidney transplantation has been shown to confer a greater survival benefit than maintenance dialysis. Extended-criteria cadaveric donors (ECD) are now considered to further expand the donor pool and to increase the number of patients receiving a transplant. Cardiovascular diseases (ischemic cardiopathy, arterial hypertension, congestive heart failure) are the major causes of increased morbidity and mortality in dialysis patients, accounting for over 50% of deaths [70]. The risk of cardiovascular disease, ten to 30 times higher in dialysis patients than in the normal population, is decreased to twice that in normal subjects after kidney transplantation. Diabetes is quite frequent in end-stage renal disease (ESRD) candidates and further increases the perioperative risk. Anemia has long been a problem in those with ESRD. The independent relative risk of mortality in dialysis patients was calculated to be 1.18 per 1.0 g/dl decrease in hemoglobin level. The use of erythropoietin has resulted in a reduction of the number of blood transfusions, and has improved quality of life, cognitive function, exercise tolerance, cardiac function, and, most importantly, survival. However, the overzealous correction of anemia, although improving uremic coagulopathy, may predispose to thrombus formation, increasing blood viscosity and decreasing erythrocyte deformability. A target hemoglobin level close to (10 to 12 g/l) is now considered a standard of care [70, 71].

Bleeding is not a major concern during kidney transplantation, if not for major surgical technical reasons. However, ESRD patients may suffer from many hemostatic abnormalities [70, 71]. Among them are abnormal platelet function and ineffective production of both FVIII and von Willebrand factor. Patients with ESRD who have regular hemodialysis may be prone to develop both thrombotic complications (ischemic heart disease, cerebral strokes, and vascular access thrombosis) [71] and a bleeding tendency because of platelet dysfunction: the latter is often multifactorial and is associated with the terminal kidney disease or is due to the use of platelet aggregation inhibitor drugs [72]. The hypercoagulable state has been associated with changes in hemostatic plasma protein factors such as lupus anticoagulant, anticardiolipin antibodies IgG and IgM, and deficiencies in protein S, protein C, and antithrombin [71]. Dialysis per se could be associated with hemostatic abnormalities. The residual heparin effect may increase bleeding tendency, but this is negligible if regional heparinization is used. Whereas thrombosis tendencies seem to be associated with recurrent platelet activation and imbalance between platelets and vascular prostaglandins, fibrinolysis might be associated with consumption of PAI-1 and increased release of tPA from the endothelium. If there is a prolonged bleeding time, dialysis is reported to be the treatment of choice [70, 71]. Preoperative dialysis improves platelet function and is the mainstay of the prevention of uremic bleeding, whereas cryoprecipitate and desmopressin have been used by some for a temporary correction. Desmopressin in particular should improve the binding of von Willebrand factor to the platelet membrane. Dynamic hemostatic monitoring by TEG/TEM might be useful to determine the type of correction. PFA-100 seems to be more appropriate to study platelet dysfunction [72].

Preoperative administration of rFVIIa to reduce/counteract the effect of platelet aggregation inhibitors (aspirin, clopidogrel) in candidates for a kidney transplant has also been reported, aiming at the reduction of the increased risk of bleeding during kidney transplantation [73]. Platelet aggregation inhibitors could lead to massive coagulation problems during surgery, because of the possible severe impact on the hemostasic profile, owing to their possible effect, which exceeds their plasma half-lives. Its use in patients with Glanzmann disease showed the potential of rFVIIa to contribute to the stabilization of the hemostatic profile in the case of impaired platelet function. Since rapid and direct antagonization of platelet aggregation antagonists is not available, rFVIIa has been proposed as an effective, safe, and rapid emergency treatment: no major complications, including thrombosis, were reported neither in this small series nor in other anecdotal kidney transplant cases [74–77]. However, according to the available literature, this latter use has to be considered with great caution: proper hemostatic assessment (TEG/TEM or with the PFA-100) has to be considered mandatory before its use.

Blood transfusion is usually unnecessary, since anemia is well tolerated. As mentioned above, the use of erythropoietin has now minimized the findings of significant anemia, which was more common in the past. In spite of having been associated in the early 1980s with improved graft survival, RBC transfusion is now kept to a minimum: it may increase the levels of alloantibodies to leukocytes antigens, potentially reducing graft survival. According to the most recent theories in transfusion (as alluded to in the previous sections), RBCs are transfused only in selected cases, when anemia is severe and paying attention more to dynamic physiologic triggers than to fixed hemoglobin values.

References

1. Moore D, Feurer I, Speroff T et al (2003) Survival and quality of life after organ transplantation in veterans and nonveterans. Am J Surg 186:476–480
2. Ortega T, Deulofeu R, Salamero et al (2009) Health-related quality of life before and after a solid organ transplantation (kidney, liver, and lung) of four Catalonia hospitals. Transpl Proc 41:2265–2267
3. Niemann CU, Eilers H (2010) Abdominal organ transplantation. Minerva Anest 76:266–275
4. Bonney GK, Aldersley MA, Asthana S et al (2009) Donor risk index and MELD interactions in predicting long-term graft survival: a single-centre experience. Transplantation 87:1858–1863
5. Rheem J, Kern B, Cooper J, Freeman RB (2009) Organ donation. Semin Liver Dis 29:19–38
6. Cameron AM, Ghobrial RM, Yersiz H, Farmer DG, Lipshutz GS, Gordon SA et al (2006) Optimal utilization of donor grafts with extended criteria a single-center experience in over 1000 liver transplants. Ann Surg 243:748–755
7. Mittler J, Pascher A, Neuhaus P, Pratschke J (2008) The utility of extended criteria donor organs in severely ill liver transplant recipients. Transplantation 86:895–896

12 Hemocoagulative Aspects of Solid Organ Transplantation

8. Sandberg WS, Raines DE (2008) Anesthesia for liver surgery and Transplantation. In: Longnecker DE, Brown DL, Newman MF, Zapol WM (eds) Anesthesiology. McGraw, New York, pp 1338–1377
9. Beebe DS, Belani KG (2008) Anesthesia for kidney, pancreas or other organ transplantation. In: Longnecker DE, Brown DL, Newman MF, Zapol WM (eds) Anesthesiology. McGraw, New York, pp 1397–1419
10. Yost CS, Niemann CU (2010) Anesthesia for organ transplantation. In: Miller RD (ed) Miller's anesthesia, 7th edn. Elsevier, Philadelphia, pp 2155–2184
11. Nussmeier NA, Hauser MC, Muhammad FS et al (2010) Anesthesia for cardiac surgical procedures. In: In: Miller RD (ed) Miller's anesthesia, 7th edn. Elsevier, Philadelphia, pp 1889–1965
12. Crespo-Leiro M, Barge-Caballero E, Marzoa-Rivas R, Paniagua-Martin MJ (2010) Cardiac transplantation. Curr Op Organ Transpl 15:633–638
13. Mehra MR, Kobashigawa J, Starling R, Russell S et al (2006) Listing criteria for heart transplantation: international society for heart and lung transplantation guidelines for the care of cardiac transplant candidates—2006. J Heart Lung Transpl 25:1025
14. Hourigan LA, Walters DR, Keck SA, Dec W (2002) HIT, a common complication in cardiac transplant candidates. J Heart Lung Transpl 21:1283–1289
15. Robinson KL, Marasco SF, Street AM (2001) Practical management of anticoagulation, bleeding and blood product support for cardiac surgery Part one: bleeding and anticoagulation issues. Heart Lung Circ 10:142–153
16. Society of Thoracic Surgeons Blood Conservation Guideline Task Force (2007) Perioperative blood transfusion and blood conservation in cardiac surgery: the Society of Thoracic Surgeons and the Society of Cardiovascular Anesthesiologists clinical practice guideline. Ann Thorac Surg 82:S27
17. Diaz Martin A, Escoresca-Ortega AM, Hernandez-Caballero C et al (2010) Considerations regarding major bleeding after cardiac transplantation. Transpl Proc 42:3204
18. Wegner JA, DiNardo JA, Arabia FA et al (2000) Blood loss and transfusion requirements in patients implanted with a mechanical circulatory support device undergoing cardiac transplantation. J Heart Lung Transplant 19(5):504–506
19. Fries D, Innerhofer P, Streif W et al (2003) Coagulation monitoring and management of anticoagulation during cardiac assist device support. Ann Thor Surg 76:1593–1597
20. Shore-Lesserson L, Manspeizer HE, DePerio M, Francis S, Vela-Cantos F, Ergin MA (1999) Thromboelastography-guided transfusion algorithm reduces transfusions in complex cardiac surgery. Anesth Analg 88:312–319
21. Ronald A, Dunning J (2005) Can the use of thromboelastography predict and decrease bleeding and blood and blood product requirements in adult patients undergoing cardiac surgery? Interact Cardiovasc Thorac Sur 4:456–463
22. Kang YG, Gaisor TA (1999) Hematologic considerations in the transplant patient. In: Sharpe MA, Gelb AW (eds) Anesthesia and transplantation. Butterworth-Heinemann, Boston, pp 363–387
23. Paradela M, González D, Parente I, Fernández R et al (2009) Surgical risk factors associated with lung transplantation. Transpl Proc 41:2218–2220
24. Gu YJ, de Haan J, Brenken UP, de Boer WJ et al (1996) Clotting and fibrinolityc disturbance during lung transplantation. Effect of low dose aprotinin. Thorac Cardiovasc Surg 112:599–606
25. Griffith BP, Hardesty RL, Trento A et al (1987) Heart lung transplantation: lesson learned and future hopes. Ann Thoracic Surg 43:6–16
26. Hunt BJ, Sack D, Yacoub MH (1992) The perioperative use of blood components during heart and heart lung transplantation. Transfusion 32:57–62
27. Peterson KL, DeCampli WM, Feeley TW, Starnes VA (1995) Blood loss and transfusion requirements in cystic fibrosis undergoing heart lung or lung transplantation. J Cardiothoracic Anesth 9:59–62

28. Murphy GJ, Reeves BC, Rogers CA et al (2007) Increased mortality, postoperative morbidity, and cost after red blood cell transfusion in patients having cardiac surgery. Circulation 116:2544–2552
29. Wang JK, Klein HG (2010) Red blood cell transfusion in the treatment and management of anaemia: the search for the elusive transfusion trigger. Vox Sang 98:2–11
30. Triulzi DJ (2002) Specialized transfusion support for solid organ transplantation. Curr Opin Hematol 9:527–532
31. Triulzi DJ, Nalesnik MA (2001) Microchimerism, GVHD, and tolerance in solid organ transplantation. Transfusion 41:419–426
32. Futier E, Robin E, Jabaudon M, Guerin R et al (2010) Central venous O_2 saturation and venous-to-arterial CO_2 difference as complementary tools for goal-directed therapy during high-risk surgery. Crit Care 14:R193
33. Orlov D, O'Farrell R, McCluskey SA et al (2009) The clinical utility of an index of global oxygenation for guiding red blood cell transfusion in cardiac surgery. Transfusion 49:682–688
34. The Society of Thoracic Surgeons and the Society of Cardiovascular Anesthesiologists blood conservation clinical practice guidelines (2011) Ann Thorac Surg 91:944–982
35. Chavez-Tapia NC, Alfaro-Lara N, Tellez-Avila F et al (2011) Prophylactic activated recombinant factor vii in liver resection and liver transplantation: systematic review and meta-analysis. PLoS ONE 6(7):e22581. doi:10.1371/journal.pone.0022581PLoSONE
36. Gandhi MJ, Pierce RA, Zhanq L, Moon MR et al (2007) Use of activated recombinant factor VII for severe coagulopathy post ventricular assist device or orthotopic heart transplant. Cardiothorac Surg 2:32
37. Gill R, Herbertson M, Vuylsteke A et al (2009) Safety and efficacy of recombinant activated factor VII: a randomized placebo-controlled trial in the setting of bleeding after cardiac surgery. Circulation 120:21–27
38. Koster A, Schirmer U (2011) Re-evaluation of the role of antifibrinolytic therapy with lysine analogs during cardiac surgery in the post aprotinin era. Curr Opin Anesthesiol 24:92–97
39. Kesten S, de Hoyas A, Chaparro C et al (1995) Aprotinin reduces blood loss in lung transplant recipients. Ann Thorac Surg 59:877–879
40. Trulock EP, Edwards LB, Taylor DO, Boucek MM, Keck BM, Hertz MI (2004) The registry of the international society for heart and lung transplantation: twenty-first official adult lung and heart-lung transplant report—2004. J Heart Lung Transpl 23:804–815
41. Balsara KR, Morowich ST, Lin SS, Davis RD et al (2009) Aprotinin's effect on blood product transfusion in off-pump bilateral lung transplantation. Interact Cardiovasc Thorac Surg 8:45–48
42. Marasco S, Pilcher D, Oto T et al (2010) Aprotinin in lung transplantation is associated with an increased incidence of primary graft dysfunction. Eur J Cardiothorac Surg 37:420–425
43. Wada H, Usui M, Sakuragawa N (2008) Haemostatic abnormalities and liver disease. Semin Thromb Hemost 34:772–778
44. Lisman T, Robert J, Porte RJ (2010) Rebalanced hemostasis in patients with liver disease: evidence and clinical consequences. Blood 116:878–885
45. Roberts LN, Patel RK, Arya R (2010) Haemostasis and thrombosis in liver disease. Br J Haematol 148:507–521
46. Tripodi A, Mannucci PM (2011) The coagulopathy of chronic liver disease. N Engl J Med 365:147–156
47. van Veen JJ, Spahn DR, Makris M (2011) Routine preoperative coagulation tests: an outdated practice? Brit J Anaesth 106:1–3
48. Amitrano L, Guardascione MA, Brancaccio V, Balzano A (2002) Coagulation disorders in liver disease. Semin Liver Dis 22:83–96
49. Lisman T, Caldwell SH, Burroughs AK (2010) Coagulation in Liver Disease Study Group. Hemostasis and thrombosis in patients with liver disease: the ups and downs. J Hepatol 53:362–371
50. Stravitz RT, Lisman T, Luketic VA et al (2011) Minimal effects of acute liver injury/acute liver failure on hemostasis as assessed by thromboelastography. J Hepatol. doi: 10.1016/j.jhep.2011.04.020

51. Boylan JF, Klinck JR, Sandler AN et al (1996) Tranexamic acid reduces blood loss, transfusion requirements, and coagulation factor use in primary orthotopic liver transplantation. Anesthesiology 85:1043–1048
52. Hannaman MJ, Hevesi ZG (2011) Anesthesia care for liver transplantation. Transpl Rev 25:36–43
53. Steadman R (2004) Anesthesia for liver transplant surgery. Anesthesiol Clin North Am 22:687–711
54. Senzolo M, Burra P, Cholongitas E, Burroughs AK (2006) New insights into the coagulopathy of liver disease and liver transplantation. World J Gastroenterol 28:7725–7736
55. Molenaar IQ, Warnaar N, Groen H et al (2007) Efficacy and safety of antifibrinolytic drugs in liver transplantation: a systematic review and meta-analysis. Am J Transpl 7:185–194
56. Massicotte L, Denault AY, Beaulieu D, Thibeaul L et al (2011) Aprotinin versus tranexamic acid during liver transplantation: impact on blood product requirements and survival. Transplantation 91:1273–1278
57. Agarwal S, Senzolo M, Melikian C et al (2008) The prevalence of a heparin-like effect shown on the thromboelastograph in patients undergoing liver transplantation. Liver Transpl 14:855–860
58. Senzolo M, Cholongitas E, Thalheimer U et al (2009) Heparin-like effect in liver disease and liver transplantation. Clin Liver Dis 13(1):43–53
59. Liu L, Niemann CU (2011) Intraoperative management of liver transplant patients. Transpl Rev (in press)
60. de Boer MT, Christensen MC, Asmussen M et al (2008) The impact of intraoperative transfusion of platelets and red blood cells on survival after liver transplantation. Anesth Analg 106:32–44
61. Pereboom IT, de Boer MT, Haagsma EB et al (2009) Platelet transfusion during liver transplantation is associated with increased postoperative mortality due to acute lung injury. Anesth Anal 108:1083–1091
62. Massicotte L, Beaulieu D, Thibeault L et al (2008) Coagulation defects do not predict blood product requirements during liver transplantation. Transplantation 85:956–962
63. Ozier Y, Tsou MY (2008) Changing trends in transfusion practice in liver transplantation. Curr Opin Organ Transpl 13:304–309
64. Dalmau A, Sabate A, Aparicio I (2009) Hemostasis and coagulation monitoring and management during liver transplantation. Curr Opin Organ Transpl 14:286–290
65. Porte RJ, Molenaar IQ, Begliomini B et al (2000) Aprotinin and transfusion requirements in orthotopic liver transplantation: a multicentre randomised double-blind study EMSALT study group. Lancet 355:1303–1309
66. Lodge JP, Jonas S, Jones RM et al (2005) Efficacy and safety of repeated perioperative doses of recombinant factor VIIa in liver transplantation. Liver Transpl 11:973–979
67. Planinsic RM, van der Meer J, Testa G et al (2005) Safety and efficacy of a single bolus administration of recombinant factor VIIa in liver transplantation due to chronic liver disease. Liver Transpl 11:895–900
68. De Gasperi A, Baudo F, De Carlis L (2005) Recombinant FVII in orthotopic liver transplantation (OLT): a preliminary single centre experience. Intensive Care Med 31(2):315–316
69. Yank V, Vaughan Tuohy C, Logan AC et al (2011) Systematic review: benefits and harms of in-hospital use of recombinant factor VIIa for off-label indications. Ann Int Med 154:529–540
70. Sarin Kapoor H, Kaur R, Kaur H (2007) Anesthesia for kidney transplantation. Acta Anaesthesiol Scand 51:1354–1367
71. Hemmens HJL (2004) Kidney transplantation: recent developments and recommendations for anesthetic management. Anesthesiol Clin North Am 22:651–662
72. Ertug Z, Celik U, Hadimioglu N, Dinckan A, Ozdem S (2010) The assessment of PFA-100 test for the estimation of blood loss in renal transplantation operation. Ann Transpl 19:46–52

73. Nampoory MRN, Das CK, Johny VK (2003) Hypercoagulability, a serious problem in patients with ESRD on maintenance hemodialysis, and its correction after kidney transplantation. Am J Kidney Dis 42:797–805
74. Hagen Loertzer H, Soukup J, Fornara P (2007) Recombinant Factor VIIa reduces bleeding risk in patients on Platelet aggregation inhibitors immediately prior to renal transplantation—a retrospective analysis. Urol Int 78:135–139
75. Gielen-Wijffels SE, van Mook WN, van der Geest S, Ramsay G (2004) Successful treatment of severe bleeding with recombinant factor VIIa after kidney transplantation. Intensive Care Med 30:1232–1234
76. Dunkley SM, Mackie F (2003) Recombinant factor VIIa used to control massive haemorrhage during renal transplantation surgery; vascular graft remained patent. Hematology 8:263–264
77. Sander M, von Heymann C, Kox W et al (2004) Recombinant factor VIIa for excessive bleeding after thrombectomy prior to kidney transplantation. Transplantation 77:1912–1913
78. Sarris GE, Smith JA, Shumway NE et al (1994) Long term results of combined heart lung transplantation. The Stanford experience. J Heart L Transpl 3:940–949
79. Sharples LD, Scott JP, Dennis C et al (1994) Risk factors for survival following combined heart lung transplantation. Transplantation 57:218–223
80. Chapman AJ, Blount AL, Davis DT Hooker RL (2011) Recombinant factor VIIa (NovoSeven RT) use in high risk cardiac surgery. Eur J Cardiothoracic Surg (in press)
81. Centro Nazionale Trapianti (2011) http://www.trapianti.ministerosalute.it. Accessed Oct 2011
82. Tisherman AS (2010) Is fibrinogen the answer to coagulopathy after massive transfusion? Critical Care 14:154
83. Nascimento B, Rizoli S, Rubenfeld G, Fukushima R, Ahmed N, Nathens A, Lin Y, Callum J (2011) Cryoprecipitate transfusion: assessing appropriateness and dosing in trauma. Transf Med 21:394–401
84. Carr JM (1989) Disseminated intravascular coagulation in cirrhosis. Hepatology 10:103–110
85. Noval Padillo J, León-Justel A, Mellado-Miras P, Porras-Lopez FD, Villegas-Duque MA, Gomez-Bravo MA, Guerrero JM (2010) Introduction of fibrinogen in the treatment of hemostatic disorders during orthotopic liver transplantation: implications in the use of allogenic blood. Transplant Proc 42:2973–2974

Antiphospholipid Antibody Syndrome

13

Marco Zambon, Davide Cappelli and Giorgio Berlot

13.1 Introduction

Antiphospholipid antibodies (APLA), first described in 1906 in a study by Wassermann et al. [1], are a heterogeneous group of autoantibodies directed against phospholipids and phospholipid-binding proteins (cofactors), such as β_2-glycoprotein 1 [2, 3]. In general, APLA are divided into two categories: lupus anticoagulants (LAC) and anticardiolipin antibodies (ACLA). A brief presentation of APLA and their laboratory testing is a natural introduction to APLA syndrome (APS).

LAC are antibodies that block the phospholipid surfaces relevant for coagulation. They reduce the coagulant potential of the plasma and prolong the clotting time in coagulation tests based on the activated partial thromboplastin time [4]. The presence of LAC is confirmed by the failure of the correction of the prolonged clotting time after a 1:1 mix with normal platelet-free plasma and of the clotting time after addition of excess phospholipids [5]. Consensus guidelines recommend screening for LAC with two or more phospholipid-dependent coagulation tests: activated partial thromboplastin time, dilute Russell's viper venom time, kaolin clotting time, dilute prothrombin time, textarin time, or taipan time [5]. Thromboelastography has been considered as a possible, quantitative stand-alone alternative for this multitude of assays. However, even a quantitative LAC assay is only partially informative in the prediction/exclusion of thrombosis in patients with APS. As explained below, this task is of great prognostic and therapeutic value. Detection of LAC can be problematic in patients receiving anticoagulant therapy because the clotting time will be

---

M. Zambon (✉)
Anesthesia and Intensive Care, Cattinara Hospital,
University of Trieste, Trieste, Italy
e-mail: Marco.zambon@gmail.com

G. Berlot (ed.), *Hemocoagulative Problems in the Critically Ill Patient*,
DOI: 10.1007/978-88-470-2448-9_13, © Springer-Verlag Italia 2012

209

prolonged. This problem can be overcome by mixing patient and normal plasma before LAC measurement [6].

ACLA are directed against a molecular congener of cardiolipin (a bovine cardiac protein), for which they share a common in vitro binding affinity. The immunoglobulin isotype may be IgG, IgM, or IgA. It is widely believed that the IgG isotype is most strongly associated with thrombosis, although this has not been tested in large prospective studies [7]. ACLA can be tested for with enzyme-linked immunosorbent assay (ELISA). ELISA for ACLA is poorly standardized and has shown poor concordance between laboratories [4]. Moreover, ACLA are reported as a titer specific to the isotype (IgG, IgM, or IgA phospholipid antibody titer), but because the accuracy and reliability of the assays are limited, consensus guidelines recommend semiquantitative reporting of results (low, medium, or high titer) [8]. ACLA do not prolong coagulation assays. In the diagnosis of APS, IgG and IgM isotypes may be considered, although the IgG isotype seems to have the strongest association with thrombosis [7].

To date, the lack of laboratory standardization and randomized trials makes finding APLA problematic. Current testing assays find APLA in up to 10% of healthy individuals as well as in 30–50% of patients with systemic lupus erythematosus (SLE) [9]. Laboratory testing for APLA is complicated because there is uncertainty about their antigenic target. Both LAC and ACLA may demonstrate specificity for β_2-glycoprotein I [10], but many other antigenic targets have been described, including prothrombin [11] and annexin V [12]. In some cases, antibodies directed against β_2-glycoprotein I rather than anionic phospholipids are believed to be causal in the syndrome [13]. In any case, testing for APLA is fundamental to evaluate the thrombotic risk that might be associated. In this regard, thrombography may help in the diagnosis and follow-up of APS [14, 15].

Although APLA may be found in up to 10% of healthy blood donors, only few healthy individuals are persistently APLA-positive at follow-up [16]. Persistent APLA positivity is unusual in healthy individuals (less than 2% of healthy blood donors initially found to have ACLA still had increased levels 9 months later) [16]. The prevalence of APLA appears to be higher among patients presenting with thrombosis (4–21%) [17, 18]. In a recent meta-analysis of 25 studies involving more than 7,000 patients, the mean odds ratio (OR) for thrombosis was 11.0 for LAC, and a weaker association was found for ACLA (approximately 1.6), for which half of the studies reviewed did not reach statistical significance [19].

13.2 Etiology, Pathogenesis, and Clinical Characteristics

The finding of persistent APLA in patients with arterial or venous thrombosis or pregnancy morbidity defines APS. APS is "primary" when it occurs alone, and is "secondary" when it is associated with other conditions (e.g., SLE). International consensus criteria for the classification of definite APS were initially published in 1991 [20] and updated in 2006 [21]. According to the Sapporo criteria, APS is present in patients with one clinical and one laboratory criterion. Clinical criteria include objectively confirmed arterial, venous, or small-vessel thrombosis, or pregnancy morbidity consisting of recurrent fetal loss before the tenth week of gestation, one or more unexplained fetal deaths at or beyond the tenth week of gestation, or premature birth due to placental insufficiency, eclampsia, or preeclampsia. Laboratory criteria include medium- or high-titer IgG or IgM ACLA or the presence of LAC on two or more occasions at least 6 weeks apart [22, 23]. These criteria do not take into account several clinical and/or laboratory features: clinical manifestations such as thrombocytopenia, valvular heart disease, nephropathy, and ischemic neurologic abnormalities [20], which are often associated with APLA. Because of their low specificity, other APLA (antiphosphatidylserine, antiphosphatidylethanolamine, antibodies against prothrombin, and antibodies against the phosphatidylserine–prothrombin complex, all frequent in patients with APS) are not included in the diagnosis [20].

Catastrophic APS (CAPS) is a variant defined in 1992 as a condition characterized by multiple vascular occlusive events, usually affecting small vessels, presenting over a short period of time, with the laboratory confirmation of the presence of APLA [24]. CAPS is characterized predominately by a diffuse thrombotic microvasculopathy, with a predilection for lung, brain, heart, kidney, skin, and gastrointestinal tract [25]. CAPS is unusual and represents less than 1% of cases [26]. The first studies published showed a mortality rate of approximately 50% [27]; however, a more recent report [25] gave a slightly reduced rate. This reduction in mortality appears to be attributable to the use of full anticoagulation, corticosteroids, plasma exchanges, and immunoglobulins as first-line therapies [25]. Multiple triggering factors may be present in the same patients (e.g., infections, anticoagulation withdrawal followed by a surgical procedure, or biopsy in patients with neoplasia and APLA). The presence of thrombotic microangiopathic anemia is a hallmark of CAPS. Differential diagnosis includes severe entities that share the same pathological process, such as thrombotic thrombocytopenic purpura, hemolytic uremic syndrome, acute disseminated intravascular coagulation, and hemolytic anemia, elevated liver enzyme level, and low platelet count syndrome [28]. The pathogenesis of catastrophic APS is not clear. In these patients, microvascular occlusions might be responsible for propagation of thrombosis as the clot continues to generate thrombin. Fibrinolysis may be decreased by an increased level of circulating plasminogen activator inhibitor type 1, and there is consumption of the natural anticoagulant proteins, such as protein C and antithrombin [29]. Furthermore, as supported by recent studies, thrombotic manifestations may be attributable to factors other than autoantibodies. In fact, although APS may be considered as an autoantibody-mediated disease, there is now evidence that APLA are necessary but not sufficient to trigger some of the clinical manifestations of the syndrome. For example, additional factors, such as mediators of the innate immunity, are now recognized to play a key role as second hit able to induce the thrombotic events in the presence of the autoantibodies. The APS scenario is also supplemented by the influence of genetically determined factors. Finally, environmental agents—in particular infectious ones—were reported to act as triggers for the production of autoantibodies cross-reacting with phospholipid-binding proteins as well as inflammatory stimuli that potentiate the APLA thrombogenic effect [30].

13.3 Thrombotic Risk

As stated above, it appears that the prevalence of APLA seems to be higher among patients with thrombosis [17, 18]. Even though APLA may be found in up to 10% of healthy individuals, in less than 2% of these healthy blood donors the positivity to APLA is persistant [16]. The mean odds ratio for thrombosis was 11.0 for LAC and 1.6 for ACLA [19].

All these data agree on the fact that the rates of morbidity and mortality are high in APS. As a consequence, awareness of the need for optimal prognostic markers in the prediction of complications of APS is growing [31]. The risk of thrombosis among healthy patients who are incidentally found to have APLA seems to be low: among 552 randomly selected blood donors, no thrombotic events were observed after 12 months of follow-up among patients found to have ACLA [16]. However, in patients with SLE, the incidence of thrombosis was not negligible: in a prospective cohort of 551 patients, of whom 49% had either LAC or ACLA, the annual incidence of thrombosis was 3.20 for LAC and 6.80 for high-titer ACLA. Patients with SLE all have the same high prevalence of thrombosis, even in the absence of APLA [9]. Information on the risk of recurrent thrombosis among patients with APLA is based on retrospective studies of untreated patients or prospective studies of untreated patients in which use of anticoagulants has been discontinued [32]. Three prospective studies showed a high risk of recurrence, ranging from 10 to 67% per year [33–35]. In a study of 412 patients with a first episode of venous thromboembolism who completed 6 months of anticoagulation, the presence of ACLA was associated with an increased risk of recurrence after discontinuation of anticoagulant therapy [33]. In retrospective studies, recurrent thrombosis was observed in 52–69% of patients during 5–6 years of follow-up, regardless of the type of antithrombotic therapy [36, 37], and the incidence of thrombosis was highest during the first 6 months after discontinuation of warfarin therapy. Interestingly, recurrent thrombosis tends to occur in the same vascular distribution as the original event. Patients with venous thrombosis generally have recurrent venous events and patients with arterial thrombosis have recurrent arterial events [36–38].

13.4 Pregnancy and APS

In a general obstetric population, the prevalence of LAC was 0.3% and the prevalence of ACLA was 2.2–9.1%, which was similar to that observed among patients who were not pregnant (5.6%) [39]. In comparison, the prevalence of

13 Antiphospholipid Antibody Syndrome

APLA appears to be higher, in the range of 4–21%, among patients presenting with thrombosis [17, 18]. Thrombosis is presumed to cause many of the pregnancy complications associated with APS. In women without SLE, a retrospective review of more than 13,000 patients found a prevalence of APLA of 20% among women with recurrent fetal loss compared with 5% in healthy women [40]. The association between APLA and fetal loss is strongest for loss occurring after 10 weeks [41]. The association between APLA and the risk of premature birth due to eclampsia or preeclampsia and intrauterine growth restriction remains controversial; studies contributing data to this area tend to be small, retrospective, and have conflicting results [42, 43].

13.5 Therapeutic Approaches

A venous thromboembolic event is often the initial manifestation of APS [26]. Initial treatment should include unfractionated or low molecular weight heparin for at least 4–5 days, overlapped with warfarin administered to achieve an international normalized ratio (INR) of 2.0–3.0 if the baseline INR is not elevated [44]. Management of anticoagulation may be complicated in patients with APLA by artifactual elevation of the INR. This effect is dependent on the type of instrument and thromboplastin that are used to measure the INR and can be avoided in most patients by simply selecting an INR reagent that is insensitive to the effect of APLA [45]. Alternatively, functional factor II or factor X level may be used to monitor the degree of oral-anticoagulant-associated suppression on the coagulation cascade [45].

High-intensity warfarin (INR 3.0–4.0) therapy is not better than moderate-intensity warfarin (INR 2.0–3.0) therapy in preventing recurrent thrombosis [46, 47]. Since the optimal duration of anticoagulation for prevention of recurrent thrombosis in patients with APS is unknown [28], it is also not known whether the absolute risk of recurrence decreases with increasing duration of anticoagulation [37].

Arterial events in APS most commonly involve the cerebral circulation, with stroke being the initial clinical manifestation in 13% of patients with APS and transient ischemic attack being the initial clinical manifestation in 7% of patients with APS [26]. The association between thrombosis, including myocardial infarction, is less well established [48].

The Antiphospholipid Antibodies and Stroke Study [49] is a subanalysis of a randomized, double-bind study [50] in which 1,770 patients with APLA were included. In this prospective cohort study, use of warfarin (INR 1.4–2.8) and aspirin (325 mg/day) was compared in the secondary prevention of stroke. Interestingly, there was no difference in the risk of thrombosis, death, or bleeding in patients treated with warfarin compared with aspirine-treated patients. Furthermore, the presence of either LAC or ACLA was not predictive of recurrent thrombotic events at 2 years. Warfarin and aspirin appeared to be equivalent for the prevention of thromboembolic complications in these patients. Thus, patients with a first ischemic stroke and a single positive APLA test result who do not have another indication for anticoagulation may be treated with aspirin (325 mg/day) or moderate-intensity warfarin (INR 1.4–2.8) [51], although aspirin is likely to be preferred for reason of simplicity. Combination of antiplatelet and anticoagulation therapy has been proposed as more effective than single antiplatelet therapy for secondary prevention in ischemic stroke patients with APS [52].

There are no adequate studies on the treatment of patients who are incidentally found to have APLA and have no previous thrombosis, except the case of patients with SLE. Consensus opinion suggests no treatment or a low dose of aspirin (81 mg/day) for asymptomatic, nonpregnant patients [53]. In these patients, use of warfarin or aspirin does not appear to be indicated because of the risk of bleeding [54, 55].

References

1. Wassermann A, Neisser A, Bruck C (1906) Eine serodiagnostische reaction bei Syphilis. Dtsch Med Wochenschr 32:745–746
2. Matsuura E, Igasrashi Y, Fujimoto M et al (1992) Heterogeneity of anticardiolipin antobodies defined by anticardiolipin cofactor. J Immunol 144:3885–3891
3. Forestiero RR, Martinuzzo ME, Kordich LC, Carreras LO (1996) Reactivity to β_2-glycoprotein I clearly differentiates anticardiolipin antibodies from anti-phospholipid syndrome and syphilis. Thromb Haemost 75:717–720
4. Triplett DA (2002) Antiphospholipid antibodies. Arch Pathol Lab Med 126:1424–1429
5. Brandt JT, Triplett DA, Alving B, Scharrer I (1995) Criteria for the diagnosis of lupus anticoagulants: an update. Thromb Haemost 74:1185–1190
6. Tripodi A, Chantarangkul V, Clerici M et al (2002) Laboratory diagnosis of lupus anticoagulant treatment. Performance of dilute Russell viper venom test and silica clotting time in comparison with Staclot LA. Thromb Haemost 88:583–586
7. Harris EN, Pierangeli SS (2002) Revisiting the anticardiolipin test and its standardization. Lupus 11:269–275
8. Harris EN (1990) Special report: the second international anti-cardiolipin standardization workshop/the Kingston Anti-Phospholipid Antibody Study (KAPS) group. Am J Clin Pathol 94:476–484
9. Long AA, Ginsberg JS, Brill-Edwards P et al (1991) The relationship of antiphospholipid antibodies to thromboembolic disease in systemic lupus erythematosus: a cross-sectional study. Thromb Haemost 66:520–524
10. Galli M, Luciani D, Bertolini G, Barbui T (2003) Anti-beta 2-glycoprotein I, antiprothrombin antibodies, and the risk of thrombosis in the antiphospholipid syndrome. Blood 102:2717–2723
11. de Groot PG, Horbach DA, Simmelink MJ et al (1998) Anti-prothrombin antibodies and their ralation with thrombosis and lupus anticoagulant. Lupus 7(Suppl 2):S32–S36
12. Satoh A, Suzuki K, Takayama E et al (1999) Detection of anti-annexin IV and V antibodies in patients with antiphospholipid syndrome and systemic lupus erythematosus. J Rheumatol 26:1715–1720
13. de Groot PG, Derksen RH (2005) Pathophysiology of the antiphospholipid syndrome. J Thromb Haemost 3:1854–1860
14. Hemker HC, Dieri RA, De Smedt E, Béguin S (2006) Thrombin generation, a function test of the haemostatic-thrombotic system. Thromb Haemost 96:553–561
15. Membre A, Wahl D, Latger-Cannard V et al (2008) The effect of platelet activation on the hypercoagulability induced by murine monoclonal antiphospholipid antibodies. Haematologica 93:566–573

13 Antiphospholipid Antibody Syndrome 215

16. Vila P, Hernandez MC, Lopez-Fernandez MF et al (1994) Prevalence, follow-up and clinical significance of the anticardiolipin antibodies in normal subjects. Thromb Haemost 72:209–213
17. Ginsberg JS, Wells PS, Brill-Edwards P et al (1995) Antiphospholipid antibodies and venous thromboembolism. Blood 86:3685–3691
18. Mateo J, Oliver A, Borrell M et al (1997) Laboratory evaluation and clinical characteristic of 2,132 consecutive unselected patients with venous thromboembolism: results of the Spanish multicentric study on thrombophilia (EMET-study). Thromb Haemost 77:444–451
19. Galli M, Luciani D, Bertolini G et al (2003) Lupus anticoagulants are stronger risk factor for thrombosis than anticardiolipin antibodies in the antiphospholipid syndrome: a systematic review of the literature. Blood 101:1827–1832
20. Wilson WA, Gharavi AE, Koike T et al (1999) International consensus statement on preliminary classification criteria for definite antiphospholipid syndrome: report of an international workshop. Arthritis Rheum 42:1309–1311
21. Miyakis S, Lockshin MD, Atsumi T et al (2006) International consensus statement on an update of the classification criteria for definite antiphospholipid syndrome (APS). J Thromb Haemost 4:295–306
22. Tincani A, Allegri F, Sanmarco M et al (2001) Anticardiolipin antibody assay: a methodological analysis for a better consensus in routine determinations: a cooperative project of the European antiphospholipid forum. Thromb Haemost 86:575–583
23. Brandt JT, Barna LK, Triplett DA (1995) Laboratory identification of lupus anticoagulants: results of the second international workshop for identification of lupus anticoagulants. Thromb Haemost 74:1597–1603
24. Asherson RA (1992) The catastrophic antiphospholipid syndrome. J Rheumatol 19:508–512
25. Bucciarelli S, Espinosa G, Cervera R et al (2006) For the CAPS registry project group (european forum on antiphospholipid antibodies): mortality in the catastrophic antiphospholipid syndrome: causes of death and prognostic factors in a series of 250 patients. Arthritis Rheum 54:2568–2576
26. Cervera R, Piette JC, Font J et al (2002) Antiphospholipid syndrome: clinical and immunologic manifestations and patterns of disease expression in a cohort of 1,000 patients. Arthritis Rheum 46:1019–1027
27. Asherson RA, Cervera R, Piette JC et al (1998) Catastrophic antiphospholipid syndrome: clinical and laboratory features of 50 patients. Medicine (Baltimore) 77:195–207
28. Dentali F, Crowther M (2010) Antiphospholipid antibodies in critical illness. Crit Care Med 38(Suppl 2):S51–S56
29. Kitchens CS (1998) Thrombotic storm: when thrombosis begets thrombosis. Am J Med 104:381–385
30. Meroni PL (2008) Pathogenesis of the antiphospholipid syndrome: an additional example of the mosaic of the autoimmunity. J Autoimmun 30:99–103
31. Espinosa G, Cervera R (2009) Morbidity and mortality in the antiphosholipid syndrome. Curr Opin Pulm Med 15:413–417
32. Hudson M, Herr AL, Rauch J et al (2003) The presence of multiple prothrombotic risk factors is associated with a higher risk of thrombosis in individuals with anticardiolipin antibodies. J Rheumatol 30:2385–2391
33. Schulman S, Svenungsson E, Granqvist S (1998) Duration of Anticoagulation Study Group: anticardiolipin antibodies predict early recurrence of thromboembolism and death among patients with venous thromboembolism following anticoagulant therapy. Am J Med 104:332–338
34. Kearon C, Gent M, Hirsh J et al (1999) A comparison of three month of anticoagulation with extended anticoagulation for a first episode of idiopathic venous thromboembolism. N Engl J Med 340:901–907
35. Kearon C, Ginsberg JS, Kovacs MJ et al (2003) Comparison of low-intensity warfarin therapy for long-term prevention of recurrent venous thromboembolism. N Engl J Med 349:631–639

36. Rosove MH, Brewer PM (1992) Antiphospholipid thrombosis: clinical course after the first thrombotic event in 70 patients. Ann Intern Med 117:303–308
37. Khamashta MA, Cuadrato MJ, Mujic F et al (1995) The management of thrombosis in the antiphospholipid-antibody syndrome. N Engl J Med 332:993–997
38. Finazzi G, Brancaccio V, Moia M et al (1996) Natural history and risk factors for thrombosis in 360 patients with antiphospholipid antibodies: a four years prospective study from the Italian Registry. Am J Med 100:530–536
39. Tsapanos V, Kanellopoulos N, Cardamakis E et al (2000) Anticardiolipin antibodies level in healthy pregnant and non-pregnant women. Arch Gynecol Obstet 263:111–115
40. Oshiro BT, Silver RM, Scott JR et al (1996) Antiphospholipid antibodies and fetal death. Obstet Gynecol 87:489–493
41. Rai RS, Clifford K, Cohen H et al (1995) High prospective fetal loss rate in untreated pregnancies of women with recurrent miscarriage and antiphospholipid antibodies. Hum Reprod 10:3301–3304
42. Branch DW, Silver RM, Blackwell JL, Reading JC, Scott JR (1992) Outcome of treated pregnancies in women with antiphospholipid syndrome: an update of the Utah experience. Obstet Gynecol 80:614–620
43. Out HJ, Bruinse HW, Christiens GC et al (1992) A prospective, controlled, multicenter study on the obstetric risk in pregnant women with antiphospholipid antibodies. Am J Obstet Gynecol 167:26–32
44. Buller HR, Agnelli G, Hull RD et al (2004) Antithrombotic therapy for venous thromboembolic disease: the seventh ACCP conference on antithrombotic and thrombolitic therapy. Chest 126:401S–428S
45. Garcia DA, Khamashta MA, Crowther MA (2007) How we diagnose and treat thrombotic manifestations of the antiphospholipid syndrome: a case-based review. Blood 110:3122–3127
46. Crowther MA, Ginsberg JS, Julian J et al (2003) A comparison of two intensities of warfarin for the prevention of recurrent thrombosis in patients with the antiphospholipid antibody syndrome. N Engl J Med 349:1133–1138
47. Finazzi G, Marchioli R, Brancaccio V et al (2005) A randomized clinical trial of high-intensity warfarin vs conventional antithrombotic therapy for the prevention of recurrent thrombosis in patients with the antiphospholipid syndrome (WAPS). J Thromb Haemost 3:848–853
48. Tenedios F, Erkan D, Lockshin MD (2005) Cardiac involvement in the antiphospholipid syndrome. Lupus 14:691–696
49. The APASS Writing Committee (2004) Antiphospholipid antibodies and subsequent thrombo-occlusive events in patients with ischemic stroke. JAMA 2004 291:576–584
50. Mohr JP, Thompson JL, Lazar RM et al (2001) A comparison of warfarin and aspirin for the prevention of recurrent ischemic stroke. N Engl J Med 345:1444–1451
51. Brey RL, Chapman J, Levin SR et al (2003) Stroke and antiphospholipid syndrome: consensus meeting Taormina 2002. Lupus 12:508–513
52. Okuma H, Kitagawa Y, Yasuda T et al (2009) Comparison between single antiplatelet therapy and combination of antiplatelet and anticoagulation therapy for secondary prevention in ischemic stroke patients with antiphospholipid syndrome. Int J Med Sci 7:15–18
53. Alagorn-Segovia D, Boffa MC, Branch W et al (2003) Prophylaxis of the antiphospholipid syndrome: a consensus report. Lupus 12:499–503
54. Erkan D, Harrison MJ, Levi R et al (2007) Aspirin for primary thrombosis prevention in the antiphospholipid syndrome: a randomized, double-bind, placebo-controlled trial in asymptomatic antiphospholipid antibody-positive individuals. Arthritis Rheum 56: 2382–2391
55. Vivaldi P, Rossetti G, Galli M, Finazzi G (1997) Severe bleeding due to acquired hypoprothrombinemia-lupus anticoagulant syndrome. Case report and review of literature. Haematologica 82:345–347

Pulmonary-Renal Syndrome

14

Marco Zambon, Davide Cappelli and Giorgio Berlot

14.1 Introduction

Pulmonary-renal syndrome is defined as the combination of diffuse alveolar haemorrhage (DAH) and glomerulonephritis [1, 2]. This syndrome is sustained by several immunologic as well as non immunologic mechanisms [3–5]. Small vessels vasculitis, characterized by a destructive inflammatory process that involves arterioles, venules and alveolar capillaries is believed to be the initial lesion in most of cases. These lesions disrupt perfusion and the continuity of the pulmonary wall, allowing blood to leak into the alveolar space [6]. Typical manifestations include a combination of diffuse alveolar infiltrate, haemoptysis (not always present), and a drop in haematocrit and/or haemoglobin level. Pathologically, aspects of capillaritis, bland haemorrhage, or diffuse alveolar damage with haemorrhage are often found. In pulmonary-renal syndrome, kidneys are usually affected by a focal proliferative glomerulonephritis [7], microscopically characterized by fibrinoid necrosis, microvascular thrombi and extensive crescent formation. At the contrary, necrotizing granulomas and small-vessel vasculitis are rare findings. The presence of interstitial infiltration, fibrosis and tubular atrophy are considered poor prognostic factors. Furthermore, the differentiation among anti-GBM disease (linear deposition of IgG), lupus and post-infectious glomerulonephritis (granular deposition of immunoglobulins and complement), and necrotic vasculitis (immune glomerulonephritis) is mostly achieved by means of immunofluorescence [8, 9].

M. Zambon (✉)
Anesthesia and Intensive Care, Cattinara Hospital, University of Trieste, Trieste, Italy
e-mail: Marco.zambon@gmail.com

G. Berlot (ed.), *Hemocoagulative Problems in the Critically Ill Patient*,
DOI: 10.1007/978-88-470-2448-9_14, © Springer-Verlag Italia 2012

217

14.2 Clinical Presentations of the Pulmonary-Renal Syndrome

The majority of pulmonary-renal syndromes are characterized by the presence of circulating anti-cytoplasmic neutrophil antibodies (ANCA). Although these antibodies are not specific of a single pathology, they are valuable in the differential diagnosis among the three major systemic vasculitis: Wegener's granulomatosis, microscopic polyangiitis and Churg–Strauss syndrome [10].

(a) Wegener's Granulomatosis

Wegener Granulomatosis (WG) is the most common ANCA-associated vasculitis, with an incidence of up to 8.5/million with a male-to-female ratio of 1:1. Although persons of any age and race may be affected, it is most common in 40–55-year aging Caucasians [11]. Clinically, WG is characterized by the upper airways involvement (e.g., sinusitis, otitis, ulcerations, bony deformities, and subglottic or bronchial stenosis), lower respiratory tract involvement (e.g., cough, chest pain, shortness of breath, and haemoptysis), and glomerulonephritis. However, at the onset of the disease, only as few as 40% of patients present with renal impairment; this ratio rise up to 90% in the course of the disease [12–14]. Ocular involvement, skin and musculoskeletal disease are also relatively common. Patients may present with alveolar, mixed, or interstitial infiltrates, nodular disease, or cavitary disease on the chest radiography [15, 16], to a higher frequency as compared to the other vasculitides. Microscopically, WG is characterized by small-vessel and medium-vessel necrotizing vasculitis and granulomatous inflammation [17, 18].

(b) Churg–Strauss Syndrome

Churg–Strauss syndrome (CSS) is a complex multi-organ disease characterized by upper and lower respiratory tract involvement, blood and tissue eosinophilia, and vasculitis. Altogether, this is a rare disease, with an incidence of 0.5–6.8 per million persons per year and a prevalence of 10.7–13 per million inhabitants [19, 20]. CSS affects all ages, but mainly adults of 30–60 years, without a significant difference between sexes [21, 22]. Today, the most widely accepted criteria for CSS diagnosis are those proposed by the American College of Rheumatology (ACR) in 1990, which include asthma, eosinophilia > 10%, sinusitis, pulmonary infiltrate, histological proof of vasculitis, and multiple mononeuritis. The presence of four out of six of these criteria simultaneously or over time is necessary to establish the diagnosis of CSS [23]. Generally, CSS enters in the differential diagnosis with other eosinophilic lung disease (i.e., chronic eosinophilic pneumonia, allergic bronchopulmonary mycosis, drug reactions, hypereosinophilic syndrome, and asthma/atopic disease), or in patients with asthma/atopy who develop significant GI disease (i.e., perforation, ischemia, and bleeding) or cardiac disease (i.e., conduction abnormalities, systolic dysfunction, or diastolic dysfunction). As mentioned above, the syndrome is characterized by its own triad of asthma, hypereosinophilia, and necrotizing vasculitis. While also pulmonary haemorrhage and glomerulonephritis may occur, they are much less common than in the other small-vessel vasculitides [24–27]. Cardiac complications (causing up to 50%

of CSS-related death), GI complications, or status asthmaticus and respiratory failure [24, 25, 28] often lead to morbidity and mortality. The most specific histological change is a particular pattern of granuloma, which is characterized by an eosinophilic core of necrosis with fibrinoid collagen degeneration surrounded by a granulomatous infiltrate composed by histiocytes, lymphocytes, and giant cells. This granuloma, which was formerly thought to be typical of the CSS (the "Churg–Strauss granuloma") was then described also in Wegener's granulomatosis, systemic lupus erythematosus, rheumatoid arthritis, lymphoproliferative disorders, and other inflammatory and infectious diseases [29]. Over the last several years, a number of case reports and case series [30, 31] have suggested an association between the use of leukotriene inhibitors (LI) and CSS, leading to different pathogenetic hypotheses: (a) the reduction of the steroids permitted by the use of LI unmasks previously an unrecognized CSS; or (b) LI by themselves promote the biological conversion of severe asthma/atopic disease toward CSS [32]. More recently, the analysis of post-marketing surveillance data and a number of patient cohorts offer no compelling evidence of a pathogenetic role for LI in the development of CSS, but rather support the "unmasking hypothesis" [33–36].

(c) Microscopic polyangiitis.

Microscopic polyangiitis (MPA), which mostly affects elderly people, is a systemic disease characterized by vasculitis involving small blood vessels, particularly the glomerular and pulmonary capillaries, and serologically by the presence of ANCA) [37–39]. MPA is clinically characterized by a multisystemic disease such as rapidly progressive glomerulonephritis (RPGN), alveolar haemorrhage, mononeuritis, and skin involvement. RPGN and pulmonary haemorrhage may be life-threatening. RPGN is essentially universal in MPA, whereas pulmonary involvement occurs in only a minority of patients (10–30%) [40–42]. In those patients who do develop lung involvement, DAH and capillaritis are the most common manifestation [42]. Joint, skin, peripheral nervous system, and GI involvement are also relatively common [41]. Pathologically, a focal, segmented necrotizing vasculitis and a mixed inflammatory infiltrate without granulomas are seen in various sites of vessels including arteries, arterioles, capillaries, and venules. The severity of the injury requires immediate treatment with immunosuppressive drugs including cyclophosphamide and corticosteroids. Many conditions (connective tissue disease, infection, malignancy, drug toxicity, sarcoidosis, and interstitial lung disease) may mimic the presentation of vasculitides. Chronic infections can be particularly misleading as they may cause both a positive ANCA response and a leukocytoclastic vasculitis, and therefore needs to be ruled out before being treated with aggressive immunosuppressive therapy which is indicated for MPA. In particular, any possible drug capable of induce vasculitis should be carefully ruled out. The laboratory testing is crucial to identify hematologic, renal, hepatic, and metabolic abnormalities. An initial screen should include: antinuclear antibodies, rheumatoid factor; testing for antiphospholipid antibodies, cryoglobulinemia, hepatitis B and C infection. These are then completed with the enzyme-linked immunosorbent assay (ELISA) for ANCAs, anti-PR3 and anti-myeloperoxidase (MPO) (see later) [43].

14.3 The Role of ANCA and Anti-Plasminogen Antibodies

As stated above, he ANCA-associated vasculitides (AAV) include WG, the MPA and the CSS [44]. To date, although the close association between AAV and ANCA suggests that they are involved in the pathogenesis of these diseases, clinical data support, but do not prove definitely, this cause-effect relationship [45]. According to the staining patterns, cytoplasmic ANCA (c-ANCA and perinuclear ANCA (p-ANCA) have been described. c-ANCAs have since been shown to primarily recognize the enzyme PR3, and their presence often suggest a diagnosis of WG, whereas p-ANCAs have been shown to interact with a number of distinct antigens, but most commonly MPO. Accordingly, specific ELISAs have been developed to determine the presence of anti-PR3 and anti-MPO antibodies. As with any test, the predictive value of these assays is based on the prevalence of disease in patient population tested, and the sensitivity and specificity of the test. Conventionally, c-ANCAs and anti-PR3 ELISA are said to have an 85–90% sensitivity and 95% specificity for generalized active WG with lower sensitivity for limited disease (approximately 60%) and disease in remission (approximately 40%) [46–52]. Conversely, p-ANCA or anti-MPO testing is less sensitive, with values of approximately 35–75% for MPA and 35–50% for CSS [49, 52–56]. False-positive testing may occur with other systemic autoimmune diseases (i.e. rheumatoid arthritis and systemic lupus erythematosus), inflammatory bowel diseases, subacute bacterial endocarditis, and other infections. It should be remembered that if these tests are not applied selectively to high-risk patient populations, their positive predictive value declines, as demonstrated by Mandl et al. [57]. As anticipated above, the combination of ANCA testing plus the use of ELISAs maximizes sensitivity in identifying patients with ANCA-associated vasculitis [49, 53, 57–59]. Then, a definitive diagnosis ultimately must be based on the accumulated data and not on ANCA/PR3/MPO testing alone. In conclusion, in the right clinical context, sensitivity and specificity of PR3-ANCA and MPO-ANCA for the AAVs are extremely high, with the possible exception of CSS [44]. In CSS, however, a primarily vasculitic disease pattern is strongly associated with MPO-ANCA, whereas a disease presentation dominated by eosinophilic tissue infiltration generally is ANCA negative [60].

Approximately 25% of AAV patients produce also anti-plasminogen antibodies [61]. These antibodies are directed against a protease, and their presence is associated with the occurrence of venous thromboembolic events (VTEs), suggesting functional interference with coagulation and/or fibrinolysis [62]. The relationship between anti-plasminogen antibodies and coagulation may also be directly relevant to glomerular injury and the evolution of fibrinoid necrosis, a hallmark lesion of AAV. In AAV, vascular injury is mediated by ANCA-induced neutrophil and monocyte activation [63] and characterized by the influx of inflammatory cells with fibrinoid necrosis affecting glomeruli and occasionally small arteries. Actually, it is possible that fibrinoid necrosis represents an aberrant repair mechanism that follow vascular injury. A recent study [61] investigated the

14 Pulmonary-Renal Syndrome

presence of anti-plasminogen antibodies in patients with AAV. The prevalence of anti-plasminogen antibodies was 24.1% in MPO-ANCA- and 24.4% in PR3-ANCA-positive patients. It was found that Anti-Plasminogen Antibodies compromise the fibrinolysis, extending his time to 50%; furthermore, there was identified an increased incidence of thromboembolic events in patients carrying these antibodies and the occurrence of anti-plasminogen antibody was associated with higher percentages of glomeruli with fibrinoid necrosis and cellular crescents, accompanied by more severely reduced renal function.

14.4 Treatment

In the earlier reports certain forms of vasculitis were uniformly fatal without therapy. For instance, several studies demonstrated that both WG and MPA, if left untreated, were fatal within weeks to months, especially among patients who presented with pulmonary-renal syndromes, gastrointestinal ischemia, or central nervous system involvement [64]. In the 1970–1980s, the outcome improved with the use of cyclophosphamide (CyP), methotrexate (MTX) and corticosteroids (CS). Nowadays, although the therapeutic options have greatly expanded, clinicians still face difficult treatment decisions when patients in remission are unable to tolerate or have contraindications to maintenance agents. The current therapy for the vasculitides relies on aggressive immunosuppression with a relevant potential of severe toxicity. Consequently, an accurate staging of disease severity is mandatory. With this aim, the European Vasculitis Study Group (EUVAS) developed a clinically useful grading system in which the patient's disease is categorized in limited, early generalized, active generalized, severe and refractory [43]. Limited disease refers to localized disease of the upper airways, without systemic symptoms, renal involvement and other target organ dysfunction. As such, therapy can often be limited to a single agent such as CS, azathioprine, or MTX. Early generalized disease is distinguished from active generalized disease according to the presence of organ dysfunction. The use of CYP associated with CS remains the first-line therapy for both classes of severity. Recently, the MTX versus CyP for "early systemic disease" trial, along with smaller studies [65–67], have reported MTX as equally effective as CyP in the induction of disease remission in patients with early generalized disease. Thus, both agents now represent acceptable first-line therapy for this group of patients and, due to the more favourable side-effect profile of MTX as compared to CyP, therapy with MTX plus CS seems preferable. No evidence supports that pulsed iv CyP may be as effective as oral CyP, which on the other hand presents fewer side effects [68]. The presence of severe renal involvement (creatinine concentration > 5.7 mg/dl), DAH, or other life-threatening disease defines the disease as severe. Although the management of patients with such grade had previously been the subject of some debate, recent studies [69, 70] have suggested that such patients should receive a combination therapy consisting of CyP, CS, and plasma exchange (PLEX). The addition of PLEX to the standard CyP plus CS regimen has been shown to be superior to high dose, pulsed IV CS in restoring renal function in patients with severe renal impairment [69, 70]. This strategy also appears to be effective for the treatment of DAH [70]. Additional therapies for patients with DAH may include activated human factor VII, which has been used to induce haemostasis with success [71, 72]. Extracorporeal membrane oxygenation (ECMO) has also been used to "buy time" in patients with severe DAH until other interventions have had a chance to work, although its use in adults remains controversial [73]. The term "refractory disease" addresses those patients no responders to cytotoxic agents, high-dose CS, or PE. The use of novel agents must be considered for patients in this class. Agents such as infliximab, rituximab, and antithymocyte globulin have all been suggested for the treatment of refractory vasculitis. Similarly, iv immunoglobulins (IvIg) have also been used in refractory vasculitis and represents another potential alternative. Among the new agents mentioned, rituximab has recently been investigated in the remission induction therapy for severe AAV.

Two randomized, controlled trials (RAVE "rituximab in ANCA-associated vasculitis" trial and RITUXVAS "randomized trial of rituximab versus cyclophosphamide in ANCA-associated vasculitis" trial) [74] examined the efficacy and safety of rituximab in AAV, as compared with CyP, the standard therapy for remission induction in these immune-mediated diseases. At present, there is concern in both trials in view of the complications observed among patients with exposure to rituximab; the high rates of adverse events detected over a relatively short treatment period warrant long-term safety studies of rituximab in vasculitides.

Current PLEX methodology involves (a) the filtration or centrifugation of blood to separate plasma from other blood constituents and (b) its replacement with colloids and/or albumin. The rationale of PLEX is that removal of large molecular weight substances will reduce further damage and possibly the reversal of the pathologic process. The ability of PLEX to remove autoantibodies, circulating immune complexes, adhesion molecules, cytokines, chemokines and other soluble mediators implicated in the development of tissue damage, has been demonstrated effective in the management of refractory systemic autoimmune diseases [75]. However, PLEX is a non-selective process that can also remove useful substances, such as coagulation factors and albumin. More selective technologies including double filtration apheresis and immunoadsorption are potentially safer and do not require large volumes of blood product replacement. PLEX is commonly associated with mild adverse events, especially electrolyte disturbance such as hypocalcaemia; the most serious adverse events secondary to PLEX are anaphylaxis, haemorrhage and transfusion-related lung injury (TRALI).

An association of PLEX with improved renal function in patients with WG presenting with creatinine above 250 μmol/l (2.9 mg/dl) is reported [76], without significant effect on mortality or relapse rates. There are no randomized controlled trials assessing PLEX in a pure MPA cohort or in renal limited vasculitis alone. Several recent case reports of MPA found prompt induction of remission with

PLEX and immunosuppression [77, 78]. A randomized controlled trial [79] from the mid-1990s found no effect of PLEX.

14.5 Conclusions

The pulmonary renal syndrome indicates how strong are the relationship between inflammation, immunology, coagulation and the occurrence of end-organ damage. As their symptoms can be elusive and non specific, they represent a challenge to the physician. The treatment includes the association of different drugs, each of them with a potential array of harmful side effects and possibly the use of plasma exchange.

References

1. Gallagher H, Kwan J, Jayne RW (2002) Pulmonary renal syndrome: a 4-years, single center experience. Am J Kidney Dis 38:42–47
2. Goodpasture EW (1919) The significance of certain pulmonary lesions to the etiology of pneumonia. Am J Med Sci 158:863–870
3. Collard HR, Schwarz MI (2004) Diffuse alveolar hemorrhage. Clin Chest Med 24:583–592
4. Wiik A (2003) Autoantibodies in vasculitis. Arthritis Res Ther 5:147–152
5. Langford C, Balow JE (2003) New insights into the immunopathogenesis and treatment of small vessel vasculitis of the kidney. Curr Opin Nephrol Hypertens 12:267–272
6. Davies DJ (2005) Small vessel vasculitis. Cardiovasc Pathol 14:335–346
7. Erlich JH, Sevastos J, Pussel B (2004) Goodpasture's disease: antiglomerular basement membrane disease. Nephrology 9:49–51
8. Lau K, Wyatt R (2005) Glomerulonephritis. Adolesc Med 16:67–85
9. Contreras G, Pardo V, Leclercq B et al (2004) Sequential therapies for proliferative lupus nephritis. N Engl J Med 350:971–980
10. Csernok E (2003) Anti-neutrophil cytoplasmic antibodies and pathogenesis of small vessel vasculitides. Autoimmun Rev 2:158–164
11. Langford C, Hoffman G (1999) Wegener's granulomatosis. Thorax 54:629–637
12. Anderson G, Coles ET, Crane M et al (1992) Wegener's granulomatosis: a series of 265 British cases seen between 1975 and 1985: a report by a sub-committee of the British Thoracic Society Research Committee. Q J Med 83:427–438
13. Fauci AS, Haynes BF, Katz P et al (1983) Wegener's granulomatosis: prospective clinical and therapeutic experience with 85 patients for 21 years. Ann Intern Med 98:76–85
14. Hoffman GS, Kerr GS, Leavitt RY et al (1992) Wgener's granulomatosis: an analysis of 158 patients. Ann Intern Med 116:448–498
15. Cordier J-F, Valeyre D, Guillevin L et al (1990) Pulmonary Wegener's granulomatosis: a clinical and imaging study of 77 cases. Chest 97:906–912
16. Reuter M, Schnabel A, Wesner F et al (1998) Pulmonary Wegener's granulomatosis: correlation between high-resolution CT findings and clinical scoring of disease activity. Chest 114:500–506
17. Travis WD, Hoffman GS, Leavitt RY et al (1991) Surgical pathology of the lung in Wegener's granulomatosis. Am J Surg Pathol 15:315–333
18. Lie JT (1990) Illustrated histopathologic classification criteria for selected vasculitic syndromes. Arthritis Rheum 33:1074–1087

19. Watts RA, Lane S, Scott DG (2005) What is known about the epidemiology of the vasculitides? Best Pract Res Clin Rheumatol 19:191–207
20. Mahr A, Guillevin L, Poissonnet M, Aymè S (2004) Prevalence of polyarteritis nodosa, microscopic polyangiitis, Wegener's granulomatosis, and Churg–Strauss syndrome in a French urban multiethnic population in 2000: a capture-recapture estimate. Arthritis Rheum 51:92–99
21. Della Rossa A, Baldini C, Tavoni A et al (2002) Churg–Strauss syndrome: clinical and serological features of 19 patients from a single Italian centre. Rheumatology (Oxford) 41:1286–1294
22. Pagnoux C, Guilpain P, Guilliven L (2007) Churg–Strauss syndrome. Curr Opin Rheumatol 19:25–32
23. Masi AT, Hunder GG, Lie JT et al (1990) The American college of rheumatology 1990 criteria for the classification of Churg-Srauss syndrome. Arthritis Rheum 33:1094–1100
24. Guillevin L, Cohen P, Gayraud M et al (1999) Churg–Strauss syndrome: a clinical study and long-term follow up of 96 patients. Medicine (Baltimore) 78:26–37
25. Guillevin L, Guittard T, Bletry O et al (1987) Systemic necrotizing angiitis with asthma: causes and precipitating factors in 43 cases. Lung 165:165–172
26. Lanham J, Elkon K, Pusey C et al (1984) Systemic vasculitis with asthma and eosinophilia: a clinical approach to the Churg–Strauss syndrome. Medicine (Baltimore) 63:65–81
27. Guillevin L, Houng Du LT et al (1988) Clinical findings and prognosis of polyarteritis nodosa and Churg–Strauss angiitis: a study in 165 patients. Br J Rheumatol 27:258–264
28. Morgan JM, Raposo L, Gibson DG (1989) Cardiac involvement in Churg–Strauss syndrome shown by electrocardiography. Br Heart J 62:462–466
29. Winkelmann R, Dicken CH (1980) The cutaneous necrotizing palisading granuloma (Churg–Strauss granuloma). Major Probl Dermatol 10:242–248
30. Weschler ME, Garpestad E, Flier SR et al (1998) Pulmonary infiltrates, eosinophilia, and cardiomyopathy following corticosteroid withdrawal in patients with asthma receiving zafirlukast. JAMA 279:455–457
31. Weschler ME, Finn D, Gunawardena D et al (2000) Churg–Strauss syndrome in patients receiving montelukast as treatment for asthma. Chest 117:708–713
32. Weller PF, Plaut M, Taggart V et al (2001) The relationship of asthma therapy and Churg–Strauss syndrome: NIH workshop summary report. J Allergy Clin Immunol 108:175–183
33. Jamaleddine G, Diab K, Tabbarah Z et al (2002) Leukotriene antagonists and the Churg–Strauss syndrome. Semin Arthritis Rheum 31:218–227
34. Keogh KA, Specks U (2003) Churg–Strauss syndrome: clinical presentation, antineutrophil cytoplasmatic antibodies, and leukotriene receptor antagonists. Am J Med 115:284–290
35. Coulter D (2000) Pro-active safety surveillance. Pharmacoepidemiol Drug Safe 9:273–280
36. Lilly CM, Churg A, Lazarovich M et al (2002) Asthma therapies and Churg–Strauss syndrome. J Allergy Clin Immunol 109:S1–S19
37. Jennette JC, Falk RJ, Andrassy K et al (1994) Nomenclature of systemic vasculitides: proposal of an international consensus conference. Arthritis Rheum 37:187–192
38. Hoffman GS, Specks U (1998) Antineutrophil cytoplasmic antibodies. Arthritis Rheum 41:1521–1537
39. Guillevin L, Durand-Gasselin B, Cevallos R et al (1998) Microscopic polyangiitis: clinical and laboratory findings in 85. Arthritis Rheum 41:1521–1537
40. Guillevin L, Durand-Gasselin B, Cevallos R et al (1999) Microscopic polyangiitis. Arthritis Rheum 42:421–430
41. Lhote F, Guillevin L (1998) Polyarteritis nodosa, microscopic polyangiitis and Churg–Strauss syndrome. Semin Respir Crit Care Med 19:27–45
42. Akikusa B, Sato T, Ogawa M et al (1997) Necrotizing alveolar capillaritis in autopsy cases of microscopic polyangiitis: incidence, histopathogenesis and relationship with systemic vasculitis. Arch Pathol Lab Med 121:144–149

14 Pulmonary-Renal Syndrome 225

43. Frankel SK, Cosgrove GP, Fischer A et al (2006) Update in the diagnosis and management of pulmonary vasculitis. Chest 129:452–465
44. Kallenberg CG, Heeringa P, Stegeman CA (2006) Mechanism of disease: pathogenesis and treatment of ANCA-associated vasculitides. Nat Clin Pract Rheumatol 2:661–670
45. Kallenberg CG (2010) Pathophysiology of ANCA-associated small vessel vasculitis. Curr Rheumatol Rep 12:399–405
46. Cohen-Tervaert JW, van der Woude FJ, Fauci AS et al (1989) Association between active Wegener's granulomatosis and anticytoplasmic antibodies. Arch Intern Med 149:2461–2465
47. Cohen P, Guillevin L, Baril L et al (1995) Persistence of antineutrophil cytoplasmic antibodies (ANCA) in asymptomatic patients with systemic polyarteritis nodosa or Churg–Strauss syndrome: follow up of 53 patients. Clin Exp Rheumatol 13:193–198
48. Gross WL (1995) Antineutrophil cytoplasmic autoantibody testing in vasculitides. Rheum Dis Clin North Am 21:987–1011
49. Hagen EC, Daha MR, Hermans J et al (1998) Diagnostic value of standardized assays for anti-neutrophil cytoplasmic antibodies in idiopathic systemic vasculitis: EC/BCR project for ANCA assay standardization. Kidney Int 53:743–753
50. Gaskin G, Savage CO, Ryan JJ et al (1991) Anti-neutrophil cytoplasmic antibodies and disease activity during long-term of 70 patients with systemic vasculitis. Nephrol Dial Transplant 6:689–694
51. Noille B, Specks U, Ludemann J et al (1989) Anticytoplasmic autoantibodies: their immunodiagnostic value in Wegener granulomatosis. Ann Intern Med 111:28–40
52. Schonermarck U, Lamprecht P, Csernok E et al (2001) Prevalence and spectrum of rheumatic disease associated with proteinase-3-antineutrophil cytoplasmic antibodies (ANCA) and myeloperoxidase-ANCA. Rheumatology (Oxford) 40:178–184
53. Choi HK, Liu S, Merkel PA et al (2001) Diagnostic performance of antineutrophil cytoplasmic antibody tests for idiopathic vasculitides: metaanalysis with a focus on myeloperoxidase antibodies. J Rheumatol 28:1584–1590
54. Cohen Tervaert JW, Goldschmeding R, Elema JD et al (1990) Association of autoantibodies to myeloperoxidase with different form of vasculitis. Arthritis Rheum 33:1264–1272
55. Cohen Tervaert JW, Goldschmeding R, Elema JD et al (1991) Antimyeloperoxidase antibodies in the Churg–Strauss syndrome. Thorax 46:70–71
56. Ara J, Mirapeix E, Rodriguez R et al (1999) Relationship between ANCA and disease activity in small vessel vasculitis patients with anti-MPO ANCA. Nephrol Dial Transplant 14:1667–1672
57. Mandl LA, Solomon DH, Smith EL et al (2002) Using antineutrophil cytoplasmic antibody testing to diagnose vasculitis. Arch Int Med 162:1509–1514
58. Russell KA, Wiegert E, Schroeder ER et al (2002) Detection anti-neutrophil cytoplasmic antibodies under actual clinical testing conditions. Clin Immunol 103:196–203
59. Csernok E, Holle J, Hellmich B et al (2004) Evaluation of capture ELISA for detection of antineutrophil cytoplasmic antibodies directed against proteinase 3 in Wegener's granulomatosis: first results from a multicentre study. Rheumatology (Oxford) 43:174–180
60. Kallenberg CG (2005) Churg-Srauss syndrome: just one disease entity? Arthritis Rheumatol 52:2589–2593
61. Berden AE, Nolan SL, Morris HL et al (2010) Anti-plasminogen antibodies compromise fibrinolysis and associate with renal histology in ANCA-associated vasculitis. J Am Soc Nephrol 21:2169–2179
62. Bautz DJ, Preston GA, Lionaki S et al (2008) Antibodies with dual reactivity to plasminogen and complementary PR3 in PR3-ANCA vasculitis. J Am Soc Nephrol 19:2421–2429
63. Heeringa P, Tervaert JW (2004) Pathophysiology of ANCA-associated vasculitides: are ANCA really pathogenic? Kidney 65:1564–1567
64. Hoffman GS (2010) Therapeutic interventions for systemic vasculitis. JAMA 304:2413–2414

65. Langford CA, Talar-Williams C, Sneller MC (2000) Use of methotrexate and glucocorticoids in the treatment of Wegener's granulomatosis: long-term renal outcome in patients with glomerulonephritis. Arthritis Rheum 43:1836–1840
66. de Groot K, Muhler M, Reinhold-Keller E et al (1998) Induction of remission in Wegener's granulomatosis with low dose methotrexate. J Rheumatol 25:492–495
67. Stone JH, Tun W, Hellman DB (1999) Treatment of non-life threatening Wegener's granulomatosis with methotrexate and daily prednisone as the initial therapy of choice. J Rheumatol 26:1134–1139
68. Rihova Z, Jancova E, Merta M et al (2004) Daily oral versus pulse intravenous cyclophosphamide in therapy of ANCA-associated preliminary single center experience. Prague Med Rep 105:64–68
69. Frasca GM, Soverini ML, Falaschini A et al (2003) Plasma exchange treatment improves prognosis of antineutrophil cytoplasmic antibody-associated crescentic glomerulonephritis: a case-control study in 26 patients from a single center. Ther Apher Dial 7:540–546
70. Klemmer PJ, Chalermskulrat W, Reif MS et al (2003) Plasmapheresis therapy for diffuse alveolar hemorrhage in patients with small vessel vasculitis. Am J Kidney Dis 42:1149–1153
71. Henke DC, Falk RJ, Gabriel DA (2004) Successful treatment of diffuse alveolar hemorrhage with activated factor VII. Ann Intern Med 140:493–494
72. Betensley AD, Yankaskas JR (2002) Factor VIIA for alveolar hemorrhage in microscopic polyangiitis. Am J Respir Crit Care Med 166:1291–1292
73. Ahmed SH, Aziz T, Cochran J et al (2004) Use of extracorporeal membrane oxygenation in a patient with diffuse alveolar hemorrhage. Chest 126:305–309
74. Jones RB, Cohen Tervaert JW, Hauser T et al (2010) Rituximab versus cyclophosphamide in ANCA-associated renal vasculitis. N Engl J Med 363:211–220
75. Casian A, Jaine D (2011) Plasma exchange in the treatment of Wegener's granulomatosis, microscopic polyangiitis, Churg–Strauss syndrome and renal limited vasculitis. Curr Opin Rheumatol 23:12–17
76. Szpirt WH, Heaf JG, Petersen J (2011) Plasma exchange for induction and cyclosporine A for maintenance of remission in Wegener's granulomatosis: a clinical randomized controlled trial. Nephrol Dial Transpl 26:206–213
77. Isoda K, Nuri K, Shoda T et al (2010) Microscopic polyangiitis complicated with cerebral infarction and hemorrhage: a case report and review in the literature. Nihon Rinsho Meneki Gakkai Kaishi 33:111–115
78. Omori K, Hoshino T, Hiramoto et al (2009) A case of hearing loss and diffuse alveolar hemorrhage associated with microscopic polyangiitis. Nihon Kokyuki Gekkai Zasshi 47:711–716
79. Guillevin L, Lhote F, Cohen P et al (1995) Cortocosteroids plus pulse cyclophosphamide and plasma exchange versus Cortocosteroids plus pulse cyclophosphamide and plasma exchange Churg–Strauss syndrome patients with factors predicting poor diagnosis: a prospective, randomized trial in sixty-two patients Churg–Strauss syndrome patients with factors predicting poor diagnosis: a prospective, randomized trial in sixty-two patients. Arthritis Rheum 38:1638–1645

Coagulation Disorders After Central Nervous System Injury

15

Lara Prisco, Mario Ganau and Giorgio Berlot

15.1 Introduction

Over the past decade new insights in our understanding of coagulation have identified the prominent role of tissue factor (TF) in the pathogenesis of coagulative disorders. As the brain is particularly rich in TF, it appears that any injury to the brain may initiate disturbances in local and systemic coagulation [1].

15.2 Subarachnoid Hemorrhage

Aneurysmal subarachnoid hemorrhage (SAH) is a serious disease with high rates of mortality (approximately 40%) and morbidity and it has an incidence of approximately eight per 100,000 [2]. In patients who survive the initial hours after aneurismal SAH, secondary cerebral ischemia and rebleeding are major causes of death and disability. Secondary cerebral ischemia occurs in approximately 25–35% of patients during the following days. Rebleeding within the first 4 weeks occurs in 40% of patients if the aneurysm is not treated and remains an important cause of death.

The major underlying cause of SAH is the rupture of an intracranial aneurysm due to local vascular structural abnormalities, whereas no direct evidence exists for any deficiency in the coagulation system in its pathogenesis. Immediately after the rupture, the leaked blood interacts with the extravascular matrix, ultimately leading to the activation of the hemostatic system.

L. Prisco (✉)
Anesthesia and Intensive Care, University of Trieste,
Cattinara Hospital, Trieste, Italy
e-mail: priscolara@gmail.com

G. Berlot (ed.), *Hemocoagulative Problems in the Critically Ill Patient*,
DOI: 10.1007/978-88-470-2448-9_15, © Springer-Verlag Italia 2012

15.2.1 Pathophysiology of Coagulative Abnormalities in SAH

In patients with SAH, the activation of coagulation and fibrinolysis correlates with delayed ischemic deficit, clinical status, case fatality, and outcome at 3 months after SAH [3, 4]. The pathogenesis of delayed ischemia remains controversial and may result from several factors, including:

1. Damage to endothelial cells, leading to the decreased production and function of natural anticoagulants and vasodilators [5]
2. The brain-TF-induced activation of coagulation, which translates to clinical manifestations of deep venous thrombosis, pulmonary embolism, and disseminated intravascular coagulation (DIC) [6]
3. The adhesion of activated platelets to the damaged vessel wall and subsequent release of vasoconstrictors, such as serotonin and thromboxane A_2, which further promote platelet aggregation [7, 8]

After rupture of an aneurysm, elevated plasma levels of either markers of thrombin generation (thrombin–antithrombin complex and prothrombin fragments 1 and 2) or particularly D-dimer are associated with a poor outcome [3, 9]. The association of D-dimer level with long-term outcome may be ascribed to the role played by plasmin not only in blood but also during tissue degradation and remodeling. It has been suggested that routine D-dimer monitoring is valuable to assess the severity of SAH, especially in patients who are sedated and intubated after SAH [10].

Following the contact between the blood that escaped from the ruptured aneurysm and TF, the pericytes provide an appropriate membrane surface for the assembly of the functional prothrombinase complex. These local effects lead to a rapid burst of thrombin and subsequent activation of fibrinolysis, which are easily measurable even in the systemic circulation. Endothelial cell damage and platelet attachment further promote the activation of coagulation. Postoperatively, correlations of hemostatic variables with clinical status are less marked, probably owing to the confounding effect of surgical stress or intervention on the hemostatic and fibrinolytic systems.

Alterations of the coagulation factors may be involved in aneurysmal SAH and its subsequent complications, but their role is far from clear. A possible higher risk of aneurysmal SAH has been suggested for a coagulation factor XIII subunit A Tyr204Phe polymorphism [11].

15.2.2 The Role of Genetic Factors in SAH-Associated Coagulative Anomalies

A direct analysis of coagulation factors in SAH patients is hampered by the early activation of the coagulation and fibrinolytic system following the hemorrhage [4]. Therefore, the evaluation of genetic factors may be a promising approach to investigate the role of coagulation factors in the development of complications

15 Coagulation Disorders After Central Nervous System Injury

after SAH. A genetic study in SAH patients suggested that the plasminogen activator inhibitor 1 gene influencing coagulation is involved in the occurrence of secondary brain ischemia [12]. The role of polymorphism in coagulation factor V, prothrombin, methylenetetrahydrofolate reductase (MTHFR), and coagulation factor XIII subunit A and subunit B genes is currently unclear. Factor V Leiden and prothrombin G20210A polymorphism are associated with increased risk of thrombosis [13], and for factor V Leiden a decreased risk of bleeding has also been demonstrated [14]. Factor V Leiden and prothrombin G20210A polymorphism may therefore be associated with a possible decreased risk of SAH, an increased risk of secondary cerebral ischemia, and possibly a decreased risk of rebleeding in SAH patients. Conversely, subunit A Val34Leu, Tyr204Phe, and Pro564Leu factor XIII polymorphisms are associated with an increased risk of bleeding [15] and may increase the risk of aneurysmal SAH and subsequent rebleeding, and possibly show a decreased risk of secondary cerebral ischemia in SAH patients. The roles of the MTHFR C677T polymorphism and the subunit B His95Arg factor XIII polymorphism in coagulation are not yet clear, but some studies have found an increased risk of thrombosis for both variants [16].

15.3 Traumatic Brain Injury

The reported incidence of clotting abnormalities in patients with traumatic brain injuries (TBI) is highly variable, ranging from 15 to 100% [17, 18]. This apparent lack of agreement primarily derives from the heterogeneity of the patients involved, the different sensitivities of the clotting tests used, and the different time frames of coagulation testing after injury.

Patients with post-TBI coagulopathy can be subdivided into two groups: the first group is represented by patients with overwhelming trauma whose severe coagulopathy is a terminal event, whereas the second group consists of patients in whom abnormal coagulative test findings are not associated with clinically significant bleedings, and whose values return to the normal range within hours [18].

In 1979, Pondaag reported on a small series of patients with TBI in whom early laboratory evidence of coagulopathy predicted poor outcome. A comprehensive review by Kaufman and Mattson [17] in 1985 suggested the mechanisms by which early coagulation abnormalities in TBI might lead to adverse outcomes. Kaufman et al. established a direct association between the severity of coagulopathy and the likelihood of adverse outcome, a relationship that was not dependent on the severity of injury alone [19]. Piek et al. [20] reviewed the Traumatic Coma Data Bank and found coagulopathy to be a significant independent predictor of an unfavorable outcome; actually, using backward elimination, stepwise logistic regression modeling, they determined that the effect of coagulopathy was second only to that of shock.

15.3.1 Pathophysiology

Owing to the presence of elevated amounts of TF in the brain, the fibrin clot initiated by the extrinsic pathway traps platelets and stimulates further thrombosis. The normal clotting process is associated with an intense inflammatory response, as a number of inflammatory mediators are released by platelets and by the coagulation network itself; in turn, these mediators promote further coagulation. In normal conditions, these procoagulant mechanisms are counterbalanced by endogenous anticoagulant substances to prevent the occurrence of an uncontrolled thrombosis.

In patients with TBI, the delicate balance outlined is disrupted by the DIC syndrome. The DIC syndrome consists of uncontrolled procoagulant activity, deposition of thrombi in small blood vessels, consumption of clotting factors, induced fibrinolysis, and the induction of a localized or systemic inflammatory response with vascular damage. The DIC syndrome can be fulminant, accompanied by uncontrolled hemorrhage, widespread necrosis, multiple organ failure, and death. In contrast, the DIC syndrome that accompanies some malignancies, allograft rejection, and the hemolytic-uremic syndrome is relatively slow in evolution and may be so mild as to be primarily a laboratory diagnosis. Then, it appears that the coagulopathy of TBI falls between these two extremes. However, the exact relation between TBI and DIC is not fully understood. Some of the confusion results from the lack of a universally recognized definition of DIC, the lack of standardized laboratory diagnosis, and the lack of uniformity in coagulation tests and timing in patients with TBI. Prominent fibrinogenolysis associated with inhibition of α_2-plasmin inhibitor activity may be unique to TBI. Coagulation and platelet activation are further accelerated by cerebral vascular endothelial damage as the direct result of TBI, as well as indirect damage through inflammation, toxins, and ischemia.

The various tests demonstrate abnormalities of variable severity and duration, most likely expressing the different phases of the DIC syndrome. The levels of D-dimer and fibrin degradation products, which reflect the first signs of hyperco-agulation and fibrinolysis, are abnormal within the minutes following TBI. Prothrombin and partial thromboplastin times are usually normal when measured within 1 h of injury, but their prolongation is evident soon thereafter, and they peak at about 6 h and return to normal values within 24 h. A similar pattern (in reverse) is seen in fibrinogen levels, reflecting the course of clotting factor consumption. The findings of these tests are rarely abnormal beyond 24–36 h after TBI, in marked contrast to the several-day duration of coagulopathy in general trauma.

15.3.2 Neurological Consequences of TBI-Induced Coagulative Abnormalities

Delayed and progressive posttraumatic hemorrhage has long been linked to abnormal clotting studies [21], but other investigations suggested ischemic complications were also present after TBI [22].

The importance of ischemia as a secondary injury in TBI was emphasized by Graham and Adams [23] in 1971. Their study revealed autopsy evidence of cerebral ischemia in over 90% of cases. Despite the introduction of aggressive management of hypoxemia, systemic hypotension, and intracranial hypertension in the ensuing years, the incidence of cerebral ischemia was not reduced. The causes of ischemia include cerebral herniation and arterial occlusion, direct blood vessel occlusion by hematoma, vasospasm, hypoxia, and hypotension, as well as elevated intracranial pressure.

However, in patients suffering from TBI the pathogenesis of many cases of cerebral ischemia is unclear. An alternative explanation for posttraumatic cerebral ischemia is the occurrence of intravascular microthrombosis (IMT), occurring as part of a local or systemic DIC. Kaufman et al. [17] presented a series of fatal head injuries complicated by a DIC and demonstrated that an IMT was present in the brain and in other organs.

Platelet aggregation and microvascular occlusions also have been reported in experimental TBI, particularly in pericontusional ischemic areas. Maeda et al. [24] stressed that IMT is the first histological change observed in the pericontusional cortex. Although clinical measurements of cerebral blood flow and neuroimaging techniques lack the resolution to confirm areas of ischemia caused by IMT, diffusion-weighted magnetic resonance imaging findings are consistent with this effect [25].

There are other mechanisms by which the DIC process can contribute to secondary brain injury, including (1) the deposition of fibrin on endothelial surfaces impairing oxygen exchange without occluding the vascular lumen and (2) the excessive release of cytokines and other inflammatory mediators as part of the process of blood coagulation directly damaging neural tissue and cerebrovascular endothelium. It has also been demonstrated that high concentrations of thrombin are directly neurotoxic [26].

15.3.3 Diagnosis and Therapy

In patients with TBI-associated coagulopathy the routine tests of blood coagulation and the thromboelastography are able to identify the underlying abnormalities, assess their severity, monitor their course, and follow the effects of the therapy.

The therapeutic goals of treatment consist in (1) contrasting hypercoagulation, (2) lysing existing clots, (3) replacing clotting factors, and (4) reversing hyperfibrinolysis:

1. *Contrasting hypercoagulation.* Hypercoagulation can be ameliorated with blockers of the coagulation network, antiplatelet agents, or anticoagulants. Coagulation blockers offer the greatest risk/benefit ratio. If given early in the course of DIC, they can ameliorate its progress. Antithrombin III levels were reported to fall following TBI [27]. Another procoagulant blocker, activated protein C, has proved more potent than antithrombin III in contrasting the DIC associated with severe sepsis. The multicenter protein C Worldwide Evaluation in Severe Sepsis (PROWESS) study confirmed a significant improvement in

outcome using recombinant activated protein C. Although it has been reported to improve outcome in experimental ischemic stroke, activated protein C has not been tested in TBI yet. Thrombin inhibitors may also reduce inflammation and edema in experimental TBI [28]. Inhibitors of activated factor X reduce IMT downstream from an experimentally occluded middle cerebral artery and improve neurological function [28].

Antiplatelet agents may also be useful to impede clot formation in stroke and TBI. The administration of a platelet-activating factor antagonist improved behavioral outcome and reduced cerebral edema in experimental TBI [29]. Maeda et al. [24] reported that this effect could be due to the reduction of the IMT in the pericontusional tissue. This resulted in improved regional cerebral blood flow and less necrosis. Prostacyclin, an inhibitor of platelet aggregation, has been shown to reduce cortical lesions in experimental TBI [30].

Anticoagulants could be harmful to TBI patients because they might cause excessive bleeding. However, low molecular weight heparin was found to reduce experimental contusion and edema, and low-dose heparin has been advocated as treatment for TBI with coagulopathy [31].

2. *Lysing existing clots.*Thrombolytic agents are extensively used in ischemic stroke. Both intravenous tissue plasminogen activator and intra-arterial urokinase plasminogen activator have been successful in clinical trials [32]. They have been recommended to treat DIC arising from trauma to sepsis. Plasmin itself (activated plasminogen) has been reported to be of benefit in experimental embolic strokes and to be neuroprotective in excitotoxic brain injury [33]. Topical tissue plasminogen activator has been successfully used to lyse an intraventricular clot in a patient with TBI [34]. The other effects of thrombolytic agents limit their potential effectiveness in TBI.

3. *Replacement of clotting factors.* The replacement of plasma clotting factors depleted by DIC, liver disease, and massive transfusion is advocated as a component of treatment. The administration of fresh-frozen plasma in TBI patients does not appear to be effective. Recombinant activated factor VII has proved useful in controlling excessive bleeding in hemophiliacs as well as in bleeding associated with trauma [35]. Its neurosurgical use has been extended to include some cases of TBI. Although it is certainly useful in replenishing consumed clotting factors, it must be cautioned that activated factor VII may have the unintended consequence of promoting IMT and cerebral ischemia during the hypercoagulation phase.

4. *Reversing hyperfibrinolysis.* Use of antifibrinolytic agents is not recommended in most types of DIC, because fibrinolysis is frequently already suppressed. Serine protease inhibitors have been proposed for ischemic stroke [36], although not for TBI. Mixed results in patients with spontaneous SAH, especially in light of the greater incidence of ischemic complications, makes the utility of antifibrinolytic agents in TBI unlikely.

15.4 Arteriovenous Fistulae

A number of reports on the surgical and endovascular treatment of cranial and spinal dural arteriovenous fistulae (DAVF) have been published in recent years. The pathogenesis of de novo DAVF remains controversial and may be different for cranial and spinal DAVF. Cranial DAVF are likely to be acquired vascular lesions. They comprise a heterogeneous group of vascular malformations with different morphologies, depending on the location of the venous recipient.

Trauma and prothrombotic genetic predispositions, along with sinus thrombosis and consequent venous hypertension, are the presumed etiological factors and may contribute to the development of at least a subgroup of cranial DAVF [37]. In 72% of parents with DAVF of the dural sinuses, signs of thrombosis were detectable at the time of the investigation; preliminary data from this study showed a significantly increased rate of the heterozygote G20210A mutation of the prothrombin gene in patients with cranial DAVF, whereas trauma and infection likely causes of spinal DAVF; these latter are fed by a radicular artery, which drains into a medullary vein and fills the coronal venous plexus of the spinal cord in a retrograde manner; actually, the arterialized blood flows through the medullary vein and determines the congestion and dilatation of the coronal venous plexus, eventually resulting in a progressive myelopathy.

15.4.1 Cranial DAVF

Several authors consider cranial DAVF to be an acquired vascular lesion possibly associated with underlying thrombophilic abnormalities [37]; experimentally, Herman et al. [38] demonstrated the formation of DAVF could be ascribed by a combination of venous thrombosis and venous hypertension.

The factor V Leiden mutation, which causes the resistance to activated protein C, is the most common risk factor for peripheral venous thrombosis and is also a cause of familial thrombophilia; moreover, the factor V Leiden mutation is also associated with cerebral venous thrombosis. Notably, the incidence of the factor V Leiden mutation has a wide range between different ethnic groups and is virtually absent in Africans, Asians, and populations with Asian ancestry such as Amerindians, Eskimos, and Polynesians [39]. Similarly, the G20210A mutation of the prothrombin gene, which leads to the production of abnormally elevated amounts of prothrombin, is another risk factor for venous thromboembolism (VTE) [13]. The role of hypercoagulopathy in the pathogenesis of cranial DAVF [37] is not uniform: 35% of patients with cranial DAVF and spinal DAVF had thrombophilic risk factors. However, a detailed analysis of data revealed that patients with cranial DAVF and spinal DAVF have differences in their genetic profile. An association of cranial DAVF and a mutation of the prothrombin gene (G20210A) was found in 24% of patients, which is approximately tenfold higher than the acknowledged incidence of 2% in the general population. The continuation of Gerlach's study with an increased number of patients confirmed the earlier analysis, which already showed the high incidence of the G20210A mutation of the prothrombin gene in patients with cranial DAVF [37]. In contrast, a factor V Leiden mutation was found in only one patient (4.0%) with cranial DAVF, which is within the range of the reported incidence of 5% in the Caucasian population [38]. Therefore, these data are in contrast to those from the studies of Kraus et al. [40], who found an increased prevalence of the factor V Leiden mutation in patients with cranial DAVF compared with age- and sex-matched controls, whereas the G20210A mutation of the prothrombin gene was not increased. This discrepancy is difficult to explain, and it is unlikely that the ethnic background differs between the two study populations.

15.4.2 Spinal DAVF

In contrast to patients with cranial DAVF, in patients with spinal DAVF the associations with genetic risk factors are not clearly determined. In a study by Jellema et al. [41] which included 40 patients with spinal DAVF, only one patient had the G20210A mutation of the prothrombin gene and none of the patients had factor V Leiden mutation. On the basis of these findings, the authors concluded that it is unlikely that prothrombotic factors are involved in the pathogenesis of spinal DAVF. Conversely, other authors who studied patients with either cranial DAVF or spinal DAVF [42] found a similar incidence of factor V Leiden mutation and G20210A mutation of the prothrombin gene. Although anticardiolipin antibodies and lupus anticoagulant are recognized risk factors for arterial and venous thromboembolic events, their prevalence in these series was negligible and they are unlikely to play any role in the pathogenesis of DAVF.

15.5 Malignancies

Thromboembolic complications are one of the most common causes of death in cancer patients. They are caused by a number of alterations of the coagulation, including hypercoagulable states, acute and chronic DIC, and primary fibrinolysis.

The fibrinolytic system is based on the action of several serine protease enzymes and their inhibitors which play a major role in different settings, including tissue development and remodeling, invasiveness, and migration of both normal and malignant cells. It also plays a key role in the lysis of fibrin strands. The incidence of thromboembolism is higher in patients with brain tumors than in those with systemic disease. Malignant gliomas are associated with a very high risk of VTE [43]. Whereas many clinical risk factors have previously been described in brain tumor patients, the risk of VTE associated with newer antiangiogenic therapies such as bevacizumab in these patients remains unclear. When VTE occurs in this patient population, concern regarding the potential for intracranial hemorrhage complicates management decisions regarding anticoagulation, and these patients have a worse prognosis than their VTE-free counterparts.

15 Coagulation Disorders After Central Nervous System Injury

Risk stratification models identifying patients at high risk of developing VTE along with predictive plasma biomarkers may guide the selection of eligible patients for primary prevention with pharmacologic thromboprophylaxis. Recent studies exploring disordered coagulation, such as increased expression of TF, and tumorigenic molecular signallng may help to explain the increased risk of VTE in patients with malignant gliomas.

References

1. Harhangi BS et al (2008) Coagulation disorders after traumatic brain injury. Acta Neurochir 150:165–175
2. Linn FHH et al (1996) Incidence of subarachnoid hemorrage. Role of region, year, and rate of computed tomography: a meta-analysis. Stroke 27:625–629
3. Fujii Y et al (1997) Serial changes of hemostasis in aneurismal subarachnoid hemorrhage with special reference to delayed ischemic neurological deficits. J Neurosurg 86:594–602
4. Nina P et al (2001) A study of blood coagulation and fibrinolytic system in spontaneous subarachnoid hemorrhage: correlation with Hunt-Hess grade and outcome. Surg Neurol 55:197–203
5. Macdonald RL (1995) Cerebral vasospasm. Neurosurgery 5:73–97
6. van der Sande JJ et al (1978) Head injury and coagulation disorders. J Neurosurg 49:357–365
7. Juvela S et al (1990) Effect of nimodipine on platelet function in patients with subarachnoid hemorrhage. Stroke 21:1283–1288
8. Ohkuma H et al (1991) Role of platelet function in symptomatic cerebral vasospasm following aneurismal subarachnoid hemorrhage. Stroke 22:854–859
9. Peltonen S et al (1997) Hemostasis and fibrinolysis activation after subarachnoid hemorrhage. J Neurosurg 87:207–214
10. Ilveskero S et al (2005) D-dimer predicts outcome after aneurysmal subarachnoid hemorrhage: no effect of thromboprophylaxis on coagulation activity. J Neurosurg 57:16–24
11. Reiner AP et al (2001) Polymorphism of coagulation factor XIII subunit A and risk of nonfatal hemorrhagic stroke in young white women. Stroke 32:2580–2586
12. Vergouwen MD et al (2004) Plasminogen activator inhibitor-1 4G allele in the 4G/5G promoter polymorphism increases the occurrence of cerebral ischemia after aneurysmal subarachnoid hemorrhage. Stroke 35:1280–1283
13. Poort SR et al (1996) A common genetic variation in the $3'$-untranslated region of the prothrombin levels and an increase in venous thrombosis. Blood 88:3698–3703
14. Donahue BS et al (2003) Factor V Leiden protects against blood loss and transfusion after cardiac surgery. Circulation 107:10003–10008
15. Anwar R et al (1999) Genotype/phenotype correlations for coagulation factor XIII: specific normal polymorphism are associated with high or low factor XIII specific activity. Blood 93:897–901
16. Komanasin N et al (2005) A novel polymorphism in the factor XIII B-subunit (His95Arg): relationship to subunit dissociation and venous thrombosis. J Thromb Haemost 3:2487–2496
17. Kaufman HH et al (1984) Clinicopathological correlations of disseminated intravascular coagulation in patients with head injury. Neurosurgery 15:34–42
18. Murshid WR, Gader AG (2002) The coagulopathy in acute head injury: comparison of cerebral versus peripheral measurements of haemostatic activation markers. Br J Neurosurg 16:362–369
19. Olson JD et al (1989) The incidence and significance of hemostatic abnormalities in patients with head injuries. Neurosurgery 24:825–832
20. Piek J et al (1992) Extracranial complications of severe head injury. J Neurosurg 77:901–907

21. Kaufman HH et al (1980) Delayed and recurrent intracranial hematomas related to disseminated intravascular clotting and fibrinolysis in head injury. Neurosurgery 7:445–449
22. Stein SC et al (1993) Delayed and progressive brain injury in closed-head trauma: radiological demonstration. Neurosurgery 32:25–30; discussion 30–31
23. Graham DI, Adams JH (1971) Ischaemic brain damage in fatal head injuries. Lancet 1:265–266
24. Maeda T et al (1997) Hemodynamic depression and microthrombosis in the peripheral areas of cortical contusion in the rat: role of platelet activating factor. Acta Neurochir Suppl 70:102–105
25. Liu AY et al (1999) Traumatic brain injury: diffusion-weighted MR imaging findings. AJNR Am J Neuroradiol 20:1636–1641
26. Lee KR et al (1996) The role of the coagulation cascade in brain edema formation after intracerebral hemorrhage. Acta Neurochir 138:396–400
27. Hoots WK (1996) Coagulation disorders in the head-injured patient. In: Narayan RK, Wilberger JE Jr, Povlishock JT (eds) Neurotrauma. McGraw-Hill, New York, pp 673–688
28. Zhang ZG et al (2001) Dynamic platelet accumulation at the site of the occluded middle cerebral artery and in downstream microvessels is associated with loss of microvascular integrity after embolic middle cerebral artery occlusion. Brain Res 912:181–194
29. Buchanan DC et al (1989) Platelet-activating factor receptor blockade decreases early posttraumatic cerebral edema. Ann N Y Acad Sci 559:427–428
30. Grande PO et al (2000) Low-dose prostacyclin in treatment of severe brain trauma evaluated with microdialysis and jugular bulb oxygen measurements. Acta Anaesthesiol Scand 44:886–894
31. Wojcik R et al (2001) Preinjury warfarin does not impact outcome in trauma patients. J Trauma 51:1147–1151
32. Alberts MJ (1998) tPA in acute ischemic stroke: United States experience and issues for the future. Neurology 51:S53–S55
33. Tsirka SE et al (1997) Neuronal death in the central nervous system demonstrates a non-fibrin substrate for plasmin. Proc Natl Acad Sci USA 94:9779–9781
34. Grabb PA (1998) Traumatic intraventricular hemorrhage treated with intraventricular recombinant-tissue plasminogen activator: technical case report. Neurosurgery 43:966–969
35. Aldouri M (2002) The use of recombinant factor VIIa in controlling surgical bleeding in non-haemophiliac patients. Pathophysiol Haemost Thromb 32:41–46
36. Vivien D, Buisson A (2000) Serine protease inhibitors: novel therapeutic targets for stroke? J Cereb Blood Flow Metab 20:755–764
37. Gerlach R et al (2003) Increased incidence of thrombophilic abnormalities in patients with cranial dural arteriovenous fistulae. Neurol Res 25:745–748
38. Herman JM et al (1995) Genesis of a dural arteriovenous malformation in a rat model. J Neurosurg 83:539–545
39. De Stefano V et al (1998) Epidemiology of factor V Leiden: clinical implications. Semin Thromb Hemost 24:367–379
40. Kraus JA et al (1998) Association of resistance to activated protein C and dural arteriovenous fistulae. J Neurol 245:731–733
41. Jellema K et al (2004) Spinal dural arteriovenous fistulae are not associated with prothrombotic factors. Stroke 35:2069–2071
42. Van Dijk JM et al (2007) Thrombophilic factors and the formation of dural arteriovenous fistulae. J Neurosurg 107:56–59
43. Jenkins EO et al (2010) Venous thromboembolism in malignant gliomas. J Thromb Haemost 8(2):221–227

Index

β_2-glycoprotein I, 141, 142, 209, 210

A

Accordingly, 111, 220
Alveolar haemorrhage, 217
ANCA, 218–222
Antibody, 32, 35, 51, 176, 184
Anticardiolipin, 138, 141, 147, 203, 209
Anticoagulants, 11, 32, 39, 44, 71, 101, 133,
141, 147
Anticoagulation, 10, 25, 38, 46–48, 71, 85,
139, 149, 171, 175, 184
Antiphospholipid, 21, 32, 51, 135, 147, 177,
209, 213
Anti-plasminogen, 220, 221
Antithrombin, 3, 6, 32, 43, 62, 63, 66–68, 78,
88, 99, 102
APC system, 135, 136, 142
APLA, 209–213
As stated above, 212, 220
Aspirin, 34, 45–47, 50, 52, 143, 146, 166, 174,
177, 187
Autoantibodies, 32, 209, 211, 212, 222
Autoimmune, 220, 222

B

Blood coagulation, 1–4, 10–12, 61, 73, 89,
120, 129

C

Catastrophic APS (caps), 211
Churg-Strauss, 218
Churg–strauss syndrome, 218
Circulating protein C, 88
Coagulation in sepsis, 86

Coagulation inhibitors, 30, 89, 99, 102
Coagulative, 114, 229
Consumption coagulopathy, 93, 103, 106, 107
Corticosteroids, 211, 219, 221
Cyclophosphamide, 219, 221

D

D-dimer, 33, 35, 87, 88, 99, 135, 144, 167, 228
Disseminated intravascular coagulation (DIC),
21, 30
Drotrecogin-α, 89
Eclampsia, 145, 213

E

Eclampsia, 145, 213
Eosinophilia, 218

F

Factor X, 32, 33, 37, 38, 75, 86, 165,
213, 232
Factors, 2, 113
Fibrinogen, 1, 3, 8, 10, 29, 31, 94, 113, 114,
118, 133, 136, 164
Fibrinolysis, 8, 10, 11, 14, 15, 80, 85, 88,
113, 129

G

Glomerulonephritis, 217–219

H

Haemorrhage, 217–219, 222
Heparin, 21, 28, 31–33, 37, 45, 47, 66, 71, 78,
170

G. Berlot (ed.), *Hemocoagulative Problems in the Critically Ill Patient*,
DOI: 10.1007/978-88-470-2448-9, © Springer-Verlag Italia 2012

237

I

Immunology, 223
Including an injury severity
    score (ISS), 112
Inflammation, 85, 89, 93, 101, 112, 117,
    218, 232
Infliximab, 222

L

LAC, 209, 210, 212, 213

M

Methotrexate, 221
Microscopic polyangiitis, 218, 219
Microvasculopathy, 211

O

Of trauma primarily occurs, 112

P

Plasma exchange, 34, 221, 223
Platelets, 1, 5–8, 12, 87, 103, 113, 129, 131,
    164
PLEX, 221–223
Postulates that, 113
Proinflammatory cytokines, 145
Pulmonary-renal, 217, 218, 221

R

Reduces, 17, 31, 39, 44, 64, 112, 115, 132, 140
Rituximab, 222

S

Sepsis, 21, 68, 85, 86, 88, 89, 94, 102,
    176, 195
Several approaches have been sofar, 115
Stroke, 31, 42, 44, 45, 49, 51, 95, 175, 213
Syndrome, 32, 50, 62, 88, 106, 137, 142, 144,
    168, 230
Systemic inflammatory response, 116, 176,
    188, 195
SIRS, 85

T

Thromboembolism, 37, 38, 45, 62, 139, 233
Thrombosis, 9, 13, 35, 39, 42, 55, 62, 95, 141,
    200, 210, 212, 233

V

Vasculitides, 218–220
Vasculitis, 95, 217, 218, 222

W

Warfarin, 40, 41, 48, 64, 184, 213
Wegener granulomatosis, 218

Printing: Ten Brink, Meppel, The Netherlands
Binding: Stürtz, Würzburg, Germany